Handbook of Functional Gastrointestinal Disorders

Medical Psychiatry

Series Editor

William A. Frosch, M.D.
Cornell University Medical College
New York, New York

1. *Handbook of Depression and Anxiety: A Biological Approach,* edited by Johan A. den Boer and J. M. Ad Sitsen
2. *Anticonvulsants in Mood Disorders,* edited by Russell T. Joffe and Joseph R. Calabrese
3. *Serotonin in Antipsychotic Treatment: Mechanisms and Clinical Practice,* edited by John M. Kane, H.-J. Möller, and Frans Awouters
4. Handbook of Functional Gastrointestinal Disorders, *edited by Kevin W. Olden*

ADDITIONAL VOLUMES IN PREPARATION

Handbook of Functional Gastrointestinal Disorders

edited by

Kevin W. Olden
University of California, San Francisco, and
St. Mary's Medical Center
San Francisco, California

Marcel Dekker, Inc. New York • Basel • Hong Kong

ISBN: 0-8247-9409-5

The publisher offers discounts on this book when ordered in bulk quantities. For more information, write to Special Sales/Professional Marketing at the address below.

This book is printed on acid-free paper.

Marcel Dekker, Inc.
270 Madison Avenue, New York, New York 10016

Current printing (last digit):
10 9 8 7 6 5 4 3 2 1

PRINTED IN THE UNITED STATES OF AMERICA

For
SYLVIA
who is always there for me

Series Introduction

The word *gut* has been a part of the English language, as it has of our bodies, for a long time. The Oxford English Dictionary's earliest citation is from about 1000 A.D., and from somewhat later (1580): "My eyes, my guts, yea, my soule, grief doth waste." We have been told that an army marches on its stomach, and that the way to a man's (and presumably to a woman's) heart is also through the stomach. In addition, we have always been aware of the close linkage between our emotions and our guts (see above quote!). A musician I know, describing his performance anxiety, told me that he spends the day of every concert in the toilet. This relationship was confirmed by the observations by William Beaumount of Alexis St. Martin and the studies by Harold Wolf of "Tom" through gastric stomas.

This new volume in the Medical Psychiatry series moves us out of the interesting and partially accurate, but simplistic and overly symbolic, explanations of the heyday of psychosomatic medicine into the new world of neurotransmitters, new imaging techniques, and psychometrics. It provides the reader with both the new basic sciences and the newest diagnostic and treatment techniques. Mastering the contents will help all of us to help some of those who need us.

William A. Frosch

Foreword

Not too long after they are exposed to clinical matters, medical students become aware that many of man's ills cannot be explained by pathology or even disturbed physiology. Correlation between the former and symptoms is usually possible. It is not difficult to understand cramping abdominal pain due to an organic obstructing structural lesion of the small or large intestine or to a diffusely inflamed colon. What of similar complaints without obstruction, inflammation, or ischemia? The complexity of such cases and the immediate frustration they can generate are quickly evident when the students meet their first patient with irritable bowel syndrome (IBS). Worse, in these patients the discomfort may go on and on for years, even decades, in contrast to the resolution of complaints in patients whose obstruction, inflammation, or ischemia has been managed correctly. Here is the rub. For the latter conditions, the patient often provides a clear history of a change from normalcy to disability, large bodies of verified experimental data exist to explain the pathophysiology of the symptoms, and we have a great deal of experience with rational therapies, also based in large part on experimental data. For these patients solid medical science dictates the course of evaluation and treatment. Not so for IBS, nor for globus, functional dysphagia, non-ulcer dyspepsia, chronic nausea, psychogenic vomiting, rumination, slow transit constipation, or noncardiac chest pain. These conditions and their attendant symptoms originate from a poorly defined anatomical area and at present we have no satisfactory pathophysiological explanations for them.

Lacking accepted understanding based on discernible pathology, physicians for centuries have put forth multiple explanations for logical questions such as: May there not be a relationship between environmental factors, particularly stress, and patients' emotional responses? What are the roles of personality, culture, and symptoms? What explains individual differences in pain threshold?

The evolution of thinking and experimentation in pursuit of the answers to such questions is recounted in this important book. The recurrent theme in almost all chapters is the widening body of knowledge that links psychosocial factors (as clearly expounded by George Engel) to gut dysfunction. Although much has been learned about these connections, it is unfortunately still not clear that the functional bowel disorders can be linked to particular patterns of neurotic behavior.

The evolution of psychosocial and psychometric evaluation of the functional GI disorders has been steady. We now know that psychiatric dysfunction and evidence of failure in psychosocial adjustment are to some extent measurable by a variety of available instruments. However, these tests are of limited use when one attempts to correlate psychiatric disorders and to define their exact role in pathophysiology and clinical behavior. Thus, although we have much information, for example, on the association of depression with functional GI disorders, we do not know exactly how depression disrupts normal function and alters perception of pain.

The deficit in understanding these disorders is not for want of observation and study. Data from measuring motility, secretions, or pressure for hours to days in functional gut syndromes are, by virtue of their relative brevity, difficult to attribute to lifelong moods, thoughts, or abberations of personality unless the findings are dramatic and reproducible, and clearly apply to a large group of patients with a clear-cut symptom complex.

Yet we have a large body of data on the pathophysiology of many of these functional GI disorders, such are as those that are presented, in general, by Camilleri and Frank in their chapter on the medical evaluation of functional disorders and, in particular, by Drossman on irritable bowel syndrome, by Wald, on chronic idiopathic constipation, and by Richter, on swallowing disorders. Walker discusses the relevant studies on factors affecting pain in the chapter on chronic abdominal pain, as do Waldholtz and Anderson in the chapter on the pathophysiology of eating disorders.

What can we do about treating these perplexing and common illnesses, which are the responsibility of primary-care physicians and gastroenterologists? Apparently a lot, even if we cannot explain how depression, anxiety, fear, or a long-delayed response to social and psychic trauma (e.g., sexual abuse in childhood) may lead to these illnesses. Perhaps, as emphasized by Norton, Davidoff and Whitehead, and Olden, Wise, and Goldberg in their fine chapters on different approaches to dealing with psychiatric aspects including self-help, and behavior modification and psychotherapy, respectively, in this volume, understanding the importance of the influence of the past on present complaints helps in planning care. Such understanding generates the empathy necessary for care of patients with chronic complaints that are frustratingly refractory to many measures.

Physician frustration caused by the absence of a sufficient scientific basis for treatment must be dealt with and overcome early in the relationship.

The authors of the chapters on management also concentrate on the need to deal with the *particular* patient. Thus, some will benefit from medical therapy and some will not, as pointed out by Sperling and McQuaid and Lydiard in their individual chapters. We have no set therapy for individuals with non-ulcer dyspepsia, dysphagia due to "nutcracker esophagus," IBS, or chronic constipation. Pharmacological therapy directed at stimulating motor function may help some, while others may be helped by drugs that inhibit it. For all, however, attention must be paid to the psychic forces at work, whether by appropriate situational therapy, carefully managed pharmacotherapy (particularly for anxiety and depression), biofeedback training, or formal psychiatric care. The physician (primary care or gastroenterologist) must attend particularly to anxiety and depression, which are most evident in my experience in those with IBS and non-ulcer dyspepsia, the two more common conditions, but often present as well in other functional GI disorders.

Where do we go from here? We should continue to investigate the psychosocial correlates, hoping that the methods of testing will be refined sufficiently that we will achieve some nosological certitude upon which to build a relationship to pathophysiological phenomena, clearing a path to intelligent psychological and pharmacological therapy. The search for a better understanding of how to measure the psychic factors at play is recounted in great detail by Naifeh in her chapter on psychometric testing in functional GI disorders and an accurate assessment of the prevalence of these disorders is given by Hom in her chapter on survey research methods. These efforts if supported will go a long way toward verifiable conclusions about the bases for these illnesses. We must never return to such speculations as Franz Alexander's about the causes of peptic ulcer and ulcerative colitis.

I was well taught by Stanley Cobb, Chester Jones, and Tom Almy in medical school and during fellowship. Hence, I have long been convinced that the mind–body relationship dominates much of the spectrum of GI disorders. Interest in it has waxed and waned, and, thanks to those such as the contributors of this book, it has waxed again. Kevin Olden and these contributors have given us an interesting account (and historical perspective) of this evolution. Perhaps more importantly, this book may point the way to understanding the relationship better. I am pleased to be associated with the effort in this small way.

Marvin H. Sleisenger, M.D.
University of California, San Francisco,
and Department of Veterans Affairs
Medical Center
San Francisco, California

Preface

The relationship between gastrointestinal disorders and emotional distress has a long and rich history in medicine. Psychosomatic gastroenterology can be said to have begun with the pioneering work by William Beaumont in 1833 with Alexis St. Martin. Beaumont's exquisite studies demonstrating the relationship between emotional distress and gastric motility and acid secretion have become a classic in medicine. The rise of psychoanalysis made a powerful and, in some ways, indelible mark on the field of psychosomatic gastroenterology. The work of Franz Alexander, George Engle, and Franz Reichsman significantly advanced our understanding of the relationship between behavior and function of the gastrointestinal tract. Unfortunately, as both the gastrointestinal and psychiatric literature became more complex, the two fields began to diverge. New technologies, such as nuclear medicine techniques that study gastric and esophageal emptying, improved techniques of measuring gastrointestinal motility, and the immense effect of fiberoptic endoscopy have enabled the gastroenterologist to measure the behavior of the luminal portion of the GI tract with great precision.

Simultaneously, in the last twenty years, there has been an explosion of knowledge in the area of brain neurotransmitters. Neuroscience has provided us with tremendous advances in our understanding of gut peptides and "brain–gut interactions." Psychiatry has been revolutionized by the development of the diagnostic classification system now represented in the *Diagnostic and Statistical Manual of Mental Disorders: DSM-IV*, 4th ed., of the American Psychiatric Association. Psychiatric conditions previously open to a variety of interpretations are now defined by criteria gathered through ongoing data collection and rigid analysis. These techniques have been recently adopted by gastroenterology at the 1988 Rome Conference to develop diagnostic criteria for functional GI disorders. Finally, great advances in development of screening instruments for this disease have led to greater accuracy in discriminating functional from organic disease at the clinical level.

This explosion in knowledge has occurred in a wide variety of settings and across many disciplines. The clinician with an interest in psychosomatic gastroenterology has found it increasingly difficult to follow and integrate these advances in a cohesive way. This task has been made more difficult by the highly multidisciplinary nature of psychosomatic gastroenterology. Behavioral scientists, including psychiatrists, have very different skills from gastroenterologists and vice versa. The significant advances made in both psychiatry and gastroenterology over the last ten years have tended to blur the increasingly artificial boundary between these two disciplines. It is clear that the contemporary practice of psychosomatic gastroenterology demands significant knowledge drawn from both arenas.

It is the purpose of this volume to present to the psychiatrist and psychologist, as well as the gastroenterologist and primary-care physician, a comprehensive review of the gastrointestinal conditions known to have a strong behavioral or psychosomatic component. It is our intention to give a comprehensive view of the latest technology used to assess these disorders, from both a gastroenterological and psychological perspective.

The wide spectrum of esophageal, gastric, and colonic disorders associated with behavioral abnormalities are reviewed in detail. Social, psychological, and neurophysiological and neurochemical correlates are presented to achieve an integrated biopsychosocial understanding of these complex disorders. Finally, psychopharmacological, behavioral, and psychotherapeutic interventions applicable to the various functional GI disorders are reviewed in detail in order to give the reader an effective set of tools.

I would like to acknowledge Drs. James Grendell, Bruce Scharschmidt, Ken McQuaid, and Terry Wright at the University of California, San Francisco, for supporting the development of the Functional Bowel Clinic. Thanks to Drs. Doug Drossman and Mike Camilleri for their invaluable mentoring and to Francis Creed, Ned Cassem, and the late Tom Hackett for demonstrating the important role psychiatry can play in the medical setting. Thanks to Mamie Lee for keeping my professional life in order no matter how busy it got. Finally, my thanks to Sylvia Hom, my wife, who always has a better idea.

It has been our goal to integrate data from a wide variety of disciplines to present an integrated multidisciplinary approach to the understanding of functional GI disorders. Physicians and other professionals who deal with patients with functional GI distress understand the suffering these patients endure. They also appreciate the significant challenges presented to the clinician who chooses to intervene in a behavioral as well as somatic way. It is our hope that this volume better equips all clinicians, regardless of specialty, to deal with these complex patients whose suffering demands our attention.

Kevin W. Olden

Contents

Contributors

Arnold E. Andersen, M.D. Professor of Psychiatry, Department of Psychiatry, University of Iowa College of Medicine, Iowa City, Iowa

Laurence A. Bradley, Ph.D. Professor of Medicine, Division of Clinical Immunology and Rheumatology, Department of Medicine, University of Alabama at Birmingham, Birmingham, Alabama

Michael Camilleri, M.D. Professor of Medicine, Mayo Medical School, and Consultant in Gastroenterology, Physiology, and Biophysics, Mayo Clinic, Rochester, Minnesota

Ann L. Davidoff, Ph.D. Assistant Professor, Department of Geriatric Medicine and Gerontology, Johns Hopkins University School of Medicine, Baltimore, Maryland

Douglas A. Drossman, M.D. Professor of Medicine and Psychiatry, Division of Digestive Diseases, University of North Carolina at Chapel Hill, Chapel Hill, North Carolina

Stuart J. Eisendrath, M.D. Professor of Clinical Psychiatry, Director, Consultation-Liaison Program, Department of Psychiatry, University of California, San Francisco, San Francisco, California

Jeffrey W. Frank, M.D. Clinical Instructor in Medicine, Division of Gastroenterology, Department of Internal Medicine, University of Colorado School of Medicine, Denver, Colorado

Richard L. Goldberg, M.D. Professor, Department of Psychiatry, Georgetown University School of Medicine, Washington, D.C.

Rafael O. Gray, M.D., M.P.H. Clinical Instructor, Department of Psychiatry, University of California, San Francisco, and Attending Psychiatrist, Kaiser Permanente, San Francisco, California

Sylvia S. Hom, M.P.H. Research Director, Division of Gastroenterology, St. Mary's Medical Center, San Francisco, California

R. Bruce Lydiard, M.D., Ph.D. Professor of Psychiatry, Department of Psychiatry and Behavioral Sciences, Medical University of South Carolina, Charleston, South Carolina

Kenneth R. McQuaid, M.D. Associate Professor of Clinical Medicine, University of California, San Francisco, and Director of Endoscopy, Veterans Affairs Medical Center, San Francisco, California

Karen H. Naifeh, Ph.D. Adjunct Associate Professor of Psychology, Department of Psychiatry, University of California, San Francisco, San Francisco, California

Nancy J. Norton, B.S. Founder and President, International Foundation for Bowel Dysfunction, Milwaukee, Wisconsin

Kevin W. Olden, M.D., F.A.C.P. Assistant Clinical Professor of Medicine (Gastroenterology) and Psychiatry, University of California, San Francisco, and St. Mary's Medical Center, San Francisco, California

Joel E. Richter, M.D. Chairman, Department of Gastroenterology, The Cleveland Clinic Foundation, Cleveland, Ohio

Richard M. Sperling, M.D. Gastroenterology Fellow, University of California, San Francisco, San Francisco, California

Arnold Wald, M.D. Professor of Medicine, Department of Medicine, University of Pittsburgh School of Medicine, and University of Pittsburgh Medical Center, Pittsburgh, Pennsylvania

Bruce D. Waldholtz, M.D. Assistant Professor, Clinical Internal Medicine, Department of Medicine, Eastern Virginia Medical School, Norfolk, Virginia

Edward A. Walker, M.D. Associate Professor, Department of Psychiatry, University of Washington, Seattle, Washington

William E. Whitehead, Ph.D. Research Professor of Medicine, Division of Digestive Diseases, Department of Medicine, University of North Carolina at Chapel Hill, Chapel Hill, North Carolina

Thomas N. Wise, M.D. Professor and Vice Chair, Department of Psychiatry, Georgetown University School of Medicine, and, Chair, Department of Psychiatry, Fairfax Hospital, Falls Church, Virginia

Handbook of Functional Gastrointestinal Disorders

1

Overview of the Integration of Gastroenterology and Psychiatry

Kevin W. Olden
University of California, San Francisco
and St. Mary's Medical Center
San Francisco, California

I. INTRODUCTION

When George Engel proposed the "biopsychosocial" model of disease, he concluded, as a foundation of the model, that all disease processes were influenced by physical, social, and psychological variables that interacted in a complex manner to produce the symptoms and end-organ damage observed by the physician (1). Likewise, physical illness can give rise to a spectrum of emotional reactions, which in turn can complicate efforts by caregivers to render treatment, as well as the ability of the patient to participate in that treatment. Few areas in medicine exemplify these principles better than the functional gastrointestinal (GI) disorders. Standing squarely at the interface between biomedical and behavioral science, the functional GI disorders have always proven to be a fascinating and challenging area of gastroenterology. For the clinician to be effective in treating patients with functional GI complaints, especially those that are refractory to standard medical treatment, an understanding of the strong interaction between psychological distress and physical symptoms is imperative.

The complex interactions among the physical, psychological, and sociocultural dimensions in an individual's life can take many forms. Patients who have endured extraordinary psychological stress such as childhood sexual abuse can develop a wide spectrum of physical and psychological disorders. Physical disorders include irritable bowel syndrome (IBS) and refractory low-back pain (2–4). An excess prevalence of psychiatric disturbance has also been shown in these patients, including depression, anxiety, personality disorders, and somatization (5,6). Disorders of sexual function are also commonly seen (7). The clinician who treats patients with functional GI disorders is thus presented with the formidable task of effectively dealing with a patient who often has a vague, ill-defined somatic complaint in the absence of any obvious structural or physiological abnormality. This can be a challenging situation for the physician. Failure to correctly evaluate psychosocial stressors and concomitant psychiatric diagnosis can result in redundant workup to uncover the cause of the complaints, poor symptom relief, and overuse of medical services.

Despite a rich body of literature documenting a strong overlap between functional GI disorders and emotional distress, clinicians often feel particularly vulnerable when dealing at the interface of these two areas of medicine. All too often, this interface can be quite perplexing if not distressing for the physician. This sense of uncertainty often leads to physicians' being frustrated and unfulfilled in their care of the patient. This discomfort stems directly from an inability to easily integrate biological, psychological, and social variables. However, physicians have not always been so ill at ease integrating biopsychosocial variables, as demonstrated throughout history. Functional gastroenterological disorders—indeed, psychosomatic medicine at large—can conveniently be said to have evolved through four distinct historical stages: ancient thinking, early psychoanalytical thinking, early psychophysiological research, and contemporary functional gastroenterology.

II. ANCIENT THINKING

Ancient societies were severely limited in their study of medicine by their lack of technological tools to investigate biological and chemical processes of the living organism. Likewise, the concept of the scientific method, with its demand for precision, would not be developed for centuries. Finally, the ancients did not have the luxury of building on the observations of those who had gone before them. This innocence, retrospectively, may be viewed as a stroke of good fortune in that ancient scholars were free to develop their own conceptual models of health and disease. A model of disease that reflected the importance of both the spirit and the mind along with the physical body in the development of illness was advocated by the ancient Greeks. Indeed, Hippocrates wrote, "It is more important to know what sort of person has a disease than to know what sort of disease a person has." Behavioral as well as physical symptoms were given great credence and reflected the spiritual/emotional roles as well as the physical roles that various organs played within the body. The concept was also strongly held by Plato, who wrote, "This is the great error of our day, that physicians separate the soul from the body." Behavioral manifestations of disease were considered both logical and understandable; the ancients were very comfortable in ascribing them as being symptomatic of physical disease and vice versa.

The major deficiency in this line of thinking was that it was based only on anecdotal observations and philosophical constructs, which resulted in conceptual models with no real supporting data. This purely philosophical approach to medicine continued up to the time of the Renaissance, when two significant developments occurred that profoundly changed the course of medicine. The first development was the practice of organ dissection and the founding of the sciences of anatomy and physiology. While these events were critical to the foundations of modern scientific medicine, the tendency to describe disease processes only in terms of their observable morphological, structural, and physiological changes began a trend that tended to dismiss psychosocial issues as being irrelevant to the development of disease. The early work of Harvey in describing the circulation of the blood, followed by Koch and Pasteur's pioneering work in bacteriology, revolutionized medicine. The by-product of this wave of discovery was a steady erosion of the perception that disease could result from psychological and social stressors.

The second development that impacted psychosomatic medicine during this period was the concept of "dualism" as proposed by mathematician-philosopher René Descartes. He advocated the concept that mind and body functioned in two completely separate spheres. Descartes believed that the cognitive functions of the body, the *res cogitans*, was completely separate from the body exclusive of the mind, the *res extensa*. However, Descartes himself retained some notion of mind–body interaction in that he believed the tiny pineal gland was the focus of mind–body communications (8). This rigid separation of mind and body, as proposed by Descartes and shaped by a number of his contemporaries, firmly established the notion of a separation of mind and body. The concept of dualism became a predominant theme of medicine for the next three centuries. The natural tendency was to focus on areas of medicine that were producing advances in knowledge and to avoid those areas that showed little advances.

Undeniably, from the seventeenth century to the present, there has been steady progress in our understanding of the biomedical dimensions of disease. The development of the scientific method of investigation, and the institution of new standards of scientific rigor such as Koch's postulates, created a strong respect for a biomedical approach to disease.

The biopsychosocial model was at a distinct disadvantage during this period. The absence of methods technologically advanced enough to accurately investigate complex functions of neurophysiology and gut physiology further perpetuated this dualistic approach to medicine. Behavioral disturbances could be described only through observations as opposed to being measured scientifically. The inability to apply a biomedical approach to behavioral illnesses led to their being reclassified essentially as moral or spiritual defects. Indeed, disorders with a complex organic basis but with primarily behaviorally based clinical signs, such as epilepsy or Huntington's chorea, were ascribed to "possession" or other acts of God or the devil. Behavioral abnormalities and physical symptoms that could not be explained by an identifiable organic lesion were relegated to nondisease status. Stigmatization of these patients led in turn to a wide variety of unfortunate consequences, including institutionalization and, in some instances, execution. What resulted universally was the exclusion of these patients from hospitals and from scientific study. A few courageous physicians tried to promote a "moral," nonstigmatizing approach to the treatment of patients with behavioral disorders. This approach was championed by Benjamin Rush in the United States and Pinel in France. Their ideas enjoyed only limited support in the nineteenth and early twentieth centuries (9).

The work of William Beaumont with his patient Alexis St. Martin in 1883 was a key event in the history of psychosomatic medicine (10). This was true for a number of reasons. First, Beaumont's work occurred at a time in history when dualism was in its ascent. Second, his work was conducted in accordance with the high scientific standards being set by Jenner, Koch, and others. Beaumont's eloquent studies documenting the relationship between behavior and emotion, and its effect on gastric secretion, struck a strong chord for an integrated psychosomatic approach to the study of gut function. The response of St. Martin's stomach secretions to his temperamental mood swings were carefully recorded and documented. Beaumont's exquisite use of the scientific method was widely acknowledged, and his astounding results were greeted with great excitement. This important use of the scientific method as applied to stress-induced changes in gut function, however, did not change the general direction of nineteenth-century medicine. The march continued toward dualism, i.e., "true" diseases that could be explained by anatomical abnormalities versus conditions that could not.

III. PSYCHOANALYTICAL THINKING

The revolution in psychiatry and psychology created by the work of Sigmund Freud and others paradoxically furthered the move toward dualism. Freud was keenly aware of the impact of emotions on the gut. Believing that oral and anal functioning were some of the most important bodily functions, he theorized that they were greatly related to psychological processes. His recognition that alimentary function was strongly influenced by psychosocial development created great interest (11). The major difficulty with the work of the early psychoanalysts was that, like that of the ancient Greeks, their work was all too often based mainly on empirical observations and theoretical speculation. Freud's concept of "conversion hysteria" stated quite forcefully the theory that psychological distress (conflict) could induce dramatic physical symptoms. Freud believed that a conversion reaction was the result of an unconscious psychological conflict expressed through dysfunction of the voluntary striated muscle innervated by the peripheral motor nerves simulated by the cerebral cortex (12). Sandor Ferenczi first applied the concept of conversion disorder to organs innervated by the autonomic nervous system. Ferenczi first proposed the concept that ulcerative colitis, and specifically the bleeding of ulcerative colitis, was the result of an "autonomic conversion disorder" (13). This concept was extended one more step when George Groddeck and S. Ely Jelliffe proposed that physical signs such as fever, jaundice, and hemorrhage could repress symptoms of unresolved "conflict" and therefore represented a conversion disorder (14).

An attempt to improve on this early psychoanalytical thinking led to the work of Franz Alexander and colleagues at the Chicago Psychoanalytic Institute. Their work, which became known as the "Chicago school," made a number of bold assertions as to the psychological basis of a wide spectrum of medical illnesses. Unlike Freud and the other early psychoanalysts, Alexander believed that psychosomatic disease resulted from the effect of prolonged psychic stress on end organs. This stress resulted from the inability of patients to resolve certain types of unconscious psychic conflict. These specific conflicts, mediated by the autonomic nervous system, led to dysfunction in certain organ systems based on the type of stress and the patient's coping style. The relationship between the inability to handle specific kinds of psychic conflict and the presumed tendency of certain types of maladaptation to produce injury to specific organs was dubbed the "specificity theory" by Alexander (15).

Alexander conceptualized seven "psychosomatic diseases": asthma, rheumatoid arthritis, thyrotoxicosis, essential hypertension, neurodermatitis, peptic ulcer disease, and ulcerative colitis. The fact that two of the seven conditions were GI disorders again demonstrated the belief that the gut was particularly sensitive to stress-induced dysfunction. The specificity theory was developed from open-ended interviews with patients who had various "psychosomatic" diseases. Again, the conclusions reached were based on work subject to extraordinary observer bias and anecdotal observation. For instance, Alexander and coworkers' description of the vulnerability of various ethnic groups to peptic ulcer were stereotypical and based on racial and religious bias. His conclusions are quite difficult to accept when viewed with our current understanding of peptic ulcer disease. Alexander's work has subsequently come under intense criticism in reviews of his methodology and conclusions. Helzer and colleagues in a controlled trial demonstrated a lack of association between premorbid psychological state and the subsequent development of either Crohn's disease or ulcerative colitis (16,17). This was particularly true of the characterization of patients with ulcerative colitis as having the "somatic manifestation of melancholia," conflicts about "sexual relationships or marital relationships," and the "frustrated tendency to carry out an obligation" (18). North and colleagues have written eloquently on this topic (19).

These events were occurring at a time when internal medicine was making dramatic advances in describing the physiological basis of disease, including ulcerative colitis and peptic ulcer disease. It became clear through the next three decades that a patient's risk of developing inflammatory bowel disease and peptic ulcer disease was influenced by a host of biological factors. These developments contrasted sharply with the psychosomatic thinking proposed by Alexander and his coworkers. The net result was the development in medicine of a strong skepticism about the importance of psychosocial variables in the development of disease. This skepticism, in turn, created a further schism between those pursuing a purely biomedical approach and those invested in a more biopsychosocial construct of disease.

IV. PSYCHOPHYSIOLOGICAL RESEARCH

Improvements in technology in the late 1940s subsequently led to a series of classic studies in gut physiology. The development of balloon catheters connected to pneumatically driven pressure recorders led, for the first time, to real-time recording of colonic luminal pressure. In 1949 Almy and colleagues (20–22) performed a series of classic experiments that documented acute changes in colonic motility in response to acute stress. In one study (23), Almy and Tulin performed sigmoidoscopy on medical-student volunteers blinded to the purpose of the study. Baseline sigmoid pressure was recorded, and the subject was then told that a "tumor" had been visualized. The changes in colonic motility induced by this acute stress were recorded. Only then was the hoax revealed to the subject and the subsequent return to a normal motility pattern documented. This classic study described for the first time the actual motility changes associated with acute emotional distress. In parallel work, William Grace, in cooperation with Harold Wolf, investigated the response of four subjects with colonic fistulas to stress and a variety of other stimuli. They, like Beaumont before them, demonstrated the effect of acute stress on gut (colonic) secretions (24). In a similar experiment, Reichsman et al. (25) measured the changes in gastric secretion induced by emotion in an infant. Their findings were similar to those of Beaumont a century earlier.

Almy's work in turn led to the work of Schuster and colleagues (26), who made significant advances in the technology and its application to the functional GI disorders. In 1961, Schuster developed an easy-to-use, technically practical method using a uniquely designed balloon to measure anorectal function. The development of the "Schuster balloon" set the stage for a series of rapid advances in the measurement of intestinal motility (Figure 1) (26). Subsequent work by Snape et al. (27) further documented thc presence of distinct motility abnormalities in patients with functional GI disorders. Building on the work of Wolf and Almy in the 1940s, Snape demonstrated the phenomenon of a distinct three-cycle-per-minute (CPM) pattern of myoelectrical rhythm in the distal colon of patients with irritable bowel syndrome (IBS). This rhythm was distinct from normals and those with non-IBS colon disease. Their finding was subsequently confirmed by Taylor and coworkers (28), who demonstrated the "motility marker" of 3-CPM contractions in both diarrhea-predominant and constipation-predominant IBS.

Whitehead and Schuster (29) measured the response of IBS patients to rectal balloon distention, and also demonstrated a slow pattern of motility similar to the findings of Snape and Taylor. However, Whitehead's patients demonstrated a greater tendency toward intermittent bursts of rapid tonic contraction in those

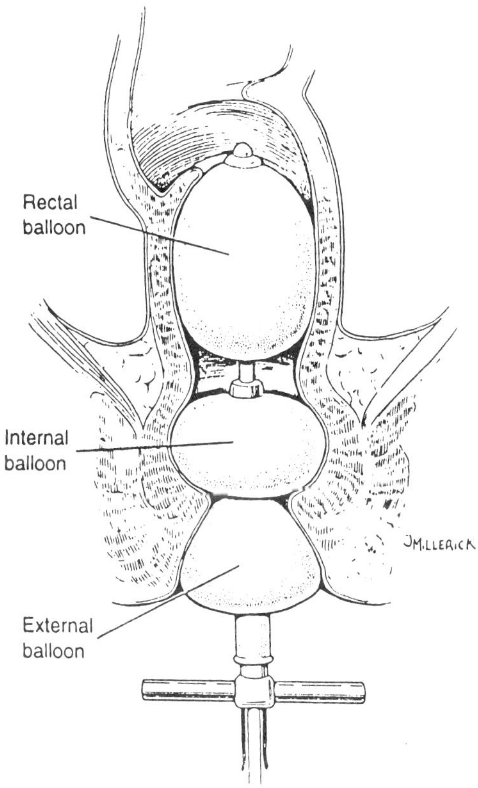

FIGURE 1 The Schuster balloon, used to evaluate anorectal function.

with diarrhea-predominant IBS. Latimer and coworkers (30) compared three groups of patients comprising normal controls, a psychoneurotic group free of bowel symptoms, and patients with IBS. The IBS patients showed similar response in the frequency and duration of contractions in the resting state. More importantly, Latimer showed that the patients with IBS and the psychoneurotic group had very similar patterns of psychological distress as well as great similarity in their pattern of colonic motility. Latimer concluded that "the similar psychological characteristics of the IBS and psychoneurotic groups . . . could be taken to support the argument that the excess of colonic contractions reported as unique to IBS may be more properly related to psychological factors" (30).

V. CONTEMPORARY PSYCHOSOMATIC GASTROENTEROLOGY

A number of forces over the last 10 to 15 yeas have led to the re-emergence of interest in the multimodal approach to functional GI disorders. Klein, in his classic 1988 article (31), documented the relative failure of a purely medical approach to the functional GI disorders. In his analysis, Klein showed quite clearly that many studies documenting "effective" treatment of functional GI complaints were based on poor diagnostic criteria, poor rating scales, poor data analysis, or other significant methodological faults. Likewise, the legacy of the psychoanalytical era showed the failure of a purely psychodynamic approach to explaining and treating functional GI disorders. These perceptions stimulated new efforts to improve our treatment approaches for these patients.

However, a number of events have altered the direction of our approach to these complex disorders. Psychiatrists have always been challenged with a situation similar to that facing physicians who study the functional GI disorders (32). Like the functional GI disorders, psychiatric disorders often have few physiological markers to aid in diagnosis and classification. Psychiatric diagnosis from its inception was based on empirical observation and classification of behavioral symptoms to develop various diagnoses (33). Emil Kraepelin was one of the first investigators to use symptom-based criteria. His textbook describing and classifying the various psychiatric disorders remains a classic in psychiatry. However, attempts by Kraepelin and others to correctly classify behavioral illness suffered from the same weaknesses that plagued the ancients. Their conclusions were based all too often on observational studies and the individual opinions of leading psychiatrists. Indeed, much of the work in the late nineteenth and early twentieth centuries in psychiatric classification was influenced by Emil Kraepelin's textbook, which was published in nine editions from 1883 to 1927 (34).

The state of psychiatric classification remained by and large the domain of individual scholars until World War II, which provided a major impetus to better classify psychiatric conditions because of the large number of veterans who emerged from the war with psychiatric problems. Multiple efforts by the Veterans Administration, the American Psychiatric Association, and others led to the creation of the *Diagnostic and Statistical Manual of Mental Disorders* (DSM-I) published in 1952. The DSM-I was the first effort by the psychiatric profession as a whole to classify psychiatric disorders (35). It was the product of a number of expert committees whose members pooled their expertise to establish common diagnostic criteria based on the standards of the day. This volume was followed by the DSM-II, which was created to bring DSM criteria into standardization with the nomenclature used by the World Health Organization in its International Classification of Diseases (ICD).

The need to classify psychiatric diagnoses on an "operational," basis—i.e., on the basis of observable behaviors—led Feighner to propose a strategy for validating diagnostic criteria. Feighner's work generated great interest in psychiatry. The "Feighner criteria" established a process for validating existing and future psychiatric diagnoses (36). In 1987, the DSM-III succeeded the DSM-II. The DSM-III differed from its predecessors in that the expert panels used, for the first time, the techniques proposed by Feighner to develop these operational definitions to classify the various mental disorders. This use of operational definitions to create and validate criteria led to a process of continuous evaluation and validation of psychiatric diagnoses. The continuous collection of data to affirm or negate the validity of specific diagnostic criteria made the DSM-III a "living document," subject to continuous revision as criteria became better defined or, in some cases, rejected as not supportable. The DSM-III Revised (DSM-IIIR), published in 1987, and most recently the DSM-IV, published in 1994, were testaments to this continuing process of validation (37,38).

Gastroenterologists have faced the same dilemma in studying the functional GI disorders. They lacked, by and large, specific biological markers to classify and distinguish the various patterns of functional GI complaints. Building on the techniques developed in psychiatry, a process was begun to categorize the wide spectrum of functional GI complaints. Since 1988, international panels of clinical investigators have convened in Rome to establish standardized criteria for the functional GI disorders, including guidelines for research and treatment (39). The so-called "Rome criteria" have provided a common point of reference for clinicians and researchers working with patients with functional GI complaints. Like their colleagues in the DSM process, the Rome working teams do not assert that their results are the final word in diagnostic classification. Rather, the Rome criteria provide a starting point for the continuing evolution of standards for diagnosis and treatment of these heterogeneous disorders.

These advances in classification have been accompanied by additional advances in our approach to psychosomatic disease. The work of Holmes and Rahe (40), who demonstrated the effect of stress and its relationship to the development of disease, led to a better understanding of "disease susceptibility." This work, which established the importance of the interaction between patients and their environment, led to new conceptual models to deal with this complex ecology. Adolph Meyer (41) championed the "psychobiological approach" of patient care, integrating the social, psychological, and environmental as well as the biological aspects of a patient's life. This approach was enlarged upon by Lipowski, who added "constitutional factors" along with past social and psychological history of the patient. George Engel (1) further developed this approach by utilizing general systems theory to create what came to be known as the *biopsychosocial model*. The potential of a multidimensional, multidisciplinary approach has been supported by recent work demonstrating the effectiveness of a combined medical and psychological approach to treating irritable bowel syndrome (42–44).

VI. FUTURE DIRECTIONS

The complex nature of the functional GI disorders requires a spectrum of skills to produce advances in their treatment. Clearly, further development in classification based on the existing Rome criteria will be undertaken. These developments can then be used in survey research to better define the epidemiology of functional GI disorders in various populations, especially across nations and cultures. The biopsychosocial model will need to be used to better define the role of psychic trauma and its relationship to the development of a functional GI disorder.

Advances in our understanding of GI motility and the basis for a drug's effect on the gut hold promise for development of more effective drug treatment for the functional GI disorders. Last but not least, advances in psychotherapeutic and other behavioral interventions will need to be developed and tested to help clinicians deal more effectively and confidently with these challenging patients.

REFERENCES

1. Engel GL. The need for a new medical model: a challenge to biomedicine. Science 1977; 196:129–136.
2. Drossman DA, Leserman J, Nachman G, et al. Sexual and physical abuse in women with functional or organic gastrointestinal disorders. Ann Intern Med 1990; 113:828–833.
3. Schofferman J, Anderson D, Hines R, et al. Childhood psychological trauma correlates with unsuccessful lumbar spine surgery. Spine 1992; 17:S138–S144.
4. Springs FE, Friedrich WN. Health risk behaviors and medical sequelae of childhood sexual abuse. Mayo Clin Proc 1992; 67:527–532.
5. Brown GR, Anderson B. Psychiatric morbidity in adult inpatients with childhood histories of sexual and physical abuse. Am J Psychiatry 1991; 148:55–61.
6. Herman JL, Perry J, Van der Kolk B. Childhood trauma in borderline personality disorder. Am J Psychiatry 1989; 146:490–495.
7. Walker EA, Katon WJ, Roy-Bryne PP, et al. Histories of sexual victimization in pa-

tients with irritable bowel syndrome or inflammatory bowel disease. Am J Psychiatry 1993; 150:1502–1506.
8. Brown TM. Cartesian dualism and psychosomatics. Psychosomatics 1989; 30:322.
9. Alexander FG, Selesnick ST. The History of Psychiatry: An Evaluation of Psychiatric Thought and Practice from Prehistoric Times to the Present. New York: Harper and Row, 1966.
10. Beaumont W. Experiments and Observations on the Gastric Juice and Physiology of Digestion. Plattsburg, NY: FP Allen, 1833.
11. Freud S. Standard Edition of the Complete Psychological Works of Sigmund Freud. London: Hogarth Press, 1953–1966.
12. Elliott G. Stress and illness. In: Cheren S, ed. Psychosomatic Medicine: Theory, Physiology and Practice. Vol 1. Madison, WI: International Universities Press, 1989.
13. Lipowski ZJ. Psychosomatic medicine: past and present. Part I: Historical background. Can J Psychiatry 1986; 31:2.
14. Lipowski ZJ. Psychosomatic medicine: past and present. Part II: Current state. Can J Psychiatry 1986; 31:8.
15. Alexander F, French T, Pollock GH. Psychosomatic Specificity. Chicago: University of Chicago Press, 1968.
16. Helzer JE, Stillings WA, Chammas S, et al. A controlled study of the association between ulcerative colitis and psychiatric diagnoses. Dig Dis Sci 1982; 27:513–518.
17. Helzer JE, Chammas S, Norland CC, et al. A study of the association between Crohn's disease and psychiatric illness. Gastroenterology 1984; 86:324–330.
18. Alexander F. Psychosomatic Medicine. New York: Norton, 1950.
19. North CS, Clouse RE, Spitznagel EL, et al. The relation of ulcerative colitis to psychiatric factors: a review of findings and methods. Am J Psychiatry 1990; 147:974–981.
20. Almy TP. Experimental studies on the irritable colon. Am J Med 1951; 9:60–67.
21. Almy TP, Kern F, Tulin M. Alterations in colonic function in man under stress. III: Experimental production of sigmoid spasm in patients with spastic constipation. Gastroenterology 1949; 12:437–449.
22. Almy TP, Kern F, Tulin M. Alterations in colonic function in man under stress. II: Experimental production of sigmoid spasm in healthy persons. Gastroenterology 1949; 12:425–436.
23. Almy TP, Tulin M. Alterations in colonic function in man under stress. I: Experimental production of changes simulating the "irritable colon." Gastroenterology 1947; 8:616–626.
24. Grace WJ, Wolf S, Wolff HG. The Human Colon. New York: Paul B Hoeber, 1951.
25. Reichsman F, Engel GL, Segal HL. Behavior and gastric secretion: the study of an infant with a gastric fistula. Psychosom Med 1955; 17:481.
26. Schuster MM, Hookman P, Hendrix TR, et al. Simultaneous manometric recording of the internal and external anal sphincteric reflexes. Bull Johns Hopkins Hosp 1965; 116:79–88.
27. Snape WJ, Carlson GM, Cohen S. Colonic myoelectric activity in the irritable bowel syndrome. Gastroenterology 1976; 70:326–330.
28. Taylor I, Darby C, Hammond P. Comparison of rectosigmoid myoelectrical activity

in the irritable colon syndrome during relapses and remissions. Gut 1978; 19:923–929.
29. Whitehead WE, Engel BT, Schuster MM. Irritable bowel syndrome: physiological and psychological differences between diarrhea-predominant and constipation-predominant patients. Dig Dis Sci 1980; 25:404–413.
30. Latimer P, Sarna S, Campbell D, et al. Colonic motor and myoelectrical activity: a comparative study of normal subjects, psychoneurotic patients and patients with irritable bowel syndrome. Gastroenterology 1981; 80:393–901.
31. Klein KB. Controlled treatment trials in the irritable bowel syndrome: a critique. Gastroenterology 1988; 95:232–240.
32. Pichot P. Nosological models in psychiatry. Br J Psychiatry 1994; 164:232–240.
33. Kendler K. Toward a scientific psychiatry nosology: strengths and limitations. Arch Gen Psychiatry 1990; 47:969–973.
34. Mack A, Forman L, Brown R, et al. A brief history of psychiatric classification from the ancients to DSM-IV. Psychiatr Clin North Am 1994; 17:515–523.
35. Kline M, Sydnor-Greenberg N, Wakefield Davis W, et al. Using field trials to evaluate changes in DSM diagnostic criteria. Hosp Community Psychiatry 1993; 44:621–623.
36. Feighner JP, Robins E, Guze SB, et al. Diagnostic criteria for use in psychiatric research. Arch Gen Psychiatry 1972; 26:57–63.
37. Diagnostic and Statistical Manual of Mental Disorders. Third Edition—Revised. Washington, DC: American Psychiatric Association, 1987.
38. Diagnostic and Statistical Manual of Mental Disorders. 4th ed. Washington, DC: American Psychiatric Association, 1994.
39. Drossman DA, Thompson WG, Talley NJ, et al. Identification of sub-groups of functional gastrointestinal disorders. Gastroenterol Int 1990; 3:159–172.
40. Holmes T, Rahe R. The social readjustment rating scale. J Psychosom Res 1967; 11:213–218.
41. Meyer A. Psychobiology: A Science of Man. Springfield, IL: Charles C Thomas, 1958.
42. Guthrie E, Creed FH, Dawson D, et al. A controlled trial of psychological treatment for the irritable bowel syndrome. Gastroenterology 1991; 100:450–457.
43. Blanchard EB, Schwartz SP. Adaptation of a multi-component treatment program for irritable bowel syndrome to a small group format. Biofeedback Self-Reg 1987; 12:63–69.
44. Svedlund J, Sjodin I, Ottosson JO, et al. Controlled study of psychotherapy in irritable bowel syndrome. Lancet 1983; ii:589–592.

2

Psychosocial Assessment of GI Symptoms

Stuart J. Eisendrath
University of California, San Francisco
San Francisco, California

Rafael O. Gray
University of California, San Francisco
Kaiser Permanente
San Francisco, California

I. INTRODUCTION

This chapter focuses on the psychosocial evaluation of the individual presenting with gastrointestinal symptoms. Many symptoms may lead to a diagnosis of an unambiguous gastrointestinal disorder. Some symptoms, however, may be less clear and have considerable diagnostic confusion as a consequence. Only when the clinician brings the psychosocial factors into focus does a clear picture of the patient's biopsychosocial condition emerge. Indeed, this condition can be seen as the focusing of the patient's biomedical disease through the lens of multiple psychosocial factors to yield what we generally regard as the patient's illness. Any two patients with the identical disease will have significantly different illnesses based on the individual psychosocial lenses each utilizes. That psychological factors influence various gastrointestinal conditions is evident (1). This chapter focuses on specific areas the clinician can explore to gather psychosocial data. This focus presumes that adequate medical evaluation of symptoms has or will be carried out as well.

II. INTERVIEW TECHNIQUES AND CONTENT FOCUS

In any history-gathering interview, it is important for the physician to start with the patient's chief complaint as the initial focus of inquiry before any psychosocial investigation takes place. For example, if the patient is complaining of abdominal pain, initial inquiry must be aimed at the pain. To do otherwise would risk alienating the patient as well as overlooking key medical information that could yield diagnostic information. By carefully listening to a patient's description of symptoms, the physician often gains valuable insights both from a biological and a psychological perspective. Adjectives used to describe symptoms convey important meaning. For example, the McGill Pain Inventory lists various pain adjectives (2). Such words as "torturing," "terrifying," and "punishing" suggest different images than "cramping," "sharp," or "deep." Similarly, a phrase such as "it feels like someone has hit me in the stomach with his fist" suggests the possibility of interpersonal significance for the symptom.

A. History of Present Illness

After the physician has gathered descriptive information from the patient abut the symptom, it is useful to gather further specific data for both medical diagnosis and psychosocial assessment. One of the most important areas to explore is the onset of the symptom. This information may have direct and obvious implications for the medical diagnosis. Psychosocially, however, this information is also a valuable source of insight. When a patient is asked, "Did anything happen or did you have any change or stress in your life at the time the symptom started?," key information may be identified. Events such as the death of a loved one or a job change often emerge with this line of questioning. Exploring these events with the patient often yields useful diagnostic information, such as a significant display of emotion. Unresolved psychological issues are often visible in this exploration. For example, a patient complaining of abdominal pain after a motor-vehicle accident in which another passenger was killed may have a posttraumatic stress disorder. In this type of situation the pain symptom may represent survivor guilt that will be hard to resolve without addressing the psychological issues involved.

B. Impact of Illness

In addition to understanding the circumstances surrounding the onset of the symptom, the physician should ask about the effects of the illness on both the patient and those around him. What does the symptom interfere with most in the patient's life? What would he be able to do if he did not have the symptom? Whom does the symptom affect most besides the patient?

These questions often lead to a clear understanding of the illness's psychological impact and significance. The physician must be careful, however, not to make etiological attributions based on this understanding. For example, even if a wife uses a symptom to chronically vent anger toward her husband, this does not mean the etiology of the symptom was the disturbed marital relationship; the illness may have arisen from purely organic roots but is being used in a sense for psychosocial purposes.

Case 1: Mr. A. was a 39-year-old bachelor with persistent difficulty in swallowing food. Full gastrointestinal evaluation including endoscopy, cine-esophagram, and esophageal manometry revealed no organic finding. When Mr. A. was asked how his symptom interfered with his life, he replied that it prevented him from getting married. He had been engaged to a woman for five years—the same amount of time his symptom had existed. He had put off marriage because of the troubling symptom since he wanted to be well if he married. Further exploration revealed he had significant conflicts about marriage. He accepted a referral to work on these conflicts while his conservative gastrointestinal follow-up continued.

C. Current Social Situation

Another important area of inquiry is the patient's current social situation. How is the illness affecting the spouse and children? Is there any particular stressor present in the family system? How has the illness affected the patient's romantic relationships? Anxiety-provoking life events have been correlated with the development of bowel symptoms in functional disorders (3,4).

Case 2: Mrs. W. was a 42-year-old woman who had a 6-month history of persistent nausea and vomiting, with a 10-pound weight loss. She had received an extensive medical evaluation without identification of any etiology. In speaking with the patient and her husband, the physician learned that the couple's only child had developed some school difficulties: she had been threatened with death by a gang and she had been receiving in-home tutoring for seven months. Referral for family counseling gradually reduced the nausea and vomiting. In this case, an investigation of the social situation led to an effective intervention.

Case 3: Mrs. C. was a 45-year-old woman who had experienced duodenal ulcer disease 20 years earlier. She had been free of symptoms until 3 months prior to her evaluation. Four months earlier, her mother had moved to another state to take care of a sister who was receiving chemotherapy for breast cancer. The patient had an extremely close relationship with her mother, whom she had seen daily until the mother moved. Despite some improvement of her symptoms with ranitidine, Mrs. C. continued to have vague medical complaints and make substantial demands on her husband for increased attention. These improved after she was referred for counseling to help her deal with the loss of her mother's support and her sister's illness.

Employment is a critical area to explore. Are there conflicts at work? How has the illness impaired job performance? Is the patient disabled or unemployed? What is the current financial situation? Is there any form of litigation involved, including workers' compensation issues? If the patient is a student, what is the effect on studies, attendance, grades, and examinations? All these factors can have important effects on the patient's illness.

D. Developmental History

The above issues involve exploration of current psychosocial issues during the patient interview. Investigating past psychosocial factors is also critical to understanding the patient. For example, asking patients whether they've ever experienced physical or sexual abuse may lead to important information. Women with pelvic and abdominal pain have a greater history of sexual abuse in childhood (5,6); this may affect their ability to tolerate normal physiological events without experiencing pain. Failure to make a psychological resolution of these traumatic expeiences often leads to a persistent somatic focus of complaints. The patient knows something is wrong in her life, but finds it difficult to directly express the trauma.

This has been researched by Drossman et al. (7) in a population of female gastroenterology clinic patients in a university-based referral practice. Almost half of the patients reported a history of physical or sexual abuse. A history of abuse was associated with increased risk in a variety of categories. These include the diagnosis of a functional disorder, chronic or recurrent abdominal or pelvic pain, multiple somatic symptoms, more lifetime surgical interventions, and a trend toward increased medical utilization.

Obtaining a sexual and physical abuse history may be intimidating for many clinicians. In the above study, only 17% had reported these events to their physician. A third had never discussed their abuse history at all. One useful technique in approaching this subject is to normalize it, for instance: "It is not unusual for patients with irritable bowel syndrome to report a history of physical or sexual abuse; has this been a problem for you?" Sexual abuse includes genital contact as well as exhibitionism, fondling, and verbal intimidation.

Another important area to explore in the patient's history is information about a symptom model—other friends or family members who had problems similar to those of the patient. If these individuals did well or had significant problems, this may affect the patient's expectations and fears about his or her own condition. Asking patients if they know anyone who had a similar problem may be very productive in understanding patient attitudes. This point is often extremely helpful when the patient is not following recommended medical treatments or not responding as expected. The source of the symptom model may also be the patient's own medical history (8).

Case 4: Mr. R. was a 50-year-old man who had recently developd ulcer disease for the first time. Despite a rather uncomplicated disease, Mr. R. was extremely anxious about his condition. When the physician asked if he had known anybody else with ulcer disease, he replied that his father had died of a perforated ulcer when 55 years old. Mr. R. responded well to educational efforts about his disease, with special attention to how his condition differed from his father's.

Case 5: Ms. W. was a 30-year-old woman who had been evaluated repeatedly for epigastric pain. No identifiable etiology had emerged despite extensive efforts. In gathering information, a psychiatric consultant learned that the patient's father had suffered for many years with alcohol-related pancreatitis, with a "pain just like mine." According to Ms. W., her father had died shortly before her pain complaints began. Her pain complaints were considered to be modeled after her father's and represented a pathological grief response to his death.

III. DIFFERENTIAL DIAGNOSIS OF PSYCHIATRIC DISORDERS

The foregoing discussion focuses on psychosocial factors that may influence the patient's illness. In addition, the presence of specific DSM-IV psychiatric diagnoses may directly impact the gastrointestinal symptoms. Appropriate psychiatric treatment is imperative. Lifetime prevalence rates of psychiatric diagnoses have been reported to range as high as 93% in one sample with irritable bowel syndrome (IBS). Those diagnosed with inflammatory bowel disease had a rate of 19%, still greater than the population at large (9). A further study suggests that it is the psychological rather than the gastrointestinal symptoms that primarily lead to a doctor visit (10).

A. Affective Disorders

One of the most common affective disorders is Major Depression (11,12). It is the most prevalent Axis I disorder and it can directly affect the gastrointestinal system in a multitude of ways. Major Depression is often associated with increased pain complaints, particularly abdominal (13). The presence of two or more pain conditions was a better predictor of Major Depression than the severity or persistence of pain (14). It is also associated with an increased incidence of both constipation and esophageal motility disorders (15,16). It may lead directly

TABLE 1 DSM-IV Criteria for a Major Depressive Episode

A. Five (or more) of the following symptoms have been present during the same 2-week period and represent a change from previous functioning; at least one of the symptoms is either (1) depressed mood or (2) loss of interest or pleasure. *Note:* Do not include symptoms that are clearly due to a general medical condition, or mood-incongruent delusions or hallucinations.
   1. Depressed mood most of the day, nearly every day, as indicated by either subjective report (e.g., feels sad or empty) or observation made by others (e.g., appears tearful). *Note:* In children and adolescents, can be irritable mood.
   2. Markedly diminished interest or pleasure in all, or almost all, activities most of the day, nearly every day (as indicated by either subjective account or observation made by others).
   3. Significant weight loss when not dieting or weight gain (e.g., a change of more than 5% of body weight in a month), or decrease or increase in appetite nearly every day. *Note:* In children, consider failure to make expected weight gains.
   4. Insomnia or hypersomnia nearly every day.
   5. Psychomotor agitation or retardation nearly every day (observable by others, not merely subjective feelings of restlessness or being slowed down).
   6. Fatigue or loss of energy nearly every day.
   7. Feelings of worthlessness or excessive or inappropriate guilt (which may be delusional) nearly every day (not merely self-reproach or guilt about being sick).
   8. Diminished ability to think or concentrate, or indecisiveness, nearly every day (either by subjective account or as observed by others).
   9. Recurrent thoughts of death (not just fear of dying), recurrent suicidal ideation without a specific plan, or a suicide attempt or a specific plan for committing suicide. The symptoms do not meet criteria for a Mixed Episode.

C. The symptoms cause clinically significant distress or impairment in social, occupational, or other important areas of functioning.

D. The symptoms are not due to the direct physiological effects of a substance (e.g., a drug of abuse, a medication) or a general medical condition (e.g., hypothyroidism).

E. The symptoms are not better accounted for by Bereavement (i.e., after the loss of a loved one), the symptoms persist for longer than 2 months or are characterized by marked functional impairment, morbid preoccupation with worthlessness, suicidal ideation, psychotic symptoms, or psychomotor retardation.

to lowered pain-tolerance levels (6). Some have hypothesized that depressive disorders may be linked to other psychiatric disorders (e.g., bulimia, panic disorder, attention-deficit disorder, obsessive-compulsive disorder) along with IBS, cataplexy, and migraine. These "affective-spectrum" disorders may be identified by response to antidepressant treatments, possibly sharing pathophysiological commonality (17).

Typically, Major Depression occurs with a lowered mood, early-morning awakening, loss of appetite and weight, lowered libido, inappropriate sense of guilt, and thoughts of death or suicide. The DSM-IV criteria are presented in Table 1. Some cases, however, will not have this typical presentation—the patient may have many signs of depression (e.g., difficult sleeping, poor appetite, and weight loss) but firmly deny any depressed mood. The individual may have what has been called a "masked depression" or a "depressive equivalent" (18,19). He or she may respond dramatically to an antidepressant yet never acknowledge that depression was experienced.

> Case 6: Mr. H. was a 68-year-old man who had lost 70 pounds over a 6-month period. Medical evaluation was unrevealing of an etiology. Despite firmly denying any feeling of depression, Mr. H. appeared flat emotionally and somewhat sullen. His wife noted that he had trouble staying asleep during the 6 months, usually awakening at 4 A.M. Although he rejected a psychiatric consultation that was offered, he accepted a trial of an antidepressant from his gastroenterologist. After starting nortriptyline, he gradually regained his lost weight and appeared more animated. His wife said that he "was his old self." He denied that he had ever been depressed but was agreeable to continuing the nortriptyline.

Major Depression may also present with atypical features. Diagnostic criteria include mood reactivity (i.e., mood brightening in response to actual or potential positive events) accompanied by two or more of the following symptoms: significant weight gain or increased appetite, hypersomnia, leaden paralysis, or chronic interpersonal rejection sensitivity. For example, with mood reactivity, a temporary positive response to the physician's encouragement may lead to an underdiagnosis of depression. Subtyping depressive syndromes has been increasingly important in guiding pharmacological treatments. Atypical depressions have been shown to respond preferentially to serotonin-specific reuptake inhibitors or monoamine oxidase inhibitors. Of course, depressions associated with a Bipolar Disorder have different treatment considerations, possibly involving lithium or an anticonvulsant alone or with an antidepressant.

Comorbid Dysthymia ("double depression") or a personality disorder should always be considered in evaluating depression. The influence of long-standing characterological factors and coping styles has been increasingly investigated (20). Episodic vomiting as a manifestation of self-mutilation has been reported as a presenting symptom for patients with Borderline Personality Disorder (21). The treatment course can be complicated and may require adjunctive behavioral or psychotherapy approaches.

There has been increasing recognition of the high prevalence of mood disorders. Studies such as the Medical Outcomes Study have revealed the need for improvement in diagnosis and treatment, especially in the primary care setting (22,23). Screening instruments designed for the primary care setting may be useful supplements for the busy clinician. An example is the PRIME-MD (Primary Care Evaluation of Mental Disorders), a 26-item patient self-report questionnaire and a brief structured clinical interview (24).

B. Psychotic Disorders

Axis I DSM-IV diagnoses other than Major Depression are also important to consider in evaluating gastrointestinal symptoms. These include the Delusional Disorders and Schizophrenias. These patients may have bizarre ideation about gastrointestinal symptoms. They should be asked what they think is causing their illness. Responses may involve paranoid beliefs about being poisoned by foreign agents. In some instances, the psychosis may be a variant of Major Depression with Psychotic Features. These individuals may have such ideas as that their bowels are being eaten up by cancer or worms, and fail to benefit from realistic reassurances to the contrary. The identification of a psychotic process is an indication for psychiatric consultation.

C. Anxiety Disorders

Another important category of Axis I DSM-IV disorders includes the anxiety disorders. Neurobiological connections between the central and the enteric nervous systems may explain the overlap between anxiety and gastrointestinal complaints (25). Sometimes these individuals focus their complaints on the gastrointestinal tract and do not spontaneously describe their anxiety (14,16).

Panic symptoms may overlap with functional gastrointestinal complaints. In the National Institute of Mental Health (NIMH) Epidemiologic Catchment Area Project, Panic Disorder patients were much more likely to endorse symptoms such as abdominal pain, nausea and vomiting, diarrhea, stomach bloating, and sickness from certain foods and constipation. A careful history will often reveal the anxious components to their symptoms, such as a sudden fear of dying or going crazy, shortness of breath, palpitations, or sweating. A positive response to antipanic medications may confirm the diagnosis (26,27). Refer to Table 2 for a list of DSM-IV panic symptoms and Table 3 for the inclusion criteria for Panic Disorder. Agoraphobia, fears of being in situations where escape may be difficult or embarassing or help unavailale, may or may not accompany a Panic Disor-

TABLE 2 DSM-IV Criteria for a Panic Attack

A discrete period of intense fear or discomfort, in which four (or more) of the following symptoms developed abruptly and reached a peak within 10 minutes:

1. Palpitations, pounding heart, or accelerated heart rate
2. Sweating
3. Trembling or shaking
4. Sensations of shortness of breath or smothering
5. Feeling of choking
6. Chest pain or discomfort
7. Nausea or abdominal distress
8. Feeling dizzy, unsteady, lightheaded, or faint
9. Derealization (feelings of unreality) or depersonalization (being detached from oneself)
10. Fear of losing control or going crazy
11. Fear of dying
12. Paresthesias (numbness or tingling sensations)
13. Chills or hot flushes

TABLE 3 DSM-IV Inclusion Criteria for Panic Disorder

Recurrent, unexpected Panic Attacks, and at least one of the attacks has been followed by 1 month (or more) of one (or more) of the following:

1. Persistent concern about having additional attacks
2. Worry about the implications of the attack or its consequences (e.g., losing control, having a heart attack, "going crazy")
3. A significant change in behavior related to the attacks

der. Questions regarding fears of being outside the home or in crowds, or avoiding travel on bridges, in tunnels, or in automobiles, airplanes, or trains are consistent with agoraphobia.

Bowel obsessions as a manifestation of Obsessive-Compulsive Disorder (OCD) or Social Phobia have been reported. (Refer to Tables 4 and 5.) These patients all described progressive functional disability as they became increasingly preoccupied with gastrointestinal symptoms. Some patients present with fears of incontinence or flatulence. Worries about the location of restrooms and excessive time spent there are also prominent. Other OCD symptoms such as checking may not be present. Antidepressants, particularly the serontonergic agents, are the treatment of choice (28–31). Monosymptomatic hypochondriasis with an olfactory reference symptom of an "anal odor" associated with disabling obsessional rituals has also been described (32). Conversely, increased IBS in OCD patients has also been reported (33).

TABLE 4 DSM-IV Inclusion Criteria for Obsessive-Compulsive Disorder

A. Either obsessions or compulsions: Obsessions as defined by (1), (2), (3), and (4):
   1. Recurrent and persistent thoughts, impulses, or images that are experienced, at some time during the disturbance, as intrusive and inappropriate and that cause marked anxiety or distress
   2. The thoughts, impulses, or images are not simply excessive worries about real-life problems
   3. The person attempts to ignore or suppress such thoughts, impulses, or images, or to neutralize them with some other thought or action
   4. The person recognizes that the obsessional thoughts, impulses, or images are a product of his or her own mind (not imposed from without as in thought insertion)

Compulsions as defined by (1) and (2):
   1. Repetitive behaviors (e.g., hand-washing, ordering, checking) or mental acts (e.g., praying, counting, repeating words silently) that the person feels driven to perform in response to an obsession, or according to rules that must be applied rigidly
   2. The behaviors or mental acts are aimed at preventing or reducing distress or preventing some dreaded event or situation; however, these behaviors or mental acts either are not connected in a realistic way with what they are designed to neutralize or prevent or are clearly excessive

B. At some point during the course of the disorder, the person has recognized that the obsessions or compulsions are excessive or unreasonable. *Note:* This does not apply to children.

C. The obsessions or compulsions cause marked distress, are time-consuming (take more than 1 hour a day), or significantly interfere with the person's normal routine, occupational (or academic) functioning, or usual social activities or relationships.

Given the abovementioned high rates of prior psychological trauma, another anxiety disorder to strongly consider is Posttraumatic Stress Disorder, in which symptoms are clustered as intrusive reexperiencing, stimuli avoidance, and hyperarousal. See Table 6 for the DSM-IV diagnostic criteria.

If anxiety is prominent but the presentation is not consistent with any of the above anxiety disorders, a final category to consider is Generalized Anxiety Disorder. The inclusion criteria are reviewed in Table 7.

D. Somatization and Conversion Disorders

Besides the above specific diagnostic categories, there is another category of individuals who present with gastrointestinal symptoms (among others); these can

TABLE 5 DSM-IV Inclusion Criteria for Social Phobia

A. A marked and persistent fear of one or more social or performance situations in which the peson is exposed to unfamiliar people or to possible scrutiny by others. The individual fears that he or she will act in a way (or show anxiety symptoms) that will be humiliating or embarrassing.
B. Exposure to the feared social situation almost invariably provokes anxiety, which may take the form of a situationally bound or situationally predisposed Panic Attack.
C. The person recognizes that the fear is excessive or unreasonable. *Note:* In children, this feature may be absent.
D. The feared social or performance situations are avoided or else are endured with intense anxiety or distress.
E. The avoidance, anxious anticipation, or distress in the feared social or performance situation(s) interferes significantly with the person's normal routine, occupational (academic) functioning, or social activities or relationships, or there is marked distress about having the phobia.
F. In individuals under age 18 years, the duration is at least 6 months.

be classified as the abnormal illness-affirming behaviors. In these conditions, the individual amplifies signs and symptoms out of proportion to the disease that is present.

One of the foremost of these conditions to consider in evaluation of the gastrointestinal patient is somatization (34). Somatization is basically the somatic expression of psychological distress without the patient's being aware of what he is doing—the process is entirely unconscious. When the somatization is a discrete loss of function such as a paralysis, it has been termed a conversion phenomena. There is usually no organic etiology discovered in the evaluation of the symptom or, if there is an organic etiology, the symptom is out of proportion to the finding.

In some cases the somatization is so widespread (involving multiple symptoms in different organ systems) that the patient qualifies for having the full-blown Somatization Disorder. Women with this disorder outnumber men by a ratio of 10:1. It is usually diagnosed by the time the patient reaches 30 years of age (35,36). Cultural factors seem to influence the type of presentation of somatization symptoms. The DSM-IV criteria reviewed in Table 8 represent the pattern most often seen in the United States. The sex ratio is also influenced by cultural factors; for instance, Greek and Puerto Rican men have higher prevalence rates than reported in U.S. samples. A physician, as opposed to a nonphysician interviewer, also seems to increase the rate of diagnosis (37).

TABLE 6 DSM-IV Diagnostic Criteria for Posttraumatic Stress Disorder

A. The person has been exposed to a traumatic event in which both of the following were present:
   1. The person experienced, witnessed, or was confronted with an event or events that involved actual or threatened death or serious injury, or a threat to the physical integrity of self or others.
   2. The person's response involved intense fear, helplessness, or horror. Note: In children, this may be expressed instead by disorganized or agitated behavior.

B. The traumatic event is persistently reexperienced in one (or more) of the following ways:
   1. Recurrent and intrusive distressing recollections of the event, incuding images, thoughts, or perceptions. Note: In young children, repetitive play may occur in which themes or aspects of the trauma are expressed.
   2. Recurrent distressing dreams of the event. Note: In children, there may be frightening dreams without recognizable content.
   3. Acting or feeling as if the traumatic event were recurring (includes a sense of reliving the experience, illusions, hallucinations, and dissociative flashback episodes, including those that occur on awakening or when intoxicated). Note: In young children, trauma-specific re-enactment may occur.
   4. Intense psychological distress at exposure to internal or external cues that symbolize or resemble an aspect of the traumatic event.
   5. Physiological reactivity on exposure to internal or external cues that symbolize or resemble an aspect of the traumatic event.

C. Persistent avoidance of stimuli associated with the trauma and numbing of general responsiveness (not present before the trauma), as indicated by three (or more) of the following:
   1. Efforts to avoid thoughts, feelings, or conversations associated with the trauma.
   2. Efforts to avoid activities, places, or people that arouse recollections of the trauma.
   3. Inability to recall an important aspect of the trauma.
   4. Markedly diminished interest or participation in significant activities.
   5. Feeling of detachment or estrangement from others.
   6. Restricted range of affect (e.g., unable to have loving feelings).
   7. Sense of a foreshortened future (e.g., does not expect to have a career, marriage, children, or a normal life span).

D. Persistent symptoms of increased arousal (not present before the trauma), as indicated by two (or more) of the following:
   1. Difficulty falling or staying asleep.
   2. Irritability or outbursts of anger.
   3. Difficulty concentrating.
   4. Hypervigilance.
   5. Exaggerated startle response.

TABLE 6 Continued

E. Duration of the disturbance (symptoms in criteria B, C, and D) is more than 1 month.
F. The disturbance causes clinically significant distress or impairment in social, occupational, or other important areas of functioning. Specify if:
Acute: if duration of symptoms is less than 3 months.
Chronic: if duration of symptoms is 3 months or more.
With Delayed Onset: if onset of symptoms is at least 6 months after the stressor.

These patients do best when treated by one primary physician who sets regular appointments for the patient; the appointments should not be symptom-contingent or the patient will need to continue the symptom production to maintain the relationship with the physician. Unless there are clearcut signs of disease, abstaining from invasive diagnostic procedures is also helpful in minimizing costs and iatrogenic complications (35).

Case 7: Mrs. L. was a 48-year-old woman who had been married 28 years. She presented to the gastroenterologist with a somewhat vague history of abdominal cramps and diarrhea alternating with periods of constipation. She had failed to respond to several measures to treat irritable bowel. Several surgical procedures had been done over a 20-year period for a variety of complaints; these include a laparotomy for fulguration of endometriosis, a hysterectomy for dysmenorrhea and men-

TABLE 7 DSM-IV Inclusion Criteria for Generalized Anxiety Disorder

A. Excessive anxiety and worry (apprehensive expectation), occurring on more days than not for at least 6 months, about a number of events or activities (such as work or school performance).
B. The person finds it difficult to control the worry.
C. The anxiety and worry are associated with three (or more) of the following six symptoms (with at least some symptoms present for more days than not for the past 6 months). *Note:* Only one item is required in children.
   1. Restlessness or feeling keyed up or on edge
   2. Being easily fatigued
   3. Difficulty concentrating or mind going blank
   4. Irritability
   5. Muscle tension
   6. Sleep disturbance (difficulty falling or staying asleep, or restless unsatisfying sleep)

TABLE 8 DSM-IV Diagnostic Criteria for Somatization Disorder

A. A history of many physical complaints beginning before age 30 years that occur over a period of several years and result in treatment being sought or significant impairment in social, occupational, or other important areasl of functioning.

B. Each of the following criteria must have been met, with individual symptoms occurring at any time during the course of the disturbance:
   1. Four pain symptoms: a history of pain related to at least four different sites or functions (e.g., head, abdomen, back, joints, extremities, chest, or rectum, during menstruation, sexual intercourse, or urination).
   2. Two gastrointestinal symptoms: a history of at least two gastrointestinal symptoms other than pain (e.g., nausea, bloating, vomiting other than during pregnancy, diarrhea, or intolerance of several foods).
   3. One sexual symptom: a history of at least one sexual or reproductive symptom other than pain (e.g., sexual indifference, erectile or ejaculatory dysfunction, irregular menses, excessive menstrual bleeding, vomiting throughout pregnancy).
   4. One pseudoneurological symptom: a history of at least one symptom or deficit suggesting a neurological condition not limited to pain (conversion symptoms such as impaired coordination or balance, paralysis or localized weakness, difficulty swallowing or lump in throat, aphonia, urinary retention, hallucinations, loss of touch or pain sensation, double vision, blindness, deafness, seizures; dissociative symptoms such as amnesia; or loss of consciousness other than fainting).

C. Either (1) or (2):
   1. After appropriate investigation, each of the symptoms in criteria B cannot be fully explained by a known general medical condition or the direct effects of a substance (e.g., a drug of abuse, a medication).
   2. When there is a related general medical condition, the physical complaints or resulting social or occupational impairment are in excess of what would be expected from the history, physical examination, or laboratory findings. The symptoms are not intentionally feigned or produced (as in Factitious Disorder or Malingering).

orrhagia, an exploratory laparotomy for lysis of adhesions, and a cholecystectomy for right-upper-quadrant pain. She also had a history of chronic headache and firbomyalgia. In getting history from the patient's husband, the physician learned that she "had been sick with one thing after another since I first knew her." The physician diagnosed her with a somatization disorder and discussed an appropriate treatment plan with her primary physician.

There are many instances, however, where an individual uses a few specific symptoms over time as part of his or her somatization, for example, recurring abdominal cramps or nausea without any identifiable organic etiology. These pains might be expected to occur with particular psychosocial stressors; if the history-gathering is meticulous, a pattern of stressors and somatization symptoms may emerge. The somatization symptoms can be considered the patient's preferred coping mechanism. There is evidence that some individuals may be biologically prone to using this type of coping mechanism and being much less inclined to talk about distressed emotions (38,39). On the other hand, adults usually do use similar coping techniques throughout their lives. Thus, if a patient is being evaluated and there is not a past history of somatizing (confirmed by previous medical records or a spouse), this history makes it extremely unlikely that the current symptom is a somatization. Adults rarely develop a coping technique de novo.

E. Hypochondriasis

Another condition similar to somatization, in terms of being unconsciously produced by the patient, is hypochondriasis. In this condition, the patient has the persistent belief that he or she has a disease; this belief is refractory to medical evaluations and reassurances by physicians. The condition often occurs in patients during their 40s or older, usually with an equal proportion of men and women. Some investigators have linked hypochondriasis to depression and recommended antidepressant-medication trials (40). Similar to patients with somatization disorder, these patients often do not recognize that any psychiatric disorder is present, so they do best when followed by one primary physician (41). This physician should adopt an attitude that is not too reassuring lest the patient feel the doctor is dismissing him; it is preferable for the physician to say that because he realizes the patient is genuinely suffering he wants to see him regularly to monitor the medical condition. As with somatization-disorder patients, hypochondriacal patients often do best with time-contingent appointments.

F. Factitious Disorder

There are two forms of abnormal illness-affirming behaviors that are consciously produced (42). Factitious disorders are consciously produced by the patient, but the motivation is unconscious. An outside observer, speculating as to why a patient would create an illness, could only guess that the patient wanted to assume the sick role for some psychological reason. Although Munchausen syndrome is the most widely recognized variant of factitious disorder (case 8), the majority of these patients are not Munchausen (43). They do not meet the Munchausen criteria of wandering, sociopathy, pseudologia fantastica (tall tales), and uninterrupted patienthood. Most patients with factitious disorder are stable geographically, have significant social networks, and often work in the health field. Although Munchausen patients are regarded as untreatable psychiatrically, other factitious disorder patients have better prognoses (44).

These patients may present to the gastroenterologist in various ways. They may take substances that simulate or actually produce illness. Other agents can be ingested that also produce symptoms, such as persistent electrolyte abnormalities. Dilution of stool samples has been reported in cases of factitious diarrhea (45). These patients can be effectively treated psychiatrically once the diagnosis has been established (46). The diagnosis often takes several years, however, because the patient's deception surprises most physicians.

> Case 8: Mr. G. was admitted to the hospital for an investigation of persistent symptoms of small-bowel obstruction. He claimed that he had had severe nausea and vomiting over the prior 12 months and requested a gastrectomy, saying that, prior to moving to the area, his former physicians had told him that was the only hope for relief from his condition. Medical history revealed that he had obtained several different surgical procedures in various parts of the country. His psychosocial history had several inconsistencies—he stated that he had a Ph.D. in neuroanatomy but he was not knowledgeable in that area. Eventually, his physicians determined that a gastrectomy would not be helpful to his medical status. They were about to suggest psychiatric treatment for factitious disorder when he abruptly left the hospital, saying he had heard of another hospital where he knew he could ge the surgery.

There are two broad approaches to the treatment of factitious physical disorders (47). One strategy is to have a primary physician and a consulting psychiatrist confront the patient in a nonpunitive way. The factitious disorder is interpreted as a cry for help and the patient is urged to enter psychiatric treatment. In another approach—one that avoids confrontation—the physician provides the patient with a face-saving way to recover without having to admit the factitious etiology. There are several variations to this technique. One mode is to offer the patient such vehicles as biofeedback or hypnosis as new ways to recover from his or her illness. A stronger approach is to utilize a double-bind. In this method, the patient is told there are two possible diagnoses: a factitious one and an organic one. If the problem is organic, it should respond to the next medical intervention (usually a minor one, such as a new medication trial). If the symptom fails to respond, the diagnosis will be of factitious etiology. The patient is thus offered alternative pathways of either improving or confirming the factitious diagnosis.

G. Malingering

In contrast to Facitious Disorder, Malingering involves an individual's consciously producing signs or symptoms of illness for conscious motivations. An outside observer could easily speculate on the individual's motivation: winning litigation, gaining disability payments, getting relief from a noxious situation. In most settings that do not involve a forensic evaluation, a true malingerer is rare. Many physicians, however, are not sensitive to the important differentiations involved and lump all abnormal illness-affirming patients into the malingerer category. This does a gross disservice to paients, because those in all the other categories produce their symptoms without knowing why, and not for secondary gain. Table 9 reviews the conscious and unconscious components of these disorders.

H. Pain Disorder Associated with Psychological Factors (Somatoform Pain Disorder)

A final category of abnormal illness-affirming behavior to consider is that of Pain Disorder Associated with Psychological Factors (Somatoform Pain Disorder in DSM-IIIR). In this category, the pain symptoms are generally regarded to be out of proportion to the disease that is present. These patients are similar to somatization patients except that their symptom is pain. Often the pain complaint has specific psychological connections that can be explored as outlined earlier in the chapter. Often, the pain complaint is modeled after a family member who had a similar pain (48,49). Indeed, if one thinks of a pain complaint arising without adequate somatic stimulant, it must be based on psychological input; the psychological input must then be related to someone with a similar pain. In other words, a psychologically derived complaint could not arise with-

TABLE 9 Abnormal Illness Behaviors

	Signs and Symptoms	
	Production	Motivation
Malingering	Conscious	Conscious
Factitious Disorder	Conscious	Unconscious
Conversion Disorder		
Hypochondriasis		
Somatization Disorder	Unconscious	Unconscious
Pain Disorder Associated with Psychological Factors		

Source: Adapted from Ref. 42.

out some model. As noted earlier, patients with Pain Disorder Associated with Psychological Factors often have a childhood history of physical and sexual abuse. They also have prominent concerns with guilt; this may be manifest with pain increasing at "positive" moments in life such as on vacation or after a job promotion.

> Case 9: Mrs. W. was a 42-year-old woman who had persistent complaints of abdominal pain. She described a "deep, cruel pain" in her epigastric region. When asked if she knew anyone else who had a similar problem, she said the pain seemed similar to the pain her father had died of with pancreatic cancer 10 years earlier. Questioned about her family and her childhood, she described it as "terrible." Her father had been sexually abusive of her and her younger sister for several years. She had married as a teenager to escape her father, but her husband had turned out to be physically abusive of her. She divorced him, but then married another man who was also physically abusive. After a second divorce, she found a third husband, who treated her well. Shortly after that marriage, however, she developed the abdominal pain. She accepted a referral for outpatient psychotherapy.

Many of these individuals will do best if managed similarly to the somatization disorder patient—regular visits with a primary physician who limits invasive procedures to those indicated by signs of disease (49). These individuals often benefit from antidepressant trials as well. Not only do the antidepressants treat the depression occurring in association with the pain, but they also may directly treat the pain via central nervous system effects (50). Tricyclic agents such as doxepin have multiple effects, including anticholinergic, serotonergic, and anti-H_2. These effects may be used advantageously with some abdominal pain patients. Similarly, the newer serotonin-specific agents such as fluoxetine tend to enhance gut motility and may be selected when this feature is important. It has also been used successfully to treat abdominal pain (50).

I. Eating Disorders

Another set of disorders that share some features with the factitious disorders are the eating disorders. These patients consciously alter their food intake, usually for motivations that are unconscious. As with factitious disorder patients, these individuals appear to act compulsively as they attempt to alter their bodily functions. They can be differentiated from factitious disorder patients by their abnormal body image—e.g., the anorexic who believes she is fat when she is actually cachexic. Physical signs of anorexia or bulimia also serve to identify these patients. Findings such as loss of tooth enamel with recurrent emesis or melanosis coli with laxative abuse may be diagnostic. These are discussed more fully in Chapter 11.

IV. SUMMARY

The psychosocial assessment of the gastrointestinal symptom may yield extraordinary amounts of information. At a minimum, this assessment will enhance the physician's understanding of the patient's illness and its impact. In some instances, this assessment will be crucial to making any successful intervention with the patient. Anything that fosters the psychosocial assessment, such as talking to the patient's spouse or primary physician, will improve the accuracy of the assessment. Once a clear understanding of the patient's biopsychosocial situation has been achieved, the path to appropriate treatment is more easily chosen.

REFERENCES

1. Folks DG, Kinney FC. The role of psychological factors in gastrointestinal conditions Psychosomatics 1992; 33:257–270.
2. Melzack R. The McGill pain questionnaire: Major properties and scoring methods. Pain 1975; I:277–299.
3. Ford MJ, McMiller P, Eastwood J, Eastwood MA. Life events, psychiatric illness and the irritable bowel syndrome. Gut 1987; 28:160–165.
4. Creed F, Craig T, Farmer R. Functional abdominal pain, psychiatric illness, and life events. Gut 1988; 29:235–242.
5. Walker E, Katon K, Harrop-Griffiths J, et al. Relationship of chronic pelvic pain to psychiatric diagnoses and childhood sexual abuse. Am J Psychiatry 1988; 145:75–80.
6. Katon W, Egan K, Miller D. Chronic pain: lifetime psychiatric diagnoses and family history. Am J Psychiatry 1985; 142:1156–1160.
7. Drossman D, Leserman J, Nachman G, et al. Sexual and physical abuse in women with functional or organic gastrointestinal disorders. Ann Intern Med 1990; 113:828–833.
8. Raskin M, Talbott JA, Myerson AT. Diagnosis of conversion reactions-predictive value of psychiatric criteria. JAMA 1966; 1966:102–106.
9. Walker, EA, Roy-Byrne PP, Katon WJ et al. Psychiatric illness and irritable bowel syndrome: A comparison with inflammatory bowel disease. Am J Psychiatry 1990; 147:1656–1661.
10. Whitehead WE, Bosmajian L, Zonderman AB, et al. Symptoms of psychologic distress associated with irritable bowel syndrome: Comparison of community and medical clinic samples. Gastroenterology 1988; 95:709–714.
11. von Ammon Cavanaugh S. Depression in the hospitalized inpatient with various medical illnesses. Psychother Psychosom 1986; 4:97–104.
12. Rodin G, Voshart K. Depression in the medically ill: an overview. Am J Psychiatry 1986; 696–705.
13. Melzack R, Wall PD. The Challenge of Pain. New York: Basic Books, 1983.
14. Dworkin SF, Von Korff M. Multiple pains and psychiatric disturbance. Arch Gen Psychiatry 1990; 47:239–244.
15. Bradley LA, McDonald JE, Richer JE. Psychophysiological interactions in the

esophageal diseases: implications for assessment and treatment. Semin Gastrointest Dis 1990; 1:5–22.
16. Nielzen S, Pettersson KI, Regnell G et al. The role of psychiatric factors in symptoms of hiatus hernia or gastric reflux. Acta Psychiatr Scand 1986; 73:214–220.
17. Hudson J, Pope H. Affective spectrum disorder: Does antidepressant response identify a family of disorders with a common pathophysiology? Am J Psychiatry 1990; 147:552–564.
18. Lesse S. Behavioral problems masking severe depression. Am J Psychother 1979; 33:41–53.
19. Blumer D, Heilbronn M. The pain-prone disorder: a clinical and psychological profile. Psychosomatics 1981; 22:395–402.
20. Drossman DA, McKee DC, Sandler RS, et al. Psychosocial factors in the irritable bowel syndrome: A multivariate study of patients and nonpatients with irritable bowel syndrome. Gastroenterology 1988; 95:701–708.
21. Johnson TM. Vomiting as a manifestation of borderline personality disorder in primary care. J Am Board Fam Prac 1993; 6:385–394.
22. Sturm R, Wells KB. How can care for depression become more cost-effective? JAMA 1995; 273:51–58.
23. Wells KB, Katon W, Rogers B, Camp P. Use of minor tranquilizers and antidepressant medications by depressed outpatients: Results of the medical outcomes study. Am J Psychiatry 1994; 151:694–700.
24. Spitzer RL, Williams J, Kroenke K, et al. Utility of a new procedure for diagnosing mental disorders in primary care: The PRIME-MD 1000 study. JAMA 1994; 272:1749–1756.
25. Clouse RE. Anxiety and gastrointestinal illness. Psychiatric Clin North Am 1988; 11:399–417.
26. Lydiard RB, Greenwald S, Weissman M, et al. Panic disorder and gastrointestinal symptoms: findings from the NIMH Epidemiologic Catchment Area project. Am J Psychiatry 1994; 151:64–70.
27. Lydiard RB, Laraia MT, Howell EF, Ballenger JC. Can panic disorder present as irritable bowel syndrome? J Clin Psychiatry 1986; 47:470–473.
28. Jenike MA, Vitagliano HL, Rabinowitz, J, et al. Bowel Obsessions responsive to tricyclic antidepressants. Am J Psychiatry 1987; 144:1347–1348.
29. Sharma V. Bowel obsessions and clomipramine. Can J Psychiatry; 1991; 36:233–234.
30. Lyketsos CG. Successful treatment of bowel obsessions with nortriptyline. Am J Psychiatry 1992; 149:573.
31. Kahne CJ, Wray RW. Clomipramine for bowel obsessions. Am J Psychiatry 19898; 146:120–121.
32. Jenike MA. Illness related to obsessive-compulsive disorder. In: Jenike MA, Baer L, Minichiello WE, eds. Obsessive-Compulsive Disorders: Theory and Management. 2nd ed. St. Louis: Mosby-Year Book, 1990:39–60.
33. Olden K, Jenike M, Baer L, Horn S. Is irritable bowel syndrome related to OCD? 146th Annual Meeting of American Psychiatric Association, San Francisco, CA, May 22–27, 1993.
34. Pilowsky I, Chapman C, Bonica J. Pain, depression and illness behavior in a pain clinic population. Pain 1977; 4:183–192.

35. Smith GR. Effectiveness of treatment for somatoform disorder patients. Psychiatric Med 1991; 9:545–558.
36. Katon W, Kleinman A, Rosen G. Depression and somatization: a review, Part I. Am J Med 1982; 72:127–247.
37. Diagnostic and Statistical Manual of Mental Disorders, 4th ed. Washington DC: American Psychiatric Press, 1994.
38. Sifneos P, Apfel-Savitz F, Frankel F. The phenomenon of alexythymia. Psychother Psychosom 1977; 28:47–57.
39. Cloninger CR, Sigvardsson S, von Knorring AL. An adoption study of somatoform disorders: II: identification of two discrete somatoform disorders. Arch Gen Psychiatry 1984; 41:863–871.
40. Kellner R. Diagnosis and treatment of hypochondriacal symptoms. Psychosomatics 1992; 33:278–289.
41. Hernandez J, Kellner R. Hypochondriacal concerns and attitudes towards illness in males and females. Int J Psychiatry Med 1992; 22:251–263.
42. Eisendrath SJ. Factitious illness: a clarification. Psychosomatics 1984; 25:110–117.
43. Reich P, Gottfried LA. Factitious disorders in a teaching hospital. Ann Intern Med 1983; 99:240–247.
44. Eisendrath SJ. Factitious physical disorders: treatment without confrontation. Psychosomatics 1989; 30:383–387.
45. Topazian M, Binder HJ. Brief report: factitious diarrhea detected by measurement of stool osmolality. New Engl J Med 1994; 330:1418–1419.
46. Engel GL. Psychogenic pain and the pain-prone patient. Am J med 1959; 26:899–918.
47. Eisendrath SJ. Factitious physical disorders. West J Med 1994; 160:177–179.
48. Eisendrath SJ, Way LW, Ostroff JW, Johanson CA. Identification of psychogenic abdominal pain. Psychosomatics 1986; 27:705–711.
49. DeVaul RA, Faillace LA. Persistent pain and illness insistence. Am J Surgery 1978; 135:828–833.
50. Eisendrath SJ. Fluoxetine management of chronic abdominal pain. Psychosomatics 1992; 33:227–229.

3

Functional GI Disorders: Classification and Epidemiology

Douglas A. Drossman
University of North Carolina at Chapel Hill
Chapel Hill, North Carolina

I. INTRODUCTION

The functional gastrointestinal (GI) disorders are defined as a ". . . variable combination of chronic or recurrent gastrointestinal symptoms not explained by structural or biochemical abnormalities" (1). The first published account of a functional GI disorder using symptoms similar to modern criteria was made 175 years ago (2), but there were only occasional reports until the middle of this century, when their systematic investigation began (3–5). Since that time, there has been a progressive increase in attention to these disorders by both the general public and clinical investigators. For example, as shown in Figure 1, over the last 15 years, the number of publications on irritable bowel syndrome (IBS) accessible through the National Library of Medicine (MEDLINE) has tripled.

There are several possible reasons for this increased interest: 1) newer investigative techniques in GI physiology (motility/visceral pain measurement), 2) recent epidemiological data (e.g., population-based studies) that indicate their high prevalence and health impact within society, 3) increasing interest in women's health issues, and 4) growing focus on a systems-oriented (biopsychosocial) and patient-centered approach toward illness and health care, with the

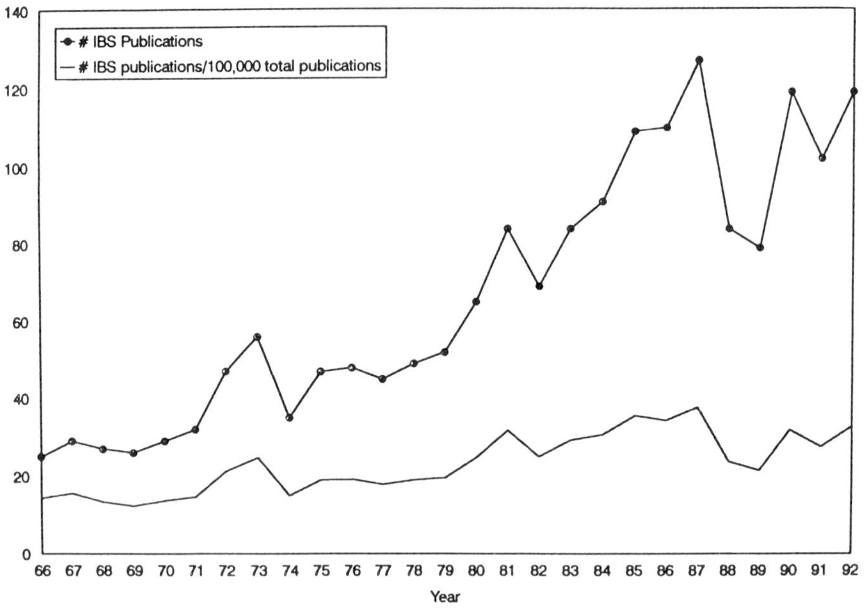

FIGURE 1 Number of publications on irritable bowel syndrome (IBS) accessible through the National Library of Medicine (MEDLINE) from 1966 to 1992. The lower line represents the number of publications about IBS adjusted for the number of total publications in the library. (From Ref. 10, © 1994. Published by Little, Brown and Company.)

functional GI disorders being most representative. Relevant to this chapter, another important reason for the increased attention to these disorders relates to the development of diagnostic classification systems. While the functional GI disorders have existed throughout history, the lack of identifiable pathology impeded their categorization as clinical entities, and some people even doubted their existence (6)! Only recently have efforts been made to define and classify the functional GI disorders, and, interestingly, the first diagnostic criteria for IBS, published in 1978 (7), just preceded the dramatic increase in research publications (Figure 1).

In this chapter I review the rationale, limitations, and process for developing a symptom-based classification for the functional GI disorders. Following this I describe the major symptom subgroups of these disorders based on the newly established multinational ("Rome") consensus criteria. Finally, I review their epidemiology, sociodemographic features, and health impact. It is anticipated that the use of these criteria will improve upon previous research efforts and clinical care by permitting the proper selection of patient groups for pathophysiological investigation and treatment.

II. RATIONALE FOR DEVELOPMENT OF SYMPTOM-BASED ("ROME") CRITERIA

The rationale for a diagnostic classification system is based on the premise that each symptom grouping "breeds true." In effect, patients fulfilling criteria for a diagnosis are presumed to be more similar to one another in their underlying pathophysiology and treatments than to those having other diagnoses. This presumption provides a framework for patient identification and investigation that can be modified as new scientific data emerge. At the least, diagnostic categories reduce the difficulties that existed in previous studies in which arbitrary selection criteria yielded mixed clinical populations (8,9).

The rationale for a classification system has three bases:

A. Regional Differences Along the Gastrointestinal Tract

Patients with functional GI disorders report a wide variety of symptoms affecting different regions of the gastrointestinal tract. While these symptoms may have in common disturbances in sensory or motor gastrointestinal function, or in the neurotransmitters and receptors affecting these functions, their target organs are frequently different. A disorder such as globus presumably results from a disturbance of upper-esophageal-sphincter function, while gallbladder dyskinesia results from a disturbance of gallbladder function, and levator syndrome from a disturbance in pelvic-floor-muscle function. This presumption permits the functional GI disorders to be separated into six regional groupings: Esophageal, Gastroduodenal, Bowel, Functional Abdominal Pain, Biliary, and Anorectal disorders. Diagnostic entities can also be subcategorized within each site. For example, IBS, functional constipation, and functional diarrhea all describe abnormalities related to the regulation of colonic function, and are subsumed under the Functional Bowel Disorder grouping.

B. Epidemiological Studies

Epidemiological studies of various functional GI disorders show similarities across social groups. For example, the frequencies of irritable bowel syndrome in England, France, and China are similar, and range from 10 to 17% (10). Within the United States, the frequencies of functional constipation (3.0%) and diarrhea (1.6%) in a national study of U.S. householders (11) using the "Rome" criteria are similar to data from the National Health Interview Survey (3.0%, and 1.2%, respectively), which used a different assessment method (12).

The rationale for symptom-based diagnostic criteria are also upheld by statistical methods such as factor analysis, which identifies groups of symptoms that aggregate into discrete clusters. For example, a factor analysis study using two community samples (13) identified an irritable bowel factor, and the symptoms for this factor were similar to those obtained by discriminant-function analysis ("Manning criteria") from a clinical population of irritable bowel patients (7).

C. Need for Symptom-Based Criteria in Clinical Care and Research

While functional GI symptoms have underlying physiological determinants, valid or clinically acceptable physiological markers do not exist, and physiological assessment remains an investigative tool that is not easily applied to clinical settings. Furthermore, physiological dysfunction does not necessarily correlate with symptoms. Since patients bring symptoms to physicians for treatment, it is clinically important to categorize them in order to characterize their underlying pathophysiology, whether due to abnormal motility, visceral sensation, psychological factors, or a combination. Symptom-based criteria simplify diagnosis and the selection of patients for research.

The use of symptom-based diagnostic criteria has already achieved worldwide acceptance, notably through the American Psychiatric Association's *Diagnostic and Statistical Manual of Mental Disorders* (DSM-IV) (14) and the American Rheumatologic Association's *Primer on the Rheumatic Diseases* (15). In both cases, biochemical (in psychiatry) or histopathological (in rheumatology) findings did not adequately classify the known clinical disorders, and a symptom-based categorization has led to new advancements in their pathophysiology and treatment.

It is also important to standardize the selection of patients for clinical trials. In previous studies with IBS, mixed patient samples (e.g., combining those with predominant diarrhea with those having predominant constipation) increased the likelihood that a medication (e.g., to control diarrhea) would not be effective (9). Symptom-based criteria allow patient groups to be targeted to the predicted effects of the treatment (i.e., to treat diarrhea or constipation). Within psychiatry, there is evidence that panic disorder is clinically distinct from generalized anxiety, and is more closely linked to depression, even though anxiety is common to both disorders. Therefore, these disorders are classified separately in DSM-IV. Using these criteria, it was found that patients with panic disorder respond better to antidepressants than patients with generalized anxiety.

III. QUALIFICATIONS AND LIMITATIONS OF SYMPTOM-BASED CRITERIA

A. Symptoms May Overlap

Since the functional GI disorders are interrelated in their pathophysiology and clinical expression, many patients will have symptoms that incorporate more than one functional GI disorder. For the purposes of research, the diagnostic criteria include statements that permit separation of subgroups. For example, if an individual has a functional bowel disorder and fulfills criteria for both IBS and functional constipation, by convention he or she is given a diagnosis of IBS.

B. Functional GI Disorders May Coexist with Other Diseases

The high prevalences of the functional GI disorders make it likely that they will coexist with other GI diseases. For example, recent attention has been paid to the coexistence of inflammatory bowel disease and IBS (16). Therefore, an increase in symptoms of diarrhea and abdominal pain in a patient with Crohn's disease may also be based on physiological (i.e., functional) disturbance rather than activation of the primary disease (16), and often they interact. By convention, diagnosis of a functional GI disorder requires that other diseases producing similar symptoms that have a known structural (e.g., Crohn's disease) or biochemical basis (e.g., lactase deficiency) be excluded. This convention is of pragmatic value for research, but it assumes that physicians will make adequate judgments in clinical practice with regard to the patient's diagnostic and treatment needs.

C. Symptoms Must Be Present for at Least 3 Months

Recent evidence supports the clinical observation that for many persons functional GI symptoms are transient (17,18). For this reason, their diagnosis as a clinical disorder requires that symptoms be present for at least 3 months (6 months for functional abdominal pain syndrome, 1 month for fecal incontinence).

D. Underlying Pathophysiology Will Vary with Diagnosis

Some functional GI disorders appear to be linked to disturbances in motility (e.g., sphincter of Oddi dysfunction, fecal incontinence, pelvic-floor dyssynergia). Others are characterized by disturbances in visceral sensation or CNS–Enteric Nervous System dysregulation (e.g., functional abdominal pain), and some appear to have both features (e.g., IBS, functional dyspepsia). These observations support the concept of pathophysiological heterogeneity for these disorders.

E. Validation Is Determined by Clinical Consensus and Future Research

Since there are no biochemical or physiological standards to diagnose the functional GI disorders, the proposed criteria are derived from clinical investigation, and are validated by the consensus of experts in the field. However, it is likely that future studies will lead to modification in the criteria as new data emerge and, much like the DSM system, a process for revision of the criteria is established. We recognize that experienced clinicians and investigators may have different diagnostic standards based on their training, experience, and personal beliefs. Still, the diagnosis of patients according to these criteria standardizes the selection of patients for research and serves as a starting point for investigative studies and treatment trials.

IV. CRITERIA DEVELOPMENT AND THE WORKING TEAM COMMITTEES

The original idea for using a consensus process to establish diagnostic criteria was initiated by Professor Aldo Torsoli, the president of the International Congress of Gastroenterology held in Rome in 1988 (Roma '88). He proposed that diagnostic criteria for IBS be established. The committee process was similar to the "Delphi" method (19), which fosters a team effort to produce consistency in opinion, or consensus (although not necessarily total agreement). After the publication of the IBS criteria (20), an ongoing process was set up to define, characterize, and establish diagnostic standards for all the functional GI disorders by committee (1). Over the last 6 years, the so-called "Rome" criteria have appeared in *Gastroenterology International* (21–25), and an expanded and updated compilation of the diagnosis, pathophysiology, and treatment of these disorders has been published in book form (26). The documents produced by these committees have involved the work of 30 members from 11 countries, in addition to 48 international consultants. As new investigative data emerge, a mechanism has been set up for these Working Team Committees to modify the diagnostic criteria and other information in future publications (27).

V. CLASSIFICATION

The functional GI disorders are listed in Table 1. The specific criteria for these disorders and their clinical features are beyond the scope of this chapter and can be found elsewhere (1,21–26). However, several general features of this classification system are to be noted: 1) the disorders are classified by organ systems, 2) as in the DSM system, most of the major categories have an "unspecified" diagnosis to include those disorders not fulfilling specific criteria, 3) adequate medical evaluation must be done to exclude other diseases (e.g., peptic ulcer disease for functional dyspepsia, inflammatory bowel disease for IBS) producing similar symptoms, and 4) the symptoms must be present for at least 3 months (1 month for functional incontinence, 6 months for functional abdominal pain).

Table 1 Functional Gastrointestinal Disorders

A. Esophageal disorders
   1. Globus
   2. Rumination Syndrome
   3. Functional Chest Pain of Presumed Esophageal Origin
   4. Functional Heartburn
   5. Functional Dysphagia
   6. Unspecified Functional Esophageal Disorder
B. Gastroduodenal disorders
   1. Functional Dyspepsia
      a. Ulcer-Like Dyspepsia
      b. Dysmotility-Like Dyspepsia
      c. Unspecified Dyspepsia
   2. Aerophagia
C. Bowel disorders
   1. Irritable Bowel Syndrome
   2. Functional Abdominal Bloating
   3. Functional Constipation
   4. Functional Diarrhea
   5. Unspecified Functional Bowel Disorder
D. Functional abdominal pain
   1. Functional Abdominal Pain Syndrome
   2. Unspecified Functional Abdominal Pain
E. Biliary disorders
   1. Gallbladder Dysfunction
   2. Sphincter of Oddi Dysfunction
F. Anorectal disorders
   1. Functional Incontinence
   2. Functional Anorectal Pain
      a. Levator Ani Syndrome
      b. Proctalgia Fugax
   3. Dyschezia
      a. Pelvic Floor Dyssynergia
      b. Internal Anal Sphincter Dysfunction
   4. Unspecified Functional Anorectal Disorder

VI. PREVALENCE, SOCIODEMOGRAPHIC FEATURES, AND HEALTH CARE IMPACT

As shown from a recent U.S. population study (11), the functional GI disorders have major social and economic impact. This section summarizes, based on this survey, the frequencies of the functional GI disorders and their sociodemographic associations and health care impact. The methods and a more detailed discussion of the findings can be found in the original publication (11).

We conducted a random stratified mailing to 8250 heads of U.S. households; 5430 responses (66%) were returned for analysis. Fifty-one percent were female, and the mean age was 49.1 years (±15.9 SD). Caucasians were the predominant respondents (96%), and the geographic distribution approximated that of the U.S. population. The household income was $35,000 or above in 47%, and 59% of the respondents were employed. Compared to the U.S. Householder population, there was a higher proportion of females (46% vs. 33%) and whites (96% vs. 86%), and a lower proportion of single household members (15% vs. 25%) among the respondents. These differences were controlled for in the analyses.

A. Frequencies of Functional GI Disorders and Health Care Use Rates

Table 2 includes the frequencies for the functional GI disorders before and after excluding subjects with self-reported structural diagnoses. It notes that the national estimate of having at least one functional GI symptom was 69%, and breaks them down by anatomical region: esophageal symptoms 42%, gastroduodenal symptoms 26%, bowel symptoms and chronic (functional) abdominal pain 44%, and anorectal symptoms 26%. The degree of overlap among the functional GI symptoms is noted in Figure 2. So, for example, of those with functional bowel symptoms, 56% also reported esophageal symptoms, 37% reported gastroduodenal symptoms, and 41% reported anorectal symptoms.

The estimated national prevalences for each specific functional GI diagnosis ranges from less than 1% (sphincter of Oddi dyskinesia) to 32% (functional abdominal bloating). These frequencies may differ from clinical prevalence rates because, for the latter, estimates are determined by who goes to the doctor. However, an epidemiological study also allows us to determine the differential frequencies of health care use. For example, functional abdominal bloating and aerophagia are two of the most prevalent diagnoses (32% and 24%, respectively), yet the rate of physician visits is low (9% and 13%), so physicians see only a small proportion of symptomatic individuals. In comparison, more painful disorders: functional chest pain, functional dyspepsia, IBS, chronic functional abdominal pain, and functional biliary pain occur relatively less frequently in the population (less than 15%), but they lead to higher rates of health care seeking (at least 40% have seen a physician). These observations are consistent with the presumption that painful symptoms are more likely to lead to physician visits (28).

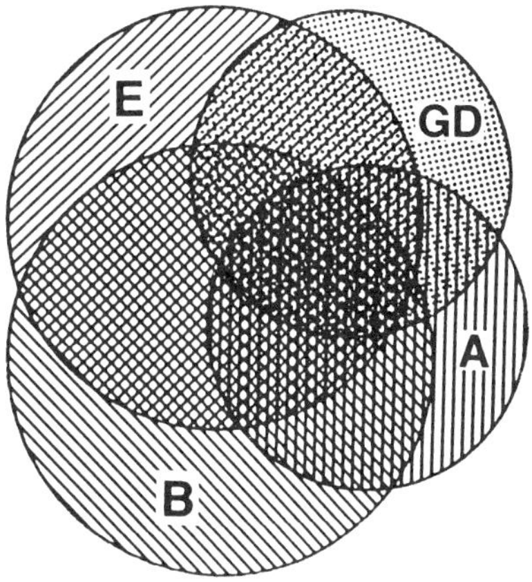

FIGURE 2 Schematic representation of frequencies of functional GI disorders and their associations among survey respondents. E = esophageal; GD = gastroduodenal; B = bowel; A = anorectal. (From Ref. 11.)

B. Sociodemographic Associations

Gender

As shown in Table 3, there is a general tendency for females to report more functional GI symptoms, including globus, functional dysphagia, IBS, functional constipation, functional abdominal pain, functional biliary pain, and dyschezia. However, females were *less likely* to report aerophagia and functional bloating. We also found that females were more likely to seek health care for functional GI disorders. For all diagnoses combined, 44.2% of females had been to physicians, compared to 34.6% of males.

Age

Table 3 also indicates frequencies of functional GI diagnoses based on age strata. When compared to respondents 45 years and over, there was a greater frequency of functional GI disorders in younger patients—for all diagnoses: age 15–34: OR 1.17, 95% CI 1.0–1.4; age 35–44: OR 1.24, 95% CI 1.1–1.5). With regard to specific diagnoses, the younger groups were more likely to report most categories of functional esophageal symptoms, aerophagia, IBS, and proctalgia fugax. However, the frequency of functional incontinence increased with age.

Other Sociodemographic Associations

There were no race-related differences except that Caucasians were less likely to report functional dyspepsia (OR 0.44, 95%CI 0.3–0.8) and functional constipa-

TABLE 2 Prevalence of Functional GI Disorders and Physician Visits Before and After Excluding Structiral Diagnoses

Functional GI symptoms	Met diagnostic criteria		Had ever seen doctor		Diagnosis after excluding self-reported structural diagnoses		
	n	%	*n*	%[a]	*n*	%	National estimate [b]
A Esophageal symptoms	2488	45.8	947	38.1	2310	42.5	41.6 (40.0–43.2)
1. Globus	680	12.5	249	36.3	679	12.5	10.4 (9.4–11.4)
2. Rumination Syndrome	592	10.9	132	22.3	578	10.6	10.4 (9.5–11.5)
3. Functional Chest Pain	736	13.6	321	43.6	693	12.8	12.5 (11.5–13.6)
4. Functional Heartburn	1770	32.6	560	31.6	1636	30.1	29.1 (27.6–30.6)
5. Functional Dysphagia	405	7.5	165	40.7	401	7.4	6.8 (6.0–7.7)
B. Gastroduodenal symptoms	1400	25.8	317	22.6	1381	25.4	26.0 (24.7–27.5)
1. Functional Dyspepsia	160	2.9	97	60.6	143	2.6	2.7 (2.3–3.3)
a. Ulcer-Like Dyspepsia	19	0.3	12	63.2	13	0.2	0.2 (0.1–0.4)
b. Dysmotility-Like Dyspepsia	60	1.1	38	63.3	55	1.0	0.9 (0.7–1.3)
c. Unspecified Dyspepsia	85	1.6	50	58.8	79	1.5	1.5 (1.2–2.0)
2. Aerophagia	1273	23.4	170	13.4	1269	23.4	23.7 (22.4–25.1)
C. Bowel symptoms	2418	44.5	555	23.0	2392	44.1	44.3 (42.8–45.9)
1. IBS	629	11.6	288	45.8	606	11.2	9.4 (8.5–10.5)
2. Functional Constipation	197	3.6	44	22.3	197	3.6	3.0 (2.5–3.6)
3. Functional Diarrhea	96	1.8	26	27.1	94	1.7	1.6 (1.3–2.1)
4. Functional Abdominal Bloating	1669	30.7	146	8.8	1667	30.7	32.1 (30.6–33.6)

D. Chronic abdominal pain	120	2.2	60	50.0	117	2.2	1.7 (1.3–2.2)
E. Functional biliary pain							
1. Sphincter of Oddi Dyskinesia	83	1.5	47	56.6	79	1.5	0.8 (0.6–1.2)
F. Anorectal symptoms	1453	26.8	241	16.6	1453	26.8	26.3 (24.9–27.7)
1. Functional Incontinence	424	7.8	80	18.9	424	7.8	7.4 (6.6–8.3)
a. Fecal Soiling	388	7.1	61	15.7	388	7.1	6.9 (6.2–7.8)
b. Gross Incontinence	36	0.7	19	52.8	36	0.7	0.3 (0.2–0.6)[c]
2. Functional Anorectal Pain	629	11.6	142	22.6	629	11.6	11.3 (10.3–12.4)
a. Levator Syndrome	357	6.6	104	29.1	357	6.6	6.0 (5.2–6.8)
b. Proctalgia Fugax	437	8.0	75	17.2	437	8.0	7.9 (7.1–8.8)
3. Dyschezia	749	13.8	102	13.6	749	13.8	13.1 (12.1–14.2)
All GI functional symptoms	3807	70.1	1509	39.64	3761	69.3	69.3 (67.8–70.8)

[a]Percentage of *n* that met diagnostic criteria.

[b]National estimated percentage using logistic regression model, adjusting for the 1990 U.S. householder population on age, gender, race, number of persons in household, and geographic area. Numbers in parentheses are the 95% confidence intervals for the estimates.

[c]Because of the low frequency, the national estimate is based only on the adjustment, using logistic regression, for age, gender, and residence geographic area.

Source: Ref: 11.

Table 3 Prevalence of Functional GI Disorders by Gender and Age (observed proportions, not national estimates)

	Gender (%)		Age[a] (%)		
	Male (*n*=2639)	Female (*n*=2791)	15–34 (*n*=1199)	35–44 (*n*=1289)	≥45 (*n*=2894)
Functional GI Symptoms					
A. Esophageal symptoms	40.7	44.3	48.3	45.8	38.7
1. Globus	8.3	16.4	16.4	13.6	10.4
2. Rumination Syndrome	9.9	11.4	14.5	10.6	9.0
3. Functional Chest Pain	12.1	13.4	18.4	13.9	9.9
4. Functional Heartburn	29.7	30.5	30.4	32.9	28.9
5. Functional Dysphagia	6.3	8.5	8.4	8.3	6.6
B. Gastroduodenal symptoms	26.8	24.1	29.4	25.1	24.0
1. Functional Dyspepsia	2.6	2.7	2.8	2.3	2.7
a. Ulcer-Like Dyspepsia	0.2	0.3	0.2	0.2	0.3
b. Dysmotility-Like Dyspepsia	0.9	1.1	1.0	1.2	0.9
c. Unspecified Dyspepsia	1.6	1.4	1.7	1.1	1.6
2. Aerophagia	24.9	22.0	26.9	23.5	21.9
C. Bowel symptoms	43.7	44.4	43.4	44.7	44.3
1. IBS	7.7	14.5	13.5	13.0	9.4
2. Functional Constipation	2.4	4.8	3.8	3.6	3.5
3. Functional Diarrhea	1.8	1.6	1.2	2.2	1.8
4. Functional Abdominal Bloating	34.3	27.3	27.7	28.9	32.9
D. Chronic abdominal pain	1.7	2.6	2.3	2.6	1.9
E. Functional biliary pain					
1. Sphincter of Oddi Dyskinesia	0.6	2.3	0.8	1.1	1.9
F. Anorectal symptoms	24.3	29.1	28.9	28.5	25.1
1. Functional Incontinence	7.9	7.7	5.7	6.4	9.2
a. Fecal Soiling	7.4	6.9	5.5	6.2	8.2
b. Gross Incontinence	0.5	0.9	0.2	0.2	1.0
2. Functional Anorectal Pain	11.1	12.1	14.6	14.0	9.3
a. Levator Syndrome	5.7	7.4	7.8	7.2	5.8
b. Proctalgia Fugax	7.7	8.3	10.5	10.1	6.2
3. Dyschezia	11.5	16.0	15.3	14.3	13.0
All GI functional symptoms	68.0	70.5	71.9	71.7	67.3

[a]48 respondents did not report age.
Source: Ref. 11.

tion (OR 0.54, 95% CI 0.3–0.9). There was a strong positive association between lower household income (relative to income >$45,000) and frequencies of functional GI disorders—the lower the household income, the greater the symptom reporting (<$15,000: OR 1.73, 95% CI 1.4–2.1; $15,000–24,999: OR 1.51, 95% CI 1.3–1.8; $25,000–34,999: OR 1.43, 95% CI 1.2–1.7). People in households containing more than one person were more likely to report functional esophageal symptoms and functional aerophagia. Compared to persons from the West, there was a greater tendency for persons from the South to report functional heartburn (OR 1.21, 95% CI 1.0–1.4), aerophagia (OR 1.43, 95% CI 1.2–1.7), and levator syndrome (OR 1.40, 95% CI 1.0–1.9). Persons from the Northeast were less likely to report functional abdominal pain (OR 0.44, 95% CI 0.2–0.9) and those from the Midwest were less likely to report functional diarrhea (OR 0.51, 95% CI 0.3–1.0). No significant association was seen between population density and reporting of functional GI disorders. Finally, persons with full- or part-time jobs were more likely to report symptoms than those not employed (OR 1.25, 95% CI 1.1–1.4).

C. Impact on Health Care

The health care impact of the functional GI disorders was evaluated in terms of: 1) inability to work or go to school and the amount of time lost and 2) frequencies of physician visits for illness in general and for functional GI symptoms.

Work Absenteeism

We report in Table 4 the proportion of subjects for each diagnosis who are "currently too sick to work or go to school," as well as "number of days in past year missed from work or school because of illness." The odds ratios are calculated against the rates for the 1625 respondents with no functional GI symptoms. The work-absenteeism rates varied from 29.4% for gross fecal incontinence to 6.3% for functional abdominal bloating, and are significantly higher for all categories than for subjects not having a functional GI diagnosis (4.2%). Similarly, the number of days absent from work varied from 50.1 days for gross fecal incontinence to 5.4 days for functional diarrhea. All functional GI diagnoses except functional diarrhea (5.4 days) were significantly higher than for subjects without a functional GI diagnosis (4.9 days). These data indicate that having a functional GI diagnosis puts one at greater risk for work absenteeism (adjusted OR 1.85, 95% CI, 1.40–2.45) and for more days missed from work (adjusted mean 8.7 ± 0.7 SE; $p < 0.003$).

Physician Visits

Table 5 shows the number of physician visits in the past year for GI and non-GI illnesses. Visits for GI symptoms were greatest for gross incontinence (3.53 vis-

TABLE 4 Work Absenteeism for Those With and Without Functional GI Disorders

	Currently too sick to work or go to school			No. of days in past year missed from work or school because of illness		
Functional GI disorder based on the Rome criteria	%[a]	OR[b]	(95% CI)[c]	Mean[b]	(Std. error)[d]	p value
Met none of the criteria (*n* = 1625)	4.2			4.9	(1.0)	
A. Esophageal symptoms	7.9	2.09	(1.55–2.81)	8.6	(0.8)	0.0026
1. Globus	11.9	3.90	(2.67–5.69)	14.9	(1.7)	0.0001
2. Rumination Syndrome	9.0	2.81	(1.87–4.23)	14.7	(1.8)	0.0001
3. Functional Chest Pain	9.9	3.20	(2.19–4.67)	12.6	(1.6)	0.0001
4. Functional Heartburn	9.1	2.26	(1.66–3.07)	9.5	(1.0)	0.0019
5. Functional Dysphagia	14.3	4.15	(2.77–6.23)	15.1	(2.1)	0.0001
B. Gastroduodenal symptoms	8.5	2.07	(1.49–2.86)	9.9	(1.1)	0.0010
1. Functional Dyspepsia	10.6	2.48	(1.32–4.67)	14.8	(3.2)	0.0035
a. Ulcer-Like Dyspepsia	15.4	3.94	(0.77–20.09)	40.7	(10.7)	0.0009
b. Dysmotility-Like Dyspepsia	13.2	3.98	(1.62–9.80)	18.2	(5.2)	0.0123
c. Unspecified Dyspepsia	8.9	1.75	(0.74–4.18)	8.8	(4.0)	0.3433
2. Aerophagia	8.5	2.11	(1.51–2.93)	9.4	(1.1)	0.0022
C. Bowel symptoms	7.9	1.95	(1.45–2.61)	9.7	(0.9)	0.0008
1. IBS	11.3	3.36	(2.29–4.94)	13.4	(1.7)	0.0001
2. Functional Constipation	12.9	4.59	(2.68–7.86)	21.9	(3.0)	0.0001
3. Functional Diarrhea	6.7	2.11	0.85–5.21)	5.4	(3.7)	0.9020

4. Functional Abdominal Bloating	6.3	1.47	(1.07–2.03)	8.0	(1.0)	0.0371
D. Chronic abdominal pain	11.2	3.45	(1.76–6.79)	11.8	(3.3)	0.0457
E. Functional biliary pain						
1. Sphincter of Oddi Dyskinesia	23.4	6.18	(3.20–11.94)	33.0	(4.8)	0.0001
F. Anorectal symptoms	9.0	2.40	(1.75–3.30)	11.7	(1.2)	0.0001
1. Functional Incontinence	13.2	2.90	(1.95–4.29)	15.1	(2.1)	0.0001
a. Fecal Soiling	11.7	2.61	(1.72–3.95)	12.3	(2.1)	0.0021
b. Gross Incontinence	29.4	6.80	(2.87–16.13)	50.1	(6.8)	0.0001
2. Functional Anorectal Pain	8.3	2.58	(1.72–3.86)	12.2	(1.6)	0.0001
a. Levator Syndrome	11.5	3.56	(2.29–5.55)	17.9	(2.3)	0.0001
b. Proctalgia Fugax	8.4	2.77	(1.76–4.35)	12.8	(2.0)	0.0003
3. Dyschezia	9.2	2.51	(1.73–3.64)	11.9	(1.6)	0.0001
All GI functional symptoms (*n* = 3677)	7.3	1.85	(1.40–2.45)	8.7	(0.7)	0.0023

[a]Observed proportions, not national estimates.
[b]ORs and least square means compared to those who did not meet any diagnostic criteria for functional GI disorder.
[c]ORs and 95% CIs adjusted by logistic regressions for gender, age, race, number of members in household, residence area, household income, population density, and employment status.
[d]Least square means, adjusted by OLS regression for gender, age, race, number of members in household, residence area, household income, population density, and employment status.
Source: Ref. 11.

TABLE 5 Physician Visits for Those With and Without Functional GI Disorders

	Functional GI disorder based on the Rome criteria GI symptoms			No. of visits to health care professionals in last year for Non-GI symptoms[a]		
	Mean[b]	(Std. error)[c]	*p* value	Mean[b]	(Std. error)[c]	*p* value
Met none of the criteria (n = 1629)	0.09	0.07)		1.77	0.29)	
A. Esophageal symptoms	0.81	(0.05)	0.0001	3.87	(0.26)	0.0001
1. Globus	1.41	(0.09)	0.0001	5.19	(0.43)	0.0001
2. Rumination Syndrome	1.39	(0.13)	0.0001	3.84	(0.26)	0.0001
3. Functional Chest Pain	1.33	(0.11)	0.0001	4.36	(0.37)	0.0001
4. Functional Heartburn	0.86	(0.06)	0.0001	3.86	(0.28)	0.0001
5. Functional Dysphagia	1.71	(0.14)	0.0001	4.09	(0.34)	0.0001
B. Gastroduodenal symptoms	1.01	(0.06)	0.0001	3.92	(0.30)	0.0001
1. Functional Dyspepsia	1.62	(0.11)	0.0001	3.67	(0.39)	0.0001
a. Ulcer-Like Dyspepsia	1.12	(0.17)	0.0001	6.04	(1.21)	0.0005
b. Dysmotility-Like Dyspepsia	2.42	(0.18)	0.0001	4.47	(0.64)	0.0001
c. Unspecified Dyspepsia	1.19	(0.08)	0.0001	3.94	(0.31)	0.0001

C. Bowel symptoms	0.81	(0.06)	0.0001	3.41	(0.17)	0.0001
1. IBS	1.64	(0.10)	0.0001	3.88	(0.23)	0.0001
2. Functional Constipation	1.40	(0.18)	0.0001	5.85	(0.47)	0.0001
3. Functional Diarrhea	1.08	(0.09)	0.0001	2.49	(0.47)	0.1510
4. Functional Abdominal bloating	0.49	(0.05)	0.0001	3.03	(0.20)	0.0001
D. Chronic abdominal pain	1.52	(0.09)	0.0001	5.66	(0.83)	0.0001
E. Functional biliary pain						
1. Sphincter of Oddi Dyskinesia	2.86	(0.13)	0.0001	7.71	(0.70)	0.0001
F. Anorectal symptoms	1.07	(0.07)	0.0001	4.12	(0.30)	0.0001
1. Functional Incontinence	1.80	(0.14)	0.0001	3.77	(0.28)	0.0001
a. Fecal Soiling	1.66	(0.15)	0.0001	3.33	(0.26)	0.0001
b. Gross Incontinence	3.53	(0.17)	0.0001	9.24	(0.92)	0.0001
2. Functional Anorectal Pain	1.44	(0.11)	0.0001	4.52	(0.45)	0.0001
a. Levator Syndrome	1.78	(0.09)	0.0001	5.70	(0.58)	0.0001
b. Proctalgia Fugax	1.43	(0.13)	0.0001	3.73	(0.38)	0.0001
3. Dyschezia	0.86	(0.09)	0.0001	3.83	(0.30)	0.0001
All GI functional symptoms (*n* = 3690)	0.77	(0.04)	0.0001	3.45	(0.19)	0.0001

Source: Ref. 11.

its) and least for functional abdominal bloating (0.49 visits). Similarly, the mean number of visits in the past year for non-GI symptoms varied from 9.29 visits for gross incontinence to 2.45 visits for functional diarrhea. Physician visits for those with functional GI diagnoses were significantly higher than for those not having this diagnosis (0.09/year for GI visits and 1.77/year for non-GI visits). These data indicate that having a functional GI diagnosis is associated with a higher rate of physician visits, for both GI (0.77 ± 0.04 SE vs. 0.09 ± 0.07; $p < 0.0001$) and non-GI (3.45 ± 0.19 SE vs. 1.77 ± 0.29; $p < 0.0001$) illness.

VII. CONCLUSION

In summary, we may conclude from these data that: 1) functional GI disorders are common, 2) persons frequently experience more than one functional GI disorder, 3) rates of health care use vary, and seem to be higher among persons with painful disorders or incontinence, 4) females are more likely to experience functional GI symptoms and to see physicians for them, 5) symptom-reporting declines with advancing age, 6) there is an association between more frequent symptom reports and lower household income, and 7) the health care impact, in terms of disability, work absenteeism, and physician visits, is considerable.

The findings support the utility of symptom-based criteria in classifying persons with functional GI disorders. Furthermore, the results indicate that these disorders are common and lead to considerable disability and costs from work absenteeism and health care visits.

REFERENCES

1. Drossman DA, Thompson WG, Talley NJ, Funch-Jensen P, Janssens J, Whitehead WE. Identification of subgroups of functional bowel disorders. Gastroenterol Int 1990; 3:159–172.
2. Powell R. On certain painful afflictions of the intestinal canal. Med Trans Royal Coll Phys 1818; 6:106–117.
3. Almy TP, Tulin M. Alterations in colonic function in man under stress: experimental production of changes simulating the "irritable colon." Gastroenterology 1947; 8:616–626.
4. Almy TP. Experimental studies on the irritable colon. Am J Med 1951; 10:60–67.
5. Chaudhary NA, Truelove SC. The irritable colon syndrome: a study of the clinical features, predisposing causes, and prognosis in 130 cases. Q J Med 1962; 31:307–322.
6. Christensen J. Heraclides or the physician. Gastroenterol Int 1990; 3:45–48.
7. Manning AP, Thompson WG, Heaton KW, Morris AF. Towards positive diagnosis of the irritable bowel. Br Med J 1978; 2:653–654.

8. Drossman DA. Clinical research in the functional digestive disorders. Gastroenterology 1987; 92:1267–1269.
9. Klein KB. Controlled treatment trials in the irritable bowel syndrome: a critique. Gastroenterology 1988; 95:232–241.
10. Drossman DA. The functional gastrointestinal disorders and their diagnosis: a coming of age. In: Drossman DA, Richter JE, Talley NJ, Thompson WG, Corazziari E, Whitehead WE, eds. The Functional Gastrointestinal Disorders: Diagnosis, Pathophysiology and Treatment. Boston: Little, Brown, 1994:1–23.
11. Drossman DA, Li Z, Andruzzi E, Temple R, Talley NJ, Thompson WG, Whitehead WE, Janssens J, Funch-Jensen P, Corazziari E, Richter JE, Koch GG. U.S. Householder Survey of Functional GI Disorders: prevalence, sociodemography and health impact. Dig Dis Sci 1993; 38:1569–1580.
12. LeClere FB, Moss AJ, Everhart JE, Roth HP. Prevalence of Major Digestive Disorders and Bowel Symptoms, 1989: Advance Data from Vital and Health Statistics. No. 212. Hyatsville, MD: National Center for Health Statistics, 1992.
13. Whitehead WE, Crowell MD, Bosmajian L, Zonderman A, Costa PTJ, Benjamin C, Robinson JC, Heller BR, Schuster MM. Existence of irritable bowel syndrome supported by factor analysis of symptoms in two community samples. Gastroenterology 1990; 98:336–340.
14. American Psychiatric Association. Diagnostic and Statistical Manual of Mental Disorders—DSM-IV. Washington, DC: American Psychiatric Association, 1994.
15. Schumaker HRJ. Primer on the Rheumatic Diseases. Atlanta: Arthritis Foundation, 1988.
16. Bayless TM. Inflammatory bowel disease and irritable bowel syndrome. Med Clin North Am 1990; 49:21–28.
17. Drossman DA, Li Z, Lockwood LS, Metz JA, Rice D, The Working Team Committees for Diagnosis of Functional GI Disorders. What factors are associated with retention of IBS symptoms? Gastroenterology 1993; 104:A499 (abstr).
18. Talley NJ, Weaver AL, Zinsmeister AR, Melton LJ. Onset and disappearance of gastrointestinal symptoms and functional gastrointestinal disorders. Am J Epidemiol 1992; 2:165–177.
19. Milholland AV, Wheeler SG, Heieck JJ. Medical assessment by a delphi group opinion technic. N Engl J Med 1973; 298:1272–1275.
20. Thompson WG, Dotevall G, Drossman DA, Heaton KW, Kruis W. Irritable bowel syndrome: guidelines for the diagnosis. Gastroenterol Int 1989; 2:92–95.
21. Thompson WG, Creed F, Drossman DA, Heaton KW, Mazzacca G. Functional bowel disorders and chronic functional abdominal pain. Gastroenterol Int 1992; 5:75–91.
22. Talley NJ, Colin-Jones D, Koch KL, Koch M, Myren O, Stanghellini V. Functional Dyspepsia: a classification with guidelines for diagnosis and management. Gastroenterol Int 1991; 4:145–160.
23. Richter JE, Baldi F, Clouse RE, Diamant NE, Janssens J, Staiano A. Functional oesophageal disorders. Gastroenterol Int 1992; 5:3–17.
24. Whitehead WE, Devroede G, Habib FI, Meunier P, Wald A. Functional disorders of the anorectum. Gastroenterol Int 1992; 5:92–108.
25. Corazziari E, Funch-Jensen P, Hogan WJ, Tanaka M, Toouli J. Working team report: functional disorders of the biliary tract. Gastroenterol Int 1993; 6:129.

26. Drossman DA, Richter JE, Talley NJ, Thompson WG, Corazziari E, Whitehead WE. The Functional Gastrointestinal Disorders: Diagnosis, Pathophysiology and Treatment. Boston: Little, Brown, 1994.
27. Drossman DA, Thompson WG, Talley NJ, Funch-Jensen P, Janssens J, Whitehead WE. Response to guest editorial. Gastroenterol Int 1991; 4:44–45.
28. Sandler RS, Drossman DA, Nathan HP, McKee DC. Symptom complaints and health care seeking behavior in subjects with bowel dysfunction. Gastroenterology 1984; 87:314–318.

4

Medical Evaluation of Functional GI Disorders

Michael Camilleri
Mayo Medical School and Mayo Clinic
Rochester, Minnesota

Jeffrey W. Frank
University of Colorado School of Medicine
Denver, Colorado

I. INTRODUCTION

Functional gastrointestinal disorders constitute almost 50% of patients seen in outpatient gastroenterology clinics in the Western world (1). These disorders are characterized by single or multiple symptoms that are unassociated with any demonstrable etiology; that is, anatomical, mucosal, and biochemical alterations are undetected.

Several symptoms may be attributable to functional gastrointestinal disorders, including dysphagia, odynophagia, chest pain, heartburn, nausea, vomiting, early satiety, bloating, abdominal pain, constipation, diarrhea, and incontinence. These symptoms arise from different regions of the digestive tract, including the esophagus, stomach, small bowel, colon, and anorectum. In general, most patients with these syndromes have a normal life expectancy, but

TABLE 1 Typical Symptoms and Syndromes of Disordered Function of the Digestive Tract

Region	Symptom	Syndrome
Pharynx	Dysphagia	Globus sensation
Esophagus	Dysphagia	Achalasia
	Chest pain	Diffuse spasm, nutcracker esophagus
	Heartburn	Reflux esophagitis
	Regurgitation	Rumination
Stomach	Nausea, vomiting	Gastroparesis
	Early satiety, heartburn	Functional dyspepsia
Small bowel	Nausea, vomiting	Irritable bowel syndrome
	Bloating, early satiety, abdominal pain, diarrhea	Chronic intestinal pseudo-obstruction
Colon	Abdominal pain, constipation	Slow-transit constipation
	Diarrhea	Irritable bowel syndrome
Anorectum	Constipation	Pelvic floor dysfunction; anismus

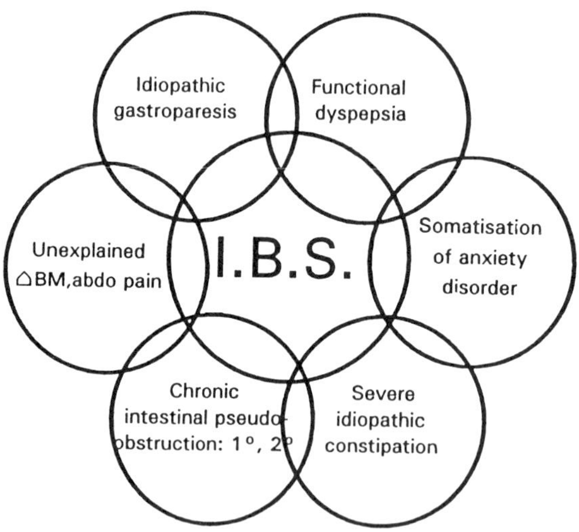

FIGURE 1 Overlap in the functional gastrointestinal disorders.

there is considerable morbidity, depending on the severity of the symptoms or syndrome in the individual patient.

Table 1 shows examples of the typical symptoms and syndromes arising at different regions of the digestive tract. Clearly, several regions may be affected and result in the same clinical manifestation (e.g., vomiting). Thus, there is overlap between different syndromes that are grouped among the functional gastrointestinal disorders (Figure 1). On the other hand, many patients present with symptoms arising from disordered function at more than one level—most commonly, dyspepsia and constipation. Extragastrointestinal smooth-muscle organs, such as the urinary bladder and bronchus, may also be involved.

This chapter focuses on the clinical approach and the use of structural and functional investigations in the evaluation of patients presenting with such symptoms. By definition, these patients are shown not to have any anatomical, mucosal, or biochemical disorders; the tests to exclude the latter mechanisms are discussed briefly.

II. COMMON MECHANISMS OF FUNCTIONAL GASTROINTESTINAL DISEASE

At least seven potential mechanisms (2) are common to functional disorders at different levels of the digestive tract. These are outlined in Table 2.

Importantly, these mechanisms are not mutually exclusive; more than one "bad actor" may play a role in the same patient. Indeed, evidence shows that excessive rectal perception of balloon distension and psychoneurotic symptoms may be present in the same patient (3). These putative mechanisms form the basis for the special tests of function that are performed in patients with suspected functional gastrointestinal disorders (2), usually after exclusion of organic disorders. On the basis of documented changes in these functions, treatment may be targeted at the nature and severity of the identified pathophysiology (2).

III. CLINICAL APPRAISAL: THE HISTORY

A careful history is essential and provides clues to the nature of the patient's complaints. As shown in Table 1, the predominant symptoms indicate to the clinician the likely region affected. It is important to specifically identify symptoms that raise suspicion of organic rather than functional disease (4); for example, significant weight loss, particularly over a short period, dysphagia to solids, and rectal bleeding necessitate a thorough search for organic disease by barium x-rays and/or endoscopy. Details that qualify the presenting symptoms are also extremely useful: the dysphagia to liquids rather than solids is indicative of achalasia; vomiting of undigested food that is recognizable more than 8 hours

Table 2 Potential Mechanisms Common to Functional Disorders of the Digestive Tract

Mechanism	Examples
Increased motility	Diarrhea-predominant IBS; spontaneous, repetitive contractions of esophageal spasm; puborectalis spasm and anismus in obstructed defecation
Decreased motility	Constipation-predominant IBS; slow-transit constipation; postprandial antral hypomotility in functional dyspepsia; weak anal-sphincter tone in incontinence
Excessive visceral perception	Irritable esphagus; functional dyspepsia (stomach and small bowel); irritable bowel syndrome (small bowel, colon, and rectum)
Impaired sensation	Rectal sensory disorder in longstanding constipation with megarectum
Endogenous irritants	Acid and bile in nonerosive reflux-like dyspepsia; bile acids in IBS with diarrhea (?)
Dietary intolerance	Aggravation of heartburn with caffeine; lactose; sucrose, and sorbitol intolerance in IBS; high-fat meals in functional dyspepsia
Psychological	Globus; functional dyspepsia; IBS; animus and puborectalis spasm; psychogenic vomiting, rumination, eating disorders

after ingestion suggests gastroparesis; nocturnal incontinence occurs when there is internal anal sphincter dysfunction; and difficulty expelling the stool, sometimes necessitating finger disimpaction and considerable straining, suggests pelvic-floor dysfunction or anismus. Just as important, the clustering of certain symptoms provides a means to positively diagnose irritable bowel syndrome, reducing the need for extensive and costly investigations. Thus, the criteria of Manning et al. (5) constitute an important clinical tool in the general evaluation of patients in the gastroenterology clinic. These symptoms include: pain at the onset of defecation, looser stools at onset of defecation, alterations of bowel movements, distention, passage of mucus, and a sense of incomplete rectal evacuation. Although there are differences in the diagnostic accuracy (6) of these symptoms, depending on gender and possibly age, the more symptoms present, the greater the accuracy, and there is general agreement (7) that a specific attempt to identify these symptoms probably leads to a more cost-effective evaluation and a reduction in the number of costly and potentially dangerous investigations performed.

Finally, patients should be interviewed at some length to determine whether there are features that suggest either a collagen-vascular disease (e.g., Raynaud's phenomenon) or an autonomic neuropathy. Thus, symptoms such as postural dizziness and abnormal sweating are indicative of a sympathetic neuroopathy, while abnormal penile erection, difficulty with emptying the bladder, recurrent urinary-tract infections, and alterations in visual accommodation when going from a bright to a dark environment suggest parasympathetic dysfunction. The past medical, surgical, and drug history will identify possible causes of the patient's symptoms, e.g., diabetes mellitus, previous vagotomy, pelvic surgery, and anithypertensive agents.

IV. CLINICAL APPRAISAL: THE PHYSICAL EXAMINATION

The main goals of examination are: 1) to exclude organic diseases such as the presence of abdominal mass, supraclavicular nodes, or rectal mass; 2) to identify features of a systemic disorder that may produce associated gastrointestinal symptoms; and 3) to identify specific evidence of a disordered motor function. The last is usually most useful in the examination of the anorectum, where excessive perineal descent, or "ballooning," or the presence of mucosal prolapse and weakness or excessive contraction of the sphincter at rest or during squeeze are specifically helpful (8). Otherwise, physical findings are relatively nonspecific, such as abdominal distention, a succussion splash, or loading of the colon with fecal material.

V. PRELIMINARY INVESTIGATIONS

Even when the symptoms are highly suggestive of a functional gastrointestinal disorder, most patients require empathetic explanation, a reasonable degree of psychosocial sensitivity (at least a caring attitude and education by the generalist or gastroenterologist), and some degree of further testing to exclude organic disease. It is not possible to generalize the precise indications for further investigations, which vary with such factors as: age, presence of "alarm" symptoms (e.g., weight loss, rectal bleeding), family history of cancer, travel history, duration of symptoms, patient's perception of the seriousness of the disorder, and the degree of investigation already performed by previous physicians consulted for the same problem. It is inevitable that many patients will consult multiple physicians. Much expense and useless anxiety for patient and doctor can be saved if the first physician attempts to make a positive diagnosis, performs a minimum of tests to exclude organic disease, and provides empathetic advice, education, and symptomatic treatment.

Following a thorough history and physical examination, what screening investigations should be performed to exclude organic disease? In a secondary or tertiary practice (2), we perform:

1. Sedimentation rate, hematology group, chemistry group, urinalysis, and sensitive TSH level
2. Barium meal or upper gastrointestinal endoscopy in patients presenting with dysphagia, dyspepsia, or vomiting
3. Flexible sigmoidoscopy in those presenting with alterations of bowel movements and barium enemas in those over 45 years of age or who have a parent or sibling with cancer of the colon
4. Stool for giardia in those presenting with diarrhea and for occult blood in those with altered bowel habits if criteria for performing barium enema are not satisfied

If all these tests are normal, we do not perform any more general investigations, but use the clinical history and examination to suggest a specific test or tests to demonstrate an altered function that would result in a specific treatment rather than the customary symptomatic treatment. For example, if the patient has intractable constipation despite increased dietary fiber, or if there are disturbances of defecation, we pursue further testing because this may lead to additional therapeutic approaches, such as osmotic laxative and prokinetic therapy in those with slow-transit constipation, or biofeedback for those with anismus or puborectalis spasm.

The role for abdominal ultrasonography is chiefly the exclusion of biliary-tract or pancreatic disease in patients presenting with upper abdominal pain or dyspepsia. In our experience, ultrasonographic detection of pathology in the biliopancreatic region is rare in the absence of other clinical features such as the indicative location, typical nature, and radiation of pain, as well as Murphy's sign. In the absence of these common features or "alarm" symptoms or signs, computed tomography of the abdomen or pelvis is unnecessary when the clinical features suggest a functional gastrointestinal disorder.

VI. RADIOGRAPHIC EVALUATION

Radiographic tests have traditionally played a prominent role in evaluation of gastrointestinal disease. With the advent and greater usage of newer methods to assess anatomic and functional aspects of the gut, the role of radiology is being challenged. In general, radiology is most helpful in delineating esophageal, colonic, and anorectal anatomy and function and in determining the lumenal anatomy of the small bowel.

Static and dynamic (video) barium esophagography (Figure 2) can be very important in evaluating the motor function of the upper and lower esophagus (9,10). In combination with manometry, diagnoses of achalasia, diffuse spasm, neuromuscular disorders, and a variety of structural disorders can be made. Lim-

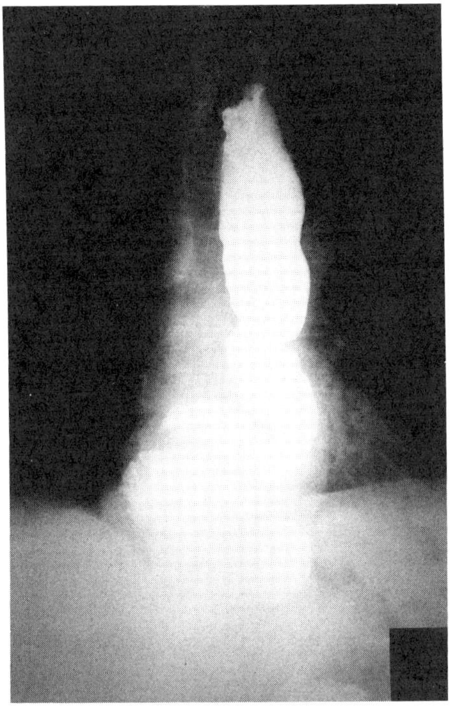

Figure 2 A barium esophagogram in a patient with classical achalasia. Note the dilated proximal esophagus and the tortuous (sigmoid) distal esophagus leading to a smooth narrowing of the lower-esophageal sphincter region.

itations include inability to detect intermittent abnormalities, variation in test performance from center to center, and variation in interpretation among skilled radiologists (11). The pharyngeal phase of swallowing is probably best delineated by a combined dynamic radiographic (12) and solid-state transducer pressure profile.

In the stomach and small intestine, radiology is more useful in ruling out structural lesions and assessing lumenal caliber than in assessing motility. Enteroclysis may be more beneficial than standard barium follow-through in evaluating the distal small bowel (13,14).

In the colon, radiography is useful to determine regional lumenal caliber to diagnose megacolon or megarectum. The radiopaque marker study is useful to measure transit (15; see below). Anorectal testing with barium, balloon, and radioisotopes can be helpful to determine structure and function (see below).

VII. TESTS OF ESOPHAGEAL FUNCTION

There are three main modalities for evaluation of esophageal functional disorders: esophageal manometry and prolonged and short reflux tests (16). Manometry is a method whereby a series of perfused catheters, with sideholes located at several levels of the esophagus, provide a pressure profile during swallowing of the contractions at different levels of the esophagus (Figure 3) (17). Alternatively, solid-state transducers can be used instead of perfused manometers (Figure 4). Diagnostic profiles are discussed elsewhere in this book. The main indications for esophageal manometry are: the evaluation of barium x-ray or endoscopy-negative dysphagia, noncardiac chest pain, and in the preoperative assessment of patients about to undergo fundoplication or other hiatal hernia repair for reflux esophagitis.

Prolonged (usually 24-hour) esophageal pH monitoring is performed by placing a small probe transnasally so that its tip is located 5 cm above the lower esophageal sphincter. A data-logger records pH and patient symptoms such as heartburn, chest pain, and cough and major events such as meal ingestion and ly-

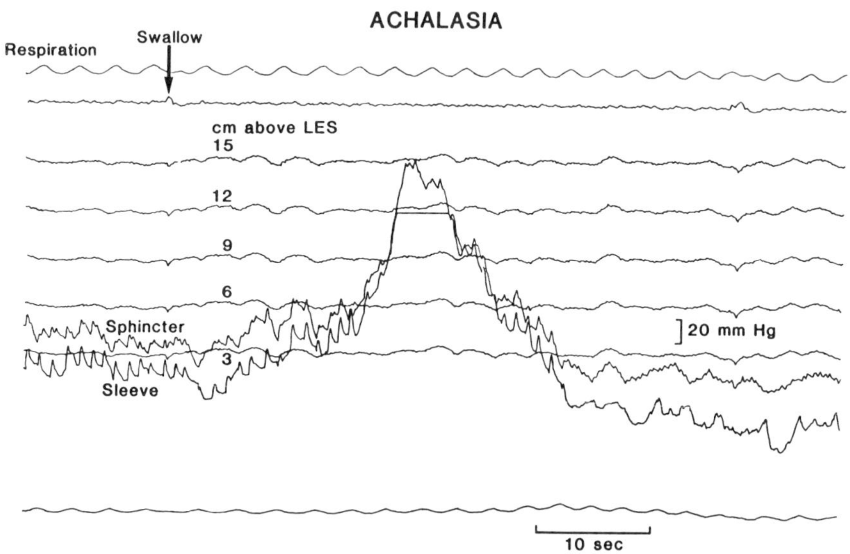

FIGURE 3 Manometric tracing showing the classic appearances of achalasia. Note that after a single wet swallow (5 ml water), there is no contractile response in the proximal, mid-, or distal esophagus. At the level of the lower esophageal sphincter, which is also monitored by a Dent sleeve, note the slight relaxation of the lower esophageal sphincter, which does not reach gastric baseline, and the prominent contraction consistent with a spastic lower esophageal sphincter.

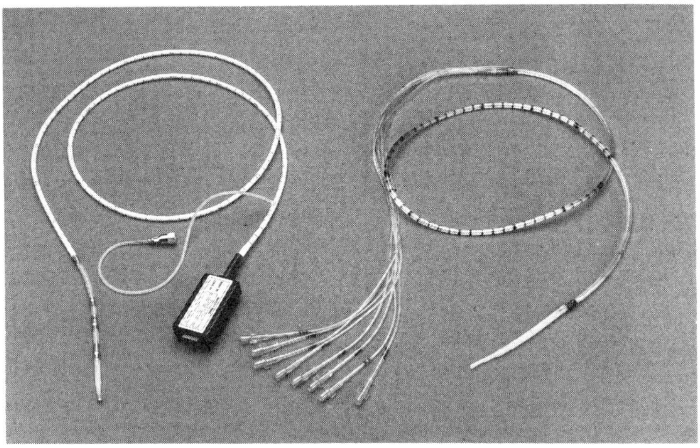

FIGURE 4 Left: solid-state catheter with pH probe at tip, four sensors 2.5 to 5.0 cm apart, electrical connection device, and separate port for infusion. Right: Polyvinyl pneumohydraulic catheter with Dent sleeve at tip, eight perfusion ports—five proximal to sleeve (3 cm apart), one within the sleeve, and one adjacent to the proximal and distal edge of the sleeve. External diameter of both catheters is 5 mm.

ing down (Figure 5). In general, most centers diagnose significant reflux when the pH is below 4 for 5.8% of the duration of the study (18). The pattern of reflux relative to major events may also help identify the nature of "reflux" symptoms. For example, repetitive short-duration drops in the esophageal pH postprandially without reportings of heartburn and the lack of occurrence of reflux in the supine position may alert the physician to the possibility of rumination syndrome. On the other hand, prolonged periods of low intraesophageal pH with slow resumption of the normal neutral or slightly alkaline pH in the esophagus suggest that esophageal clearance mechanisms are impaired. These observations complement the manometric demonstration of the weakness of antireflux functions and may be useful in practice because they may permit selection of patients for prokinetic as well as antiacid secretory drugs.

A third test, employed in some laboratories, involves placement of a pH probe in the distal esophagus, and then performance of maneuvers that raise intra-abdominal pressure (e.g., Valsalva and Muller's maneuvers, abdominal compression, coughing) prior to and following the instillation of 300 ml of 0.1 N hydrochloric acid into the stomach. This is a short, laboratory-based provocative test. Regrettably, the relative accuracies of prolonged pH monitoring and this short reflux test are unknown; however, there is an inherent advantage of a short, supervised test with objective maneuvers. Nevertheless, it must be stressed that

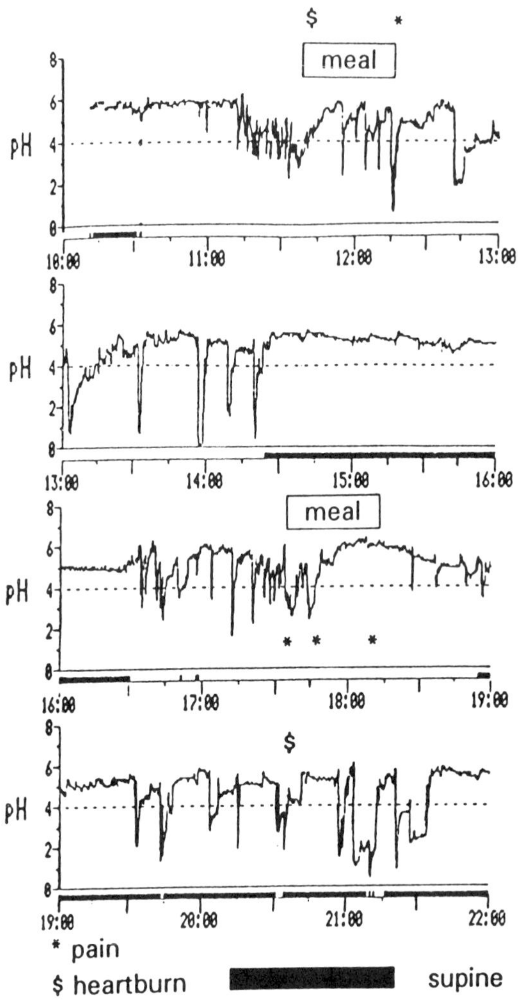

FIGURE 5 A prolonged pH-monitoring study demonstrating repetitive episodes of gastroesophageal reflux associated with low intraesophageal pH and concomitant symptoms.

many patients with negative endoscopy for esophagitis have positive short or prolonged reflux tests and respond to specific antiacid secretory treatment.

Other esophageal function tests include balloon distension to detect those patients with visceral hypersensitivity who present with noncardiac chest pain or the "irritable esophagus" (19).

VIII. DIETARY TOLERANCE TESTS (BREATH TESTS)

Carbohydrate-substrate breath tests can be utilized to detect certain disaccharide intolerances, of which lactose intolerance is the most common (20). These methods take advantage of the fact that relatively few anaerobic bacteria populate the proximal bowel in health; these bacteria are found in high numbers in the colon, where carbohydrates are fermented to hydrogen, methane, and carbon dioxide. Hydrogen is absorbed and exhaled within minutes of reaching the colon and can be measured in the breath. Patients who are intolerant of carbohydrates develop symptoms such as bloating, borborygmi, or diarrhea, and an increase in breath hydrogen from baseline of > 10 ppm can be documented for a sustained period of time (21).

Breath-hydrogen tests have been proposed as surrogates for measuring intestinal transit and bacterial overgrowth. In these cases, a nonabsorbable carbohydrate such as lactulose or baked beans can be administered by mouth, and the time taken to achieve a sustained elevation from baseline of > 10 to 20 ppm of breath hydrogen provides a measure of the orocecal transit time. If lactulose is given in the fasting period, without a caloric meal to induce a pattern of motility consistent with the postprandial state, there is great variability in orocecal transit time. This is due to the fact that the substrate is ingested during one of the various phases of the migrating motor complex (22). Less variability occurs in healthy volunteers when lactulose is given with a caloric meal (23); however, gastric emptying may have an impact on the measurement of orocecal transit, and hence these terms do not provide reliable measurements of small bowel transit.

There are difficulties in interpretation of breath-hydrogen tests. Early peaks may result from oral bacteria metabolizing the substrate, or from the sudden delivery of previously ingested carbohydrates to the colon. Similarly, bacterial overgrowth in the small bowel may metabolize the substrate and result in a peak in breath hydrogen. This is particularly relevant when breath testing is used in patients with significant small bowel dysmotility. Conversely, hyperventilation or exercise during the test or cigarette smoking may erroneously reduce or increase breath hydrogen, respectively (24). Previous ingestion of antibiotics or bowel cleansing will alter colonic bacteria, mitigating the accuracy of breath-hydrogen tasks. Lack of hydrogen production occurs in 6% of the population, and lower hydrogen excretion is found in those who are also methane producers (25). Finally, the accuracy of breath tests for detecting bacterial overgrowth is reduced in severe gastrointestinal motility disorders, probably due to lack of delivery of the substrate to the overgrowing bacteria (26).

In conclusion, breath tests are infrequently required in clinical practice, and then only when diagnoses are elusive or when objective data are absolutely necessary in the evaluation of a patient with presumed functional disease. They are better in detecting dietary intolerance than as measures of small-bowel transit.

IX. RADIOPAQUE MARKER TRANSIT

A simple, cost-effective method to evaluate colonic transit in patients with chronic constipation involves ingestion of radiopaque markers 20 rings of radiopaque tubing) on 3 successive days, and taking an abdominal radiograph on the fourth day (15). A simple calculation allows an overall assessment of right, left, and rectosigmoid colon transit times (1.2 x number of markers in each region = mean transit time in hours through that region) (Figure 6).

X. SCINTIGRAPHY

Noninvasive measurement of increased or decreased motility in different regions of the digestive tract is most accurately achieved by scintigraphy (27). In

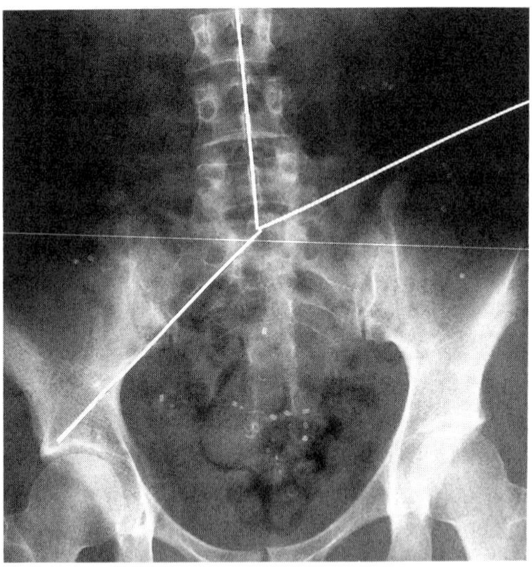

FIGURE 6 Abdominal radiograph showing radiopaque markers in three segments of the colon: right colon, left colon, and rectosigmoid. (From Ref. 27.)

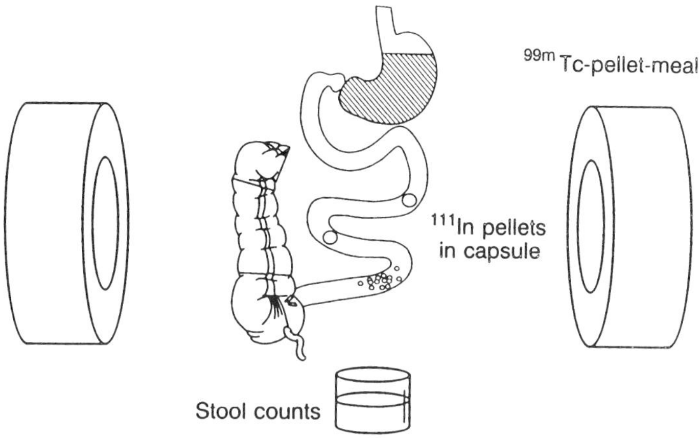

FIGURE 7 Scintigraphic method for combined measurement of gastric, small-bowel, and colonic transit. Note use of different istotopes to label pellets that are incorporated in meal and in methacrylate-coated capsule. (From Ref. 27.)

our practice, we have developed (28) and utilized a test for measuring transit of nondigestible solid particles ingested with a meal (for stomach and small-bowel transit); simultaneously, particles radiolabeled with a different isotope are placed in a delayed-release medication capsule that dissolves in the distal ileum, delivering isotope to the ascending colon for measurement of colonic transit (Figure 7). Scans taken immediately after ingestion of a meal, and 2, 4, 6, and 24 hours later, provide evidence for accelerated or delayed transit through stomach, small bowel, or colon (29). Such quantitative studies also indicate the severity of the problem and help the clinician select pharmacological or other therapy (e.g., colonic resection) for the patient not responding to initial therapies. They also provide an objective measure for follow-up of the problem. These tests have been reviewed in detail elsewhere (27).

XI. GASTRODUODENOJEJUNAL-PRESSURE PROFILES

Using multilumen perfused manometric tubes or solid-state transducers, a pressure profile of the stomach and small bowel is obtained in the fasting and postprandial periods. Five classes of pathological pressure profiles have been identified (30) and are summarized in Table 3, and examples are shown in Figure 8.

It is necessary to obtain such pressure recordings only when the clinical diagnosis or prognosis are in doubt, or when empirical or symptomatic treatment does not provide sufficient symptom relief. It is our practice to have documented evidence of a transit disorder [e.g., by scintigraphy (27) or pres-

TABLE 3 Pathological Pressure Profiles

Process	Pressure profile	Disease example
Obstructive	Simultaneous prolonged contractions; postprandial clustered contractions	Strictures, internal hernia
Myopathic	Low-amplitude pressure profile	Systemic sclerosis, amyloidosis
Neuropathic	Incoordinated normal-amplitude profile in antrum and/or small bowel	Autonomic neuropathy
Antral hypomotility	Reduced frequency of postprandial antral contractions	Vagotomy, diabetic gastroparesis
Small-bowel clusters	Propagated clustered contractions	IBS

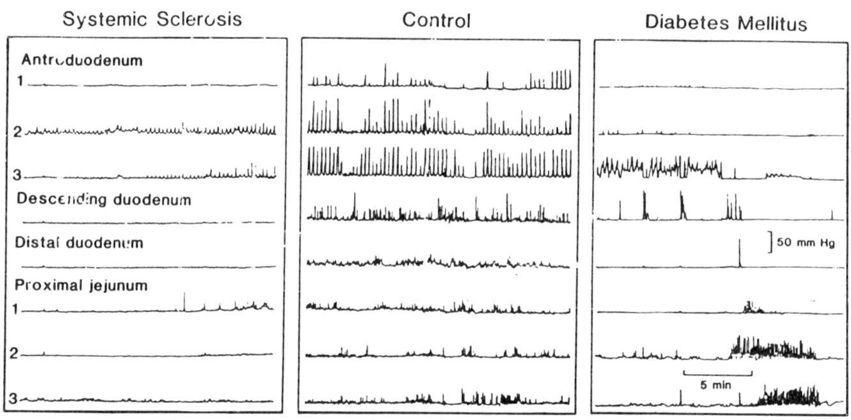

FIGURE 8 Manometric profiles of the stomach, duodenum, and jejunum in the postprandial period. Note the sustained but irregular contractile activity in the stomach and small intestine characteristic of the fed pattern in a healthy individual (control panel). In contrast, a patient with a myopathic disorder such as systemic sclerosis demonstrates low amplitude of contractions at all levels, whereas the patient with a neuropathic disorder demonstrates postprandial antral hypomotility (lanes 1 and 2), a prominent pyloric tonic and phasic pressure activity (lane 3), and the persistence of cyclical motor activity following the meal without generation of an irregular fed pattern. (From Ref. 43.)

ence of food in the stomach after overnight fast] prior to embarking on this invasive assessment of motility. Other centers perform either a laboratory-based 5-hour study or an ambulatory 24-hour evaluation (31) using solid-state transducers. One advantage of the stationary approach is that it enables careful monitoring of the distal antrum postprandially that cannot be reproducibly achieved by ambulatory monitoring. The major advantage of the ambulatory approach is that it provides a thorough analysis of interdigestive migrating motor complexes in the small bowel; these complexes may be absent during about one-third of the 3-hour-fasting observations as performed in our laboratory. On balance, our opinion is that the laboratory-based test, which does not depend heavily on evaluation of the migrating motor complexes to identify pathophysiological pressure profiles, appears to be preferable because it provides better postprandial assessment and control of the conditions of the study. To date, the only diseases known to significantly alter the frequency of the migrating motor complexes—systemic sclerosis (32) and vagotomy (33)—are easily identified during a shorter, laboratory-based study.

XII. COLONIC MEASUREMENTS OF MOTILITY

Apart from transit of radiopaque markers and scintigraphy, several methods have been proposed to evaluate colonic contractility, including: intraluminal EMG (34), colonic manometry (35,36), and measurement of tone (37) with a barostatic balloon (an inflated balloon in which the pressure is clamped, and changes in volume of the balloon reflect contractions of the colon). Figure 9 shows an example of abnormal colonic tone in a patient with an organic, hormonal diarrhea, but similar studies in functional disorders are currently being undertaken in several centers. These are all currently regarded as research tools that may be applied in the future, particularly to evaluate colonic motor function prior to subtotal colectomy in patients with intractable, slow-transit constipation (38).

XIII. ANORECTAL TESTING

The literature is replete with tests for evaluating anorectal function (39). In our clinical practice, the ones that are most useful in the initial evaluation of patients with suspected anorectal dysfunction are:

1. Anorectal manometry, in which a 1-cm station pull-through of manometric sideholes evaluates resting and squeezing pressures of the anal sphincters (Fig. 10).
2. Determination of the volume within a rectal balloon that is first perceived, and the volume that induces the urge to defecate (indices of

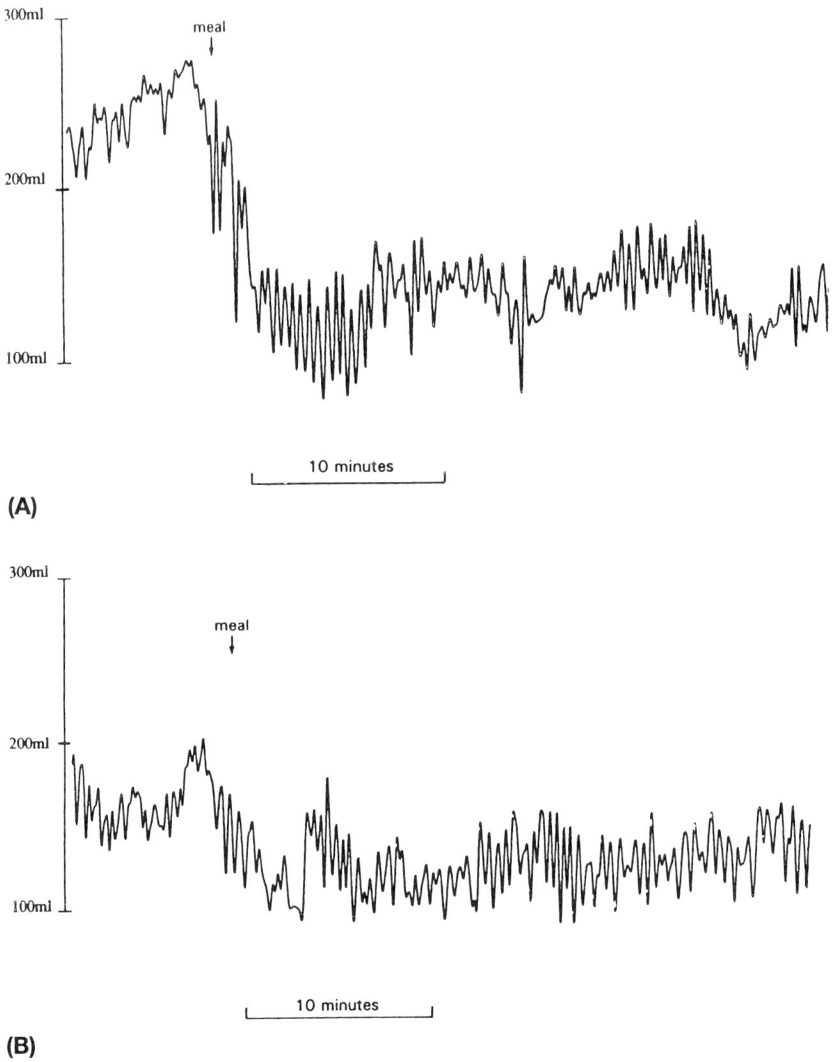

FIGURE 9 Fluctuations in the barostatic volume during 10 minutes of fasting and 30 minutes postprandially in (A) a patient with the carcinoid syndrome and diarrhea and (B) a normal subject. Note the similarity in the phasic fluctuations of volume in the two examples. In contrast, there is a postprandial reduction in volume that signifies increased colonic tone. However, the decrease in barostatic volume is clearly more marked in the tracing from the patient (panel A). (Reproduced by permission of the *New England Journal of Medicine* from Ref. 44.)

sensation); the volume that stimulates the rectoanal inhibitory reflex is also a useful parameter (absent in Hirschsprung's disease).

3. A rectal balloon-expulsion test, in which the ability to expel a 50-ml balloon from the rectum is assessed.
4. Rectal compliance, a measure of the stiffness of the rectal wall determined by the change in pressure with increments in the volume of an intrarectal balloon.

All these tests can be performed as part of a 30-minute outpatient test. If these tests show abnormal function, it may be necessary to pursue further evaluations such as anorectal ultrasonography or defecating proctography to identify sphincter or rectal-wall defects (e.g., rectocele) and neurological tests such as sphincter or puborectalis electromyography and pudendal-nerve-terminal motor latency.

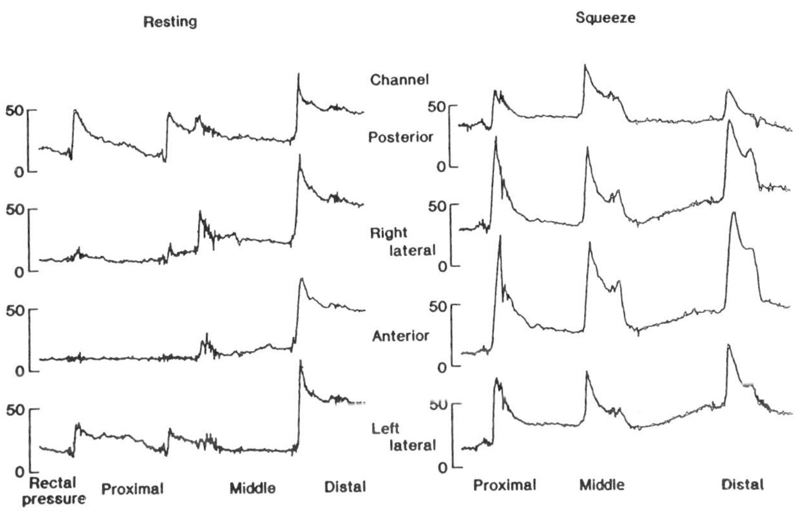

FIGURE 10 Anorectal manometry using a pull-through technique with manometric sensors at three levels of the anorectum. This profile, in a patient with progressive systemic sclerosis, shows the low amplitude of the internal anal-sphincter contractions during resting and, in contrast, the normal amplitude of the contractions of the sphincter during squeeze. It is estimated that the internal anal sphincter contributes to 85% of the resting pressure in the anal canal, whereas the external anal sphincter, which is under voluntary control, provides for augmentation of the sphincter tone during squeeze.

TABLE 4 Autonomic Function Tests

Test	Examples
Sympathetic adrenergic function	Orthostatic change in BP; orthostatic change in plasma norepinephrine
Sympathetic cholinergic function	Quantitative sudomotor axon reflex test
Thoracic vagal function	EKG R-R interval response to deep breathing
Abdominal vagal function	Plasma pancreatic polypeptide response to modified sham feeding

XIV. AUTONOMIC-FUNCTION TESTING

In severe functional disorders, diseases associated with autonomic dysfunction and in patients with positive features suggesting dysautonomy on systems review, it is sometimes helpful to assess the autonomic nervous system (40–42), chiefly for prognostic and diagnostic purposes rather than for therapeutic indications.

The most common tests performed in our practice are outlined in Table 4. These tests have been reviewed in detail elsewhere (40), and an example is shown in Figure 11.

XV. INTEGRATED APPROACH TO THE EVALUATION OF PATIENTS WITH SUSPECTED FUNCTIONAL GASTROINTESTINAL DISORDERS

As stated previously, the practicing clinician needs to develop strategies that incorporate positive diagnosis, exclusion of organic disease, empirical trials, focused evaluation of function based on predominant symptoms, and more detailed evaluation and specific treatment for those with intractable symptoms. We have previously published (2) our algorithm for patients with suspected irritable bowel syndrome and predominant pain, diarrhea, or constipation. This algorithm is reproduced in Figure 12. Our approach is similar in patients presenting with upper-abdominal or dyspeptic symptoms (Figure 13).

XVI. SUMMARY

Functional gastrointestinal diseases are frequently encountered by the generalist and the gastroenterologist, and may even present initially to psychologists or psychiatrists as a major somatization of underlying psychiatric disorder. They need to be identified positively by the clinician, and, after a limited series of tests to exclude organic disease, they can be efficiently managed with education, reassurance, empathy, and focused as well as symptomatic treatment. In a minority of cases, the disorder of function results from a significant disorder of the smooth muscle or a disturbance of the neural control, enteric, or extrinsic nerves. These can be identified by special testing, and noninvasive strategies are increasingly available for this purpose. The last decade has seen an explosion in modalities to improve our diagnostic abilities. Armed with a positive approach, common sense, empirical trials, and a modicum of focused tests, it is possible to

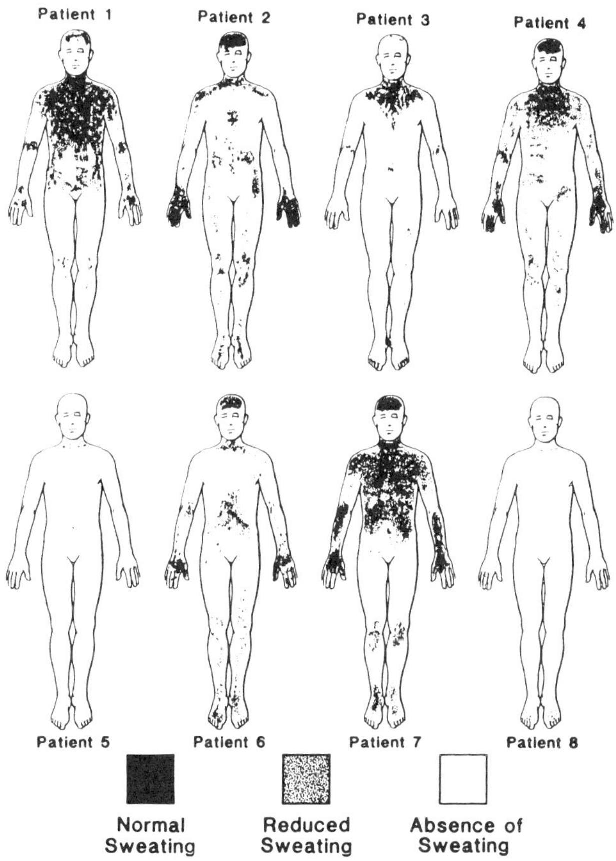

Figure 11 Thermoregulatory sweat test in a series of patients with functional gastrointestinal disorders and an idiopathic autonomic neuropathy. Note the areas of anhidrosis shown by the surface that is not shaded in each individual. (From Ref. 41.)

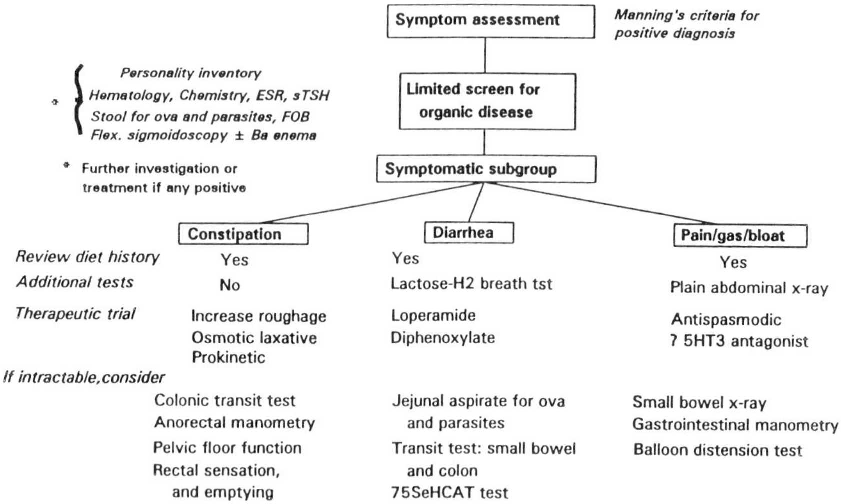

FIGURE 12 Algorithm for the management of irritable bowel syndrome and its subgroups. (Adapted from Ref. 2.)

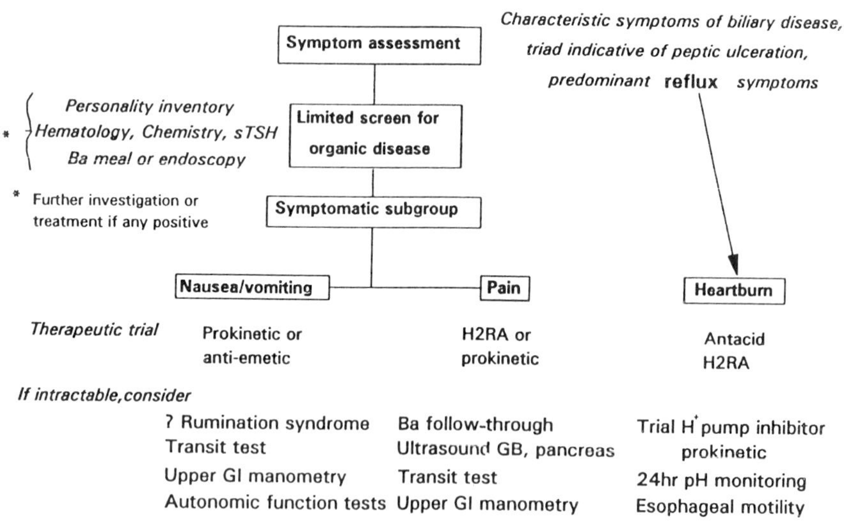

FIGURE 13 Algorithm for the management of dyspepsia.

efficiently evaluate and manage most patients with functional gastrointestinal diseases. In the future, it is hoped that availability of better drugs targeted at the underlying pathophysiological mechanisms will provide further symptomatic relief for these common and often distressing problems.

ACKNOWLEDGMENTS

We wish to thank Mrs. Cindy Stanislav for typing and preparing this chapter.

REFERENCES

1. Lennard-Jones JE. Functional gastrointestinal disorders. N Engl J Med 1983; 308:431–435.
2. Camilleri M, Prather CM. The irritable bowel syndrome: mechanisms and a practical approach to management. Ann Intern Med 1992; 116:1001–1008.
3. Prior A, Maxton DG, Whorwell PJ. Anorectal manometry in irritable bowel syndrome: differences between diarrhoea and constipation predominant subjects. Gut 1990; 31:458–462.
4 Kruis W, Thieme CH, Weinzierl M, Schüssler P, Holl J, Paulus W. A diagnostic score for the irritable bowel syndrome: its value in the exclusion of organic disease. Gastroenterology 1984; 87:1–7.
5. Manning AP, Thompson WG, Heaton KW, Morris AF. Towards positive diagnosis of the irritable bowel syndrome. Br Med J 1978; ii:653–654.
6. Smith RC, Greenbaum DS, Vancouver JB, Henry RC, Reinhart MA, Greenbaum RB, Dean HA, Mayle JE. Gender differences in Manning Criteria in the irritable bowel syndrome. Gastroenterology 1991; 100:591–595.
7. Thompson WG, Dotevall G, Drossman DA, Heaton KW, Kruis W. Irritable bowel syndrome: guidelines for the diagnosis. Gastroenterol Int 1989; 2:92–95.
8. Camilleri M. Four patients with intractable constipation. Gastrointest Diseases Today 1993; 2:7–15.
9. Ott DJ. Radiologic evaluation of esophageal dysphagia. Curr Probl Diagn Radiol 1988; 17:1–33.
10. Jones B, Donner M. Examination of the patient with dysphagia. Radiology 1988; 167:319–326.
11. Ekberg O, Nylander G, Fork F-T, Sjöberg S, Birch-Jensen M, Hillarp B. Interobserver variability in cineradiographic assessment of pharyngeal function during swallow. Dysphagia 198; 3:46–48.
12. Dodds WJ, Stewart ET, Logemann JA. Physiology and radiology of the normal oran and pharyngeal phases of swallowing. AJR 1990; 154:953–963.
13. Nolan DJ, Gourtsoyiannis NC. Crohn's disease of the small intestine: a review of the radiologic appearances in 100 consecutive patients examined by a barium infusion technique. Clin Radiol 1980; 31:597–603.
14. Chernish SM, Maglinte DDT, O'Conner K. Evaluation of the small intestine by en-

teroclysis for Crohn's disease. Am J Gastroenterol 1992; 87:696–701.
15. Metcalf AM, Phillips SF, Zinsmeister AR, MacCarty RL, Beart RW, Wolff BG. Simplified assessment of segmental colonic transit. Gastroenterology 1987; 92:40–47.
16. Castell DO, Richter JE, Boag Dalton C. Esophageal Motility Testing. New York: Elsevier, 1987.
17. Arndorfer RC, STef JJ, Dodds WJ, Linahan JH, Hogan WJ. Improved infusion system for intraluminal esophageal manometry. Gastroenterology 1977; 73:23–27.
18. Richter JE, Bradley LA, DeMeester TR, Wu WC. Normal 24-hour ambulatory esophageal pH values: influence of study center, pH electrode, ages and gender. Dig Dis Sci 1992; 37:849–856.
19. Peters L, Maas L, Petty D, Dalton C, Penner D, Wu W, Castell D, Richter J. Spontaneous noncardiac chest pain: Evaluation by 24-hour ambulatory esophageal motility and pH monitoring. Gastroenterology 1988; 94:878–886.
20. Newcomer AD, McGill DB. Irritable bowel syndrome: role of lactase deficiency. Mayo Clin Proc 1983; 58:339–341.
21. Rumessen JJ, Gudmand-Hoyer E. Functional bowel disease: malabsorption and abdominal distress after ingestion of fructose, sorbitol and fructose-sorbitol mixtures. Gastroenterology 1988; 95:694–700.
22. DiLorenzo C, Dooley CP, Valenzuela JE. Role of fasting gastrointestinal motility in the variability of gastrointestinal transit time assessed by hydrogen breath test. Gut 1991; 32:1127–1130.
23. LaBrooy SJ, male P-J, Beavis AK, Misiewicz JJ. Assessment of the reproducibility of the lactulose H_2 breath test as a measure of mouth to caecum transit time. Gut 1983; 24:893–896.
24. Thompson DG, Binfield P, DeBelder A, O'Brien J, Warren S, Wilson M. Extraintestinal influences on exhaled breath hydrogen measurements during the investigation of gastrointestinal disease. Gut 1985; 26:1349–1352.
25. Cloarec D, Bornet F, Gouilloud S, Barry JL, Salim B, Galmiche JP. Breath hydrogen response to lactulose in healthy subjects: relationship to methane producing status. Gut 1990; 31:300–304.
26. Valdovinos MA, Camilleri M, Thomforde GM, Frie C. Reduced accuracy of ^{14}C-D-xylose breath test for detecting bacterial overgrowth in gastrointestinal motility disorders. Scand J Gastroenterol 1993; 28:963–968.
27. von der Ohe MR, Camilleri M. Measurement of small bowel and colonic transit: indications and methods. Mayo Clin Proc 1992; 67:1169–1179.
28. Proano M, Camilleri M, Phillips SF, Brown ML, Thomforde GM. Transit of solids through the human colon: regional qualification in the unprepared bowel. Am J Physiol 1990; 258:G856–G862.
29. Camilleri M, Zinsmeister AR. Towards a relatively inexpensive, noninvasive, accurate test for colonic motility disorders. Gastroenterology 192; 103:36–42.
30. Camilleri M. Study of human gastroduodenojejunal motility: applied physiology in clinical practice. Dig Dis Sci 1993; 38:785–794.
31. Kellow JE, Gill RC, Wingate DL. Prolonged ambulant recordings of small bowel motility demonstrate abnormalities in the irritable bowel syndrome. Gastroenterology 1990; 98:1208–1218.

32. Rees WDW, Leigh RJ, Christofides ND, Bloom SR, Turnberg LA. Interdigestive motor activity in patients with systemic sclerosis. Gastroenterology 1982; 83:575–580.
33. Fich A, Neri M, Camilleri M, Kelly KA, Phillips SF. Stasis syndromes following gastric surgery: clinical and motility features of sixty symptomatic patients. J Clin Gastroenterol 1990; 12:505–512.
34. Bueno L, Fioramonti J, Ruckebusch Y, Frexinos J, Coulom P. Evaluation of colonic myoelectrical activity in health and functional disorders. Gut 1980; 21:480–485.
35. Bazzocchi G, Ellis J, Villanueva-Meyer J, Reddy SN, Mena I, Snape WJ Jr. Effect of eating on colonic motility and transit in patients with functional diarrhea. Gastroenterology 1991; 101:1298–1306.
36. Bazzocchi G, Ellis J, Villaneuva-Meyer J, Jing J, Reddy SN, Mena I, Snape WJ Jr. Postprandial colonic transit and motor activity in chronic constipation. Gastroenterology 1990; 98:686–693.
37. Steadman CJ, Phillips SF, Camilleri M, Haddad A, Hanson R. Variation of muscle tone in the human colon. Gastroenterology 1991; 101:373–381.
38. DiLorenzo C, Flores AF, Reddy SN, Snape WJ Jr, Bazzocchi G, Hyman PE. Colonic manometry in children with chronic intetinal pseudo-obstruction. Gut 1993; 34:803–807.
39. Pemberton JH. Anorectal and pelvic floor disorders: putting physiology into practice. J Gastroenterol Hepatol 1990; 5:127–143.
40. Camilleri M. Disorders of gastrointestinal motility in neurologic diseases. Mayo Clin Proc 1990; 65:825–846.
41. Camilleri M, Fealey RD. Idiopathic autonomic denervation in eight patients presenting with functional gastrointestinal disease: A causal association? Dig Dis Sci 1990; 35:609–616.
42. Bharucha AE, Camilleri M, Low PA, Zinsmeister AR. Autonomic dysfunction in gatrointestinal motility disorders. Gut 1993; 34:397–401.
43. Camilleri M. Medical treatment of chronic intestinal pseudo-obstruction. Practical Gastroenterol 1991; 15:10–22.
44. von der Ohe MR, Camilleri M, Kvols LK, Thomforde GM. Motor dysfunction of the small bowel and colon in patients with the carcinoid syndrome and diarrhea. N Engl J Med 1993; 329:1073–1078.

5

Psychometric Testing in Functional GI Disorders

Karen H. Naifeh
University of California, San Francisco
San Francisco, California

I. INTRODUCTION

Research over the past 40 years has shown that psychiatric disorders may play an important role in the presentation of functional gastrointestinal (GI) disorders. In early studies, clinincal judgment alone was used to detect the presence of psychiatric disorders, but soon a need was recognized for greater standardization and quantification to answer the important questions arising about prevalence, etiology, and treatment. Psychometric tests therefore began to be used as a means of measuring the coexistence of psychiatric disorders in patients with defined functional GI disorders. An examination of the literature reveals three main foci of studies. The first is prevalence. Another focus has been to determine whether psychiatric illness could be causative of functional GI disease or whether the two simply coexist. The third focus has been on adequate management of the patient who might have psychiatric symptoms as part of the clinical picture and for whom the treatment of the psychiatric symptoms, whether or not they are of etiological importance, will enhance treatment of the functional GI disorder.

The term *psychometric test* refers to a wide variety of questionnaires aimed at measuring some aspect of psychological functioning. In this chapter the focus is on tests aimed at measuring psychopathology or impaired psychological functioning. Psychometric tests in large part have the advantage of being easily self-administered or administered by office personnel, and provide quantitative information, although there is variability from test to test in terms of their accuracy in comparison to trained clinical diagnosis. Three general classes of tests are considered here: structured psychiatric interviews, personality tests, and tests measuring one, a few, or multiple psychopathological symptoms. The structured psychiatric interviews require special psychiatric training to administer and are filled out by the interviewer during the course of the interview with the patient. They were developed in order to standardize psychiatric diagnostic interviews with patients so as to obtain greater agreement on diagnosis among different interviewers for research purposes; examples are the Diagnostic Interview Schedule (DIS) and the Structured Clinical Interview for Diagnosis (SCID). Personality tests, rather than measuring more transient psychopathological symptoms, measure the relatively enduring aspects of a person's personality structure, i.e., the way a person interacts with his or her environment and other people. Psychopathological symptom questionnaires were developed for the most part to provide a relatively fast, standardized measure of the symptom or symptoms in question, for either research or clinical use. The majority of such measures are patient self-report measures and require little training on the part of the user to administer and score. Exceptions tend to be the multiple-symptom or multiple-category tests. Most of the psychometric tests covered in this chapter are copyrighted, and must be purchased from the company holding the copyright. Also important to keep in mind is that the more complex tests, such as the Minnesota Multiphasic Personality Inventory (MMPI), require adequate training in psychological assessment techniques of anyone administering or interpreting the results of the test. This is usually limited to psychologists and psychiatrists who meet the training criteria.

The development of psychometric tests involves a process of establishing the reliability of the test, that is, how *consistently* it measures what it is designed to measure. The validity—the *extent* to which the test actually measures what it was designed to measure—is also part of psychometric-test development. Finally, tests are administered to various groups of people (standardization groups) to establish criteria for scoring. When using a particular test, it is important to be sure that the patients to which the test will be administered are similar to standardization groups for that test; otherwise the scores obtained cannot be interpreted as outlined in the test's manual. For example, if a test has been standardized only on college students, then interpreting the scores of a middle-aged mechanic with irritable bowel syndrome (IBS) based on the scores of the standardization group would lead to erroneous conclusions.

The first section of this chapter is devoted to a review of the literature on the use of psychometric tests in functional GI disorders; the second section includes descriptions and evaluations of a variety of psychometric tests that have been used or are recommended for use with patients with functional GI disorders.

II. USE OF PSYCHOMETRIC ASSESSMENT IN STUDIES OF FUNCTIONAL GI DISORDERS

A. Irritable Bowel Syndrome

In considering IBS, it is important to keep in mind that most studies before 1990 were hampered by vague inclusion criteria. Only recently have precise diagnostic criteria been devised—the Rome criteria—which have helped to obviate this inconsistency. For this reason, although many of the studies considered here have addressed "IBS," they are referred to in the context of this discussion as functional GI complaints.

The earliest studies of functional GI disorders suggested a relationship between personality and/or psychiatric factors and functional GI complaints. Almy and Tulin (1) showed alterations in colonic function in response to stress which simulated the "irritable colon." A study by Chaudhary and Truelove (2) in 1962 directly demonstrated a relationship between functional GI complaints and psychological factors. This early study used only an unstructured psychiatric interview and had no control group; nevertheless, they reported that one or more psychological factors were present in four of five patients (80%). Their conclusion was that psychological factors were preeminent in the genesis of irritable bowel syndrome. Hislop (3), in a study of 67 patients with functional GI complaints and an equal number of normal controls, reported an association of "IBS" with an increased prevalence of psychological disorders of anxiety and depression, which when treated resulted in alleviation of the "IBS" symptoms. No psychometric tests were used; rather, he used relatively unstructured interviews.

A third study using only psychiatric interviews was done by Liss and colleagues (4) in 1973. Based on their findings that psychiatric illness occurred commonly among patients with functional GI disorders and that most of them experienced an onset of psychiatric symptoms prior to GI symptoms, they concluded that the symptoms of "irritable colon" are often related to a diagnosable psychiatric illness. They were the first to use a structured research interview (devised by the authors) for determining psychiatric diagnosis in this population. Twenty-five patients were studied; there was no control group. In a 1976 study using a structured psychiatric interview [adapted from Feighner et al. (6)], Young and colleagues (5) found that 72% of "IBS" patients had psychiatric illness, with hysteria and depression being the most prevalent, whereas only 18%

of normal controls had psychiatric illness. They further reported that the primary physician made an accurate psychiatric assessment in only 28% of the "IBS" patients. While Feighner's criteria have been called into question (55), this study was important in pointing to the importance of the physician's being aware of a patient's psychiatric illness in order to provide effective treatment and spare the patient needless medications, hospitalizations, and surgery.

Psychometric tests began to be used more commonly to explore in a more systematic and quantitative manner the connection between functional GI complaints and personality factors or psychopathology, either specific disorders or more globally. A second focus was to assess the effects on functional GI complaints of treatment of the psychopathology if present. Early studies using standardized psychometric tests tended to use personality tests, which measure relatively enduring traits, and psychological symptom scales rather unsystematically and interchangeably. Hill and Blendis (7), in 1967, were among the first to use a standardized psychometric test in studies of functional GI disorders. They used the Eysenck Personality Inventory (8) to study a group of 27 patients with nonorganic abdominal pain, six of whom were diagnosed with irritable colon syndrome. They found that patients scored significantly higher for neuroticism than a group of 19 peptic ulcer patients, and that the symptoms of patients with functional GI disorders often began in a setting of bereavement or some other upheaval in their lives. A third finding was that six (22%) of the patients with functional GI disorders were depressed when seen, and that treatment for depression was followed by disappearance of pain. In 1974, Palmer and colleagues (9) also used the Eysenck Personality Inventory (8) and the Crown-Crisp Experiential Index (10), a British psychometric test measuring psychoneurotic symptoms, to study 41 patients with functional GI complaints. Two control groups were used in this study; one contained 25 patients with psychoneurotic illness, the other, 25 subjects from the general population. They found that the patients with functional GI complaints were significantly more neurotic and less extroverted according to the Eysenck Personality Inventory than their normal population sample and comparable to the psychoneurotic sample, and also scored higher on the Crown-Crisp Questionnaire in all categories except hysteria than did the normal population. They concluded that patients suffering from functional GI complaints have a moderate degree of psychoneurotic disorder in the form of both a neurotic personality structure and the presence of psychoneurotic symptoms. Welgan et al. (11) also found significantly higher scores on the MMPI (12) subscales of hypochondriasis, hysteria, and depression in patients with "IBS" than a normal control group.

Gomez and Dally (13), in an uncontrolled study of 96 patients complaining of recurrent and persistent abdominal pain, used the Eysenck Personality Inventory (8) and the Hamilton Depression Scale (14). Organic disorders as a cause of symptoms were found in only 15% of patients. In the remainder, they found a high prevalence of depression, chronic tension, and hysteria—psychological factors that the authors felt accounted for abdominal pain. A problem with the study was the assumption that all patients who did not have an organic cause for their pain had a psychiatric illness, and the investigators' use of "clinical judgment" rather than standardized criteria for classification of subjects into categories of psychiatric disorder. Of note, however, is their report that over half the patients responded favorably after 6 months to psychiatric management, with a decrease in both IBS and depressive symptoms. The authors concluded that psychiatric assessment has a place in the evaluation of functional GI complaints and should not be considered simply a last resort. Gomez and Dally also included Paykel's Schedule of Life Events in the study. Like Hill and Blendis (7), they found an excess of bereavements in the preceding 12 months among the depressed patients with functional GI disorders. There was an increase in family conflicts in those with increased tension states and IBS. MacDonald and Bouchier (15) used the Hysteroid-Obsessoid Questionnaire, a British measure of hysteria and obsessive-compulsive symptoms, and the General Health Questionnaire (16), a British measure of psychiatric symptoms. This was an uncontrolled study investigating the presence of psychiatric illness in 32 patients with nonorganic gastrointestinal symptoms, including "IBS," constipation, and diarrhea. Of these, seven were diagnosed as depressed, six with anxiety neurosis, one with hysteria, one with obsessional personality, and one with bereavement reaction.

Later studies using control groups reported conflicting results: A study by Welch and colleagues (17) compared "IBS" patients to a control group with GI disorders other than "IBS." They used the British Crown-Crisp Inventory (10) and the Zung Self-Rating Depression Scale (18). Unlike Hill and Blendis, they found no differences between the two patient groups on any of the psychological measures, although both groups had elevations in phobic and somatization-scale scores as compared to a normal control group. They offered no hypotheses to account for the psychological similarities of the two patient groups, but encouraged attention to psychological needs of both "IBS" and other GI patients.

A controlled psychometric assessment of depression and functional GI complaints is that of Rose and colleagues (19). They used the short form of the Beck Depression Inventory (BDI) (20) to establish the number of patients suffering from depression among new referrals to a general medical and gastrointestinal clinic, and to a general surgical clinic, and to see whether the depression scores affected the readiness of the clinician to prescribe antidepressants. They found that the proportion of patients diagnosed clinically as being depressed increased with the severity of their depression as rated by the BDI. Sixty-four percent of the patients in the medical clinic presenting with functional GI complaints were diagnosed as depressed, whereas 19% of 75 surgical patients were diagnosed as depressed. The authors pointed out that even in their study, undertaken by interested clinicians, only two-thirds of severely depressed patients were diagnosed and treated. A study by Kumar and colleagues (21) did not find a higher incidence of depression in their IBS group as compared to another GI-disorder group and a normal control group; however, they did find a greater incidence of anxiety and obsession. The British General Health Questionnaire (16) and the Crown-Crisp Questionnaire (10) were used. The groups were quite small (10, 12, and 18 patients), making their findings somewhat questionable. Schwarz et al. (22) found higher depression and anxiety scores in 121 IBS patients than in 46 inflammatory bowel disease patients or 45 normal controls. The Spielberger State-Trait Anxiety Inventory (STAI) (23), the Beck Depression Inventory (20), the MMPI (12), and the Holmes and Rahe Life Events Scale (24) were used. Contrary to earlier studies, there were no differences between groups on the Life Events Scale.

Fowlie and colleagues (25) used a placebo-controlled trial of fiber supplementation in the treatment of IBS to study the relationship between outcome and anxiety and depression as measured by the British Delusions-Symptoms-States Inventory (26). There were no differences in treatment outcome between the fiber-supplementation group ($n = 25$) and the placebo group ($n = 24$). A low initial depression score was a better predictor of improvement than any other parameter. They concluded that IBS is best considered a response produced by the interaction of three factors: "soma, psyche, and circumstance."

Finally, a very large study by Longstreth and Wolde-Tsadik (27) of the prevalence, demographics, and clinical correlates of IBS in HMO patients undergoing a routine health appraisal used the Zung Depression Inventory (18) and the STAI (23) for psychological measurements (see Table 1). Depression was strongly associated with IBS-type symptoms and showed a strong linear increase, with higher depression scores being associated with more severe IBS symptoms. State and trait anxiety scores were also significantly elevated in both IBS groups, but did not differ according to IBS symptom severity.

Table 1 Prevalence, Demographics, and Clinical Correlates of IBS in HMO Patients

	n	*n*%	*n* and % with Zung score 50>[a]	State anxiety (mean)[b]	Trait anxiety (mean)[b]
Severe Symptoms	45	4%	4/40 (10%)	36.8	40.8
Mild/moderate Symptoms	202	16%	14/164 (8.5%)	35.5	37.8
No symptoms	1017	80%	22/835 (2.6%)	31.1	33.4

[a]*p* lt 0.0005 (association test and linear trend test).
[b]*p* lt 0.0001 (ANOVA).
Source: Ref. 27.

Although some authors (28) have questioned the value of personality data to the treating physician, Bergeron and Monto (29) disagreed based on their findings from a study of personality patterns seen in individuals with IBS. Using the MMPI to produce individual profiles for each of 82 patients, they used Q-factor analysis, resulting in four subgroupings of personality types: 1) inadequate dependency, 2) somatization of affect, 3) reactive depression, and 4) anger and denial. The authors felt that personality descriptions would provide more information to gastroenterologists about their patients than simple one-dimensional measures such as anxiety and depression. Of the four personality types described within the IBS group, the authors recommended psychotherapy only for type 3, the reactive depression. They felt that the first two types would be too defensive and therefore other types of therapeutic approaches would be necessary. Patients of the fourth type would be unsuitable for psychotherapy because of their oppositional attitude toward authority figures. Bergeron and Monto saw the MMPI as an instrument that can give the primary-care physician information about how to more effectively treat patients with functional GI disorders.

Use of Psychological Instruments to Measure Treatment Effects

For the most part, studies involving treatment of psychological disorders associated with IBS (3,7,13) have not been controlled. Of the few that were, a double-blind study of IBS and depression by Heefner and colleagues (30) utilizing desipramine and placebo found that 11 of 17 patients were depressed according to ratings on the Zung Self-Rating Depression Scale (18) and that, of the depressed patients receiving drug treatment, 60% showed improvement, whereas 64% of the placebo-treated depressed patients showed improvement in depression scores. There was a somewhat greater degree of improvement in patients receiving desipramine than in those receiving placebo, although the differences did not reach statistical significance. The authors concluded that tricyclic antidepressant therapy may be appropriate only in those patients for whom depression is an important component of IBS. Lancaster-Smith and colleagues (31) used the British General Health Questionnaire (16) to determine psychoneurotic morbidity in IBS patients, and then performed a double-blind, randomized, placebo-controlled comparison of treatment with a combined anxiolytic antidepressant (Motipress, which is 30 mg nortriptyline with 1.5 mg fluphenazine). They found a significantly better effect of Motipress than placebo on diarrhea and abdominal pain. The quantitative nature of the General Health Questionnaire data also allowed the investigators to do correlational studies, the results of which suggested that there is no direct relationship between psychoneurotic illness and IBS, but the presence of the former has an adverse effect on the short-term outcome of the bowel disorder.

An uncontrolled study by Wise and colleagues (32) evaluated the efficacy of group therapy for patients with IBS using the SCL-90 (33) and the Locus of

Control Scale (34). Immediately following group therapy, the group's psychological distress levels as measured by the SCL-90 were significantly lower in a number of dimensions, and the group's locus of control tended to shift from an external orientation to a more internal locus at the 6-month follow-up. Additionally, the more externally located IBS patients on the Locus of Control Scale tended to have significantly higher SCL-90 scores on most of the scales; that is, a more external locus of control in these patients was associated with greater psychological symptomatology. There was, however, no measure of improvement in IBS symptoms.

Psychophysiological Studies

In the 1980s, there was a series of studies that looked for sensory or motor abnormalities in IBS and the relationship between those, if present, and psychological test scores. Whitehead and colleagues (35) reported a study in which patients with different irritable bowel symptoms were compared to normal subjects to determine whether subtypes of IBS could be distinguished on the basis of colonic motility or psychological test scores. The psychological test used was the SCL-90 (33). They found that patients with IBS showed significantly elevated levels on the psychological traits of anxiety, interpersonal sensitivity, depression, hostility, and somatization of affect as compared to normal controls. However, they found no significant trait differences between IBS patients with diarrhea and those with constipation. There was also no *correlation* between amount of psychopathology and either colonic motility or severity of symptoms. They concluded that, although there is a co-occurrence between psychopathology and both symptom severity and amount of colonic motility for the whole group of IBS patients, there is no *causal* connection such that greater psychopathology creates greater symptom severity. They therefore disagreed with the conclusions of an earlier study by Latimer (36) that colonic motor dysfunction is not specific to "IBS" and that "IBS" patients are psychoneurotics who become preoccupied with one psychophysiological response. A 1981 study by Latimer and colleagues (37) corroborated the earlier findings of no significant difference between normal controls, "IBS" patients, and a psychoneurotic group of patients without bowel symptoms, on measures of either myoelectrical activity or motor activity of the colon. Findings from the STAI (23), the Beck Depression Inventory (20), and the Eysenck Personality Inventory (8) revealed similar psychological characteristics in the two groups. They concluded that the excess of colonic contractions reported as unique to "IBS" may be more properly related to psychological factors, as they were found to be equally excessive in the pure psychoneurotic group.

A study by Campbell and colleagues (38) in 1984 assessed the relationship between personality and gastrointestinal motility, using the Eysenck Personality Inventory (8) and the STAI (23) as their measures of personality and psychological symptoms. They found a highly significant *inverse* correlation between the duration of regular cycles of contractile activity and 1) a predisposition to anxiety and 2) neuroticism as assessed on the Eysenck Personality Inventory. They concluded that asymptomatic personality traits, particularly those predisposing to anxiety or neuroticism, can influence motility of the human colon. Kingham and Dawson (39) found that balloon distension of the small or large intestine mimicked their customary pain in 22 patients with right-upper-quadrant pain. The authors used the Hamilton Rating Scale for Depression (40) to assess depression in these patients; they found that depression was present in 14 of the 22 patients studied, and that the eight patients with continuous pain had more marked depression. They speculated whether depression predisposes to intractable functional abdominal pain or vice versa, and concluded that the vicious cycle of depression and functional abdominal pain will not be broken until the depression is treated.

Using a similar physical test—balloon distension of the rectosigmoid colon—but measuring tolerance for the pain produced, Whitehead and colleagues (41) assessed the presence of sensory abnormalities in 16 IBS patients and two control groups: 25 lactose malabsorbers and 18 asymptomatic controls. They found a lower tolerance for balloon-distension pain but not for non-gut pain stimuli in the IBS patients. Anxiety and depression scores were significantly elevated in IBS patients, but, as in the study by Whitehead et al. (35), there was no correlation between degree of sensory abnormality and any of the psychological traits measured. This was in line with their earlier findings regarding motor activity and psychological traits, and contrary to those of Latimer et al. (36,37). Thus, all the studies seem to agree that psychopathology is present, but there are conflicting views as to whether physiological abnormalities or psychopathology account for IBS symptoms.

In a study with a focus on pain tolerance rather than physiology per se, Cook and colleagues (42) tested the hypothesis that the increased levels of psychological symptomatology in IBS patients is accounted for by a reduced tolerance of pain. They measured pain thresholds, and used the Eysenck Personality Inventory, the STAI, and the Beck Depression Inventory to measure psychological symptomatology in a group of IBS patients, Crohn's disease patients, and normals. They found a higher pain threshold in both Crohn's disease and IBS patients as compared to the normal control group, no differences between groups on the four scales of the Eysenck Personality Inventory, significantly higher scores for depression as compared to normals in the IBS and Crohn's disease groups, and marginally higher scores for trait anxiety in both IBS and Crohn's disease patients. They concluded that, given the higher threshold for pain in IBS patients, their pain reports should not be disregarded and seem to have no relationship to the increased psychological symptomatology in this group.

Effect of Care-Seeking

A 1985 study by Welch and colleagues (43) took the first quantitative look at psychoneurotic symptomatology in a group of patients with functional GI disorders who sought medical treatment and another group who did not. Using the SCL-90, the authors found that patients with functional GI complaints were psychologically similar to nonpatients with functional GI complaints, and that both groups showed more somatic distress than normal controls. However, this study also found that the measures of anxiety, depression, obsession-compulsion, and interpersonal sensitivity were similar in both groups with IBS and in the normal control group, unlike earlier studies that have shown those measures to be higher in patients with IBS than in normal controls. A later study by Drossman and colleagues (44), using the MMPI, Profile of Mood States (POMS) (45), Life Experiences Survey (LES) (46), and Illness Behavior Questionnaire (47), found that a group of 72 IBS patients had a higher proportion of abnormal personality patterns, greater illness behaviors, and lower positive stressful life events scores than a group of 82 IBS nonreporters and a group of 84 normal subjects. They concluded that the psychological factors previously attributed to IBS are associated with patient status rather than IBS per se, and that the psychosocial factors contributing to patient status need to be evaluated and treated in these patients. Slightly different findings were reported by Greenbaum and colleagues (48): Their IBS nonreporters (n = 20) had intermediate degrees of depression, hypochondriasis, and hysteria as compared to IBS patients (n = 23) and normal controls (n = 19) on the MMPI, the Beck Depression Inventory, and the Zung Self-Rating Depression Scale.

Finally, Whitehead and colleagues (49), using the Hopkins Symptom Checklist (33), the NEO Personality Inventory (50), and the MMPI, found that women who met restrictive criteria for IBS (n = 16) but had not consulted a physician had no more symptoms of psychological distress than normal controls (n = 46), whereas both patients with lactose malabsorption (n = 23) and those with IBS (n = 10) had significantly more psychological symptoms than either of the above groups. The psychological symptoms included somatization, obsession-compulsion, interpersonal sensitivity, depression, anxiety, hostility, phobia, and paranoia. These authors concluded that symptoms of psychological distress are unrelated to IBS but influence which of those persons with IBS will consult a doctor.

Life Events

Although earlier studies had speculated about the role of life stress in IBS (1,7), Craig and Brown (51,52) were the first to use a quantitative questionnaire in a controlled study of the role of stressful life events in the etiology of IBS. Using the Life Events and Difficulty Schedule (LEDS) (53), they found that 57% of the

79 IBS patients studied had experienced a severely threatening event prior to the onset of symptoms, compared with 23% of the 56 patients with an organic diagnosis and a comparison group of 135 subjects with no gastrointestinal disorder. The authors noted that the majority of severe events in the functional group involved losses and disappointments, and did not appear to differ in content from those known to produce depression. They concluded that stressful life events are of etiological importance in the development of IBS.

IBS vs. Other Stress-Related Disorders

Blanchard and colleagues (54) compared psychological measures of patients with IBS to those of patients with a different stress-related disorder—in this case, tension headaches and migraine headaches—as well as normal controls. They used a number of types of psychological instruments: the MMPI, the Beck Depression Inventory, the STAI, and the Holmes and Rahe Life Events Scale. Their most striking and consistent finding was that, on almost all the 17 measures studied, the means were ordered such that IBS patients scored higher than tension-headache sufferers, who in turn scored higher than migraineurs, who scored higher than the normal volunteers. The IBS patients had elevated scores on the hypochondriasis, hysteria, and depression subscales of the MMPI, on both subscales of the STAI, on the Beck Depression Inventory, and on the Life Events Scale. Their conclusions were that there is no pattern of psychological symptoms or traits that is idiosyncratic to IBS, merely a difference in the level of psychological symptomatology, and that there may be a common core of distress-disturbance that takes slightly different forms, perhaps due to physiological predispositions or early socialization experiences.

In summary, the connection between functional bowel symptoms and psychopathology, stressful life events, and/or certain personality patterns has been examined in a large variety of ways in the last 40 years. Psychometric tests have played a valuable role in these investigations. At present, the consensus seems to be that psychopathology is not a necessary factor in the etiology of IBS, nor does it correlate with the severity of acute physical symptoms of IBS. However, it is present in a large percentage of those seeking treatment for the disorder, and in a smaller percentage or a lesser degree in those not seeking treatment. Further, many authors point out that treatment of psychological distress is an important component that can favorably affect clinical management of the disorder. For those interested in further reading, Creed and Guthrie (55) also reviewed the literature on psychological factors in IBS, with close attention to the methodology involved. They concluded that as of 1981 there were problems with many studies: no or inappropriate control groups, use of unreliable psychiatric measures or inappropriate use of reliable measures, and/or improper interpretation of findings. According to Creed and Guthrie, well-done studies indicated that psychiatric illness occurs in approximately 50% of clinic attenders, that untreated psychiatric illness impairs the response to conventional treatment, that persistent clinic attendance may be due to the presence of psychiatric disorder, and that, while it cannot be assumed that the "neurotic patient" does not have organic disease, the gastroenterologist should not overinvestigate patients with IBS.

B. Inflammatory Bowel Disease

Although IBD has an organic basis, earlier in this century when there was little understanding of its pathophysiology IBD was thought to be the physical manifestation of a certain pattern of personality traits characterized by a deep psychological attachment to a caretaking figure, passivity, compliance, overconscientiousness, perfectionism, and an inability to be angry or aggressive (56). This view was pioneered by Franz Alexander at the Chicago Psychoanalytic Institute and his colleagues; they postulated that IBD was the result of an intrapsychic conflict that ultimately resulted in "organ neurosis" in the form of IBD (57). The lack of understanding of the pathophysiology of IBD during those years, coupled with the emotional distress of the patients and the relief of emotional suffering provided by psychoanalytic intervention, led to the general acceptance of their theory. The research supporting these views was largely anecdotal, based on unstructured interviews, and uncontrolled or poorly controlled. Later adequately controlled and blinded studies have found little evidence for either greater psychopathology or personality patterns unique to IBD. Advances in identifying the pathophysiology of both Crohn's disease and ulcerative colitis, plus effective medical treatment for IBD, also showed that medical intervention alone can effectively treat IBD. Olden (58) provides a very good biopsychosocial perspective on IBD.

Of the earlier studies of psychological aspects of IBD using psychometric tests, a study by McMahon and colleagues (59) is an example of inadequate controls. While they used healthy siblings as a control for differences in family background, they failed to control for the effects of chronic medical illness. Even so, they found no differences between IBD patients and their healthy siblings on the Profile of Mood States (45) and the Martin-Jacobs Ego Strength Scale (60), and differences on only two of the MMPI scales—hypochondriasis and hysteria, both of which are heavily loaded with questions about physical symptoms. West (61) found a group of 56 ulcerative colitis patients to be significantly *less* psychologically disturbed on nine MMPI variables than a group of 122 patients with various psychosomatic diagnoses such as hypertension, eczema, headache, and mucous colitis. The ulcerative colitis group showed a moderately elevated pattern in the depression, hypochondriasis, and hysteria scales of the MMPI, a pattern common in medical patients in general.

The two studies by Helzer and colleagues (62,63) on 50 ulcerative colitis patients and 50 Crohn's disease patients, respectively, used carefully matched control groups with chronic medical illness of non-GI origin. They used structured psychiatric interviews, the Eysenck Personality Inventory and the Paykel Life Events Inventory (51). They found no difference in the frequency of diagnosable psychiatric disorders in either the ulcerative colitis or the Crohn's disease groups as compared to controls. When psychiatric illness was present, there was no evidence that a flareup of psychiatric illness preceded a flareup of the IBD. Personality profiles on the Eysenck were similar in IBD and control groups, and there was no correlation between the frequency of stressful life events in the 6 months prior to interview and the severity of IBD at the time of interview.

In research on IBS, IBD patients have often been used as a control group of patients with GI disorders having an organic basis. In this context they have been found to be less anxious than IBS patients using different anxiety measures: the Institute for Personality and Ability Testing (IPAT) Anxiety Scale and the STAI (64,22). However, IBD patients have been found to be significantly more alexithymic (66). Alexithymia is a concept introduced by Sifneos (67) to describe an impoverished fantasy and inner imaginative life. Fava and Pavan (66) postulate that this constriction in experiencing emotions and poverty of fantasy life leaves such persons unable to express psychological symptomatology, and that this may act permissively in the genesis of the illness.

Although IBD is not a "functional disorder," there are certainly psychological sequelae of living with this chronic debilitating disease. The methodological damage done by Alexander and his colleagues, resulting in the misdiagnosis and faulty psychiatric conceptualizations of IBD patients, was considerable, and should not be forgotten in our attempts to treat these biopsychosocially complex patients.

C. Constipation

Idiopathic constipation has also been associated with psychological distress. Tucker and colleagues (68), using the MMPI in a study of constipation, reported evidence that greater stool output tended to occur in persons who were more socially outgoing, more energetic and optimistic, and less anxious, and who described themselves in favorable terms. They found that personality factors were as important as dietary factors in predicting stool output in normal male volunteers. In an MMPI study of idiopathic constipation, Devroede et al. (69) found higher scores on hypochondriasis, hysteria, control, and low-back-pain scales, and concluded that women with constipation of a colonic origin had a different personality pattern than a group of arthritic women. A prospective study by Wald and colleagues (70) used the Hopkins Symptom Checklist to study patients with severe idiopathic constipation. They found that patients with normal transit times demonstrated significantly higher scores for psychological distress in the global symptom index and in nine of the clinical subscales than did those with slow-transit constipation or normal control subjects. They concluded that different therapeutic approaches may be required: a behaviorally and psychologically based approach for the former group and an approach focused on modification of disordered colonic transit for the latter group.

A British study (71) of patients with fecal incontinence and chronic constipation was designed to ascertain whether surgery had any effect on parameters of anxiety and depression and to identify whether patients who did badly after surgery could be identified preoperatively. Using the Hospital Anxiety and Depression Scale (HAD) (72) and the General Health Questionnaire (GHQ) (16), they found that constipated patients had significantly higher HAD depression scores than did controls, and that those who were improved with surgery had significantly lower preoperative HAD anxiety scores and depression scores as compared to those who were not improved with surgery. Similarly, those with incontinence who did poorly after surgery had significantly higher HAD anxiety scores and higher HAD depression scores than those who obtained benefit from the surgery. That is, patients who had high levels of anxiety or depression did not benefit from surgery. This study in particular underscores the need to assess patients psychologically prior to surgery for incontinence or constipation. It is also important to note, with regard to treatment of constipation and fecal incontinence, that there is an 80% success rate for biofeedback treatment for these disorders (73).

D. Globus Pharyngeus (Hystericus)

One of the first studies of the association of globus with psychopathology was that of Lehtinen and Puhakka (74). They used structured psychiatric interviews, the Holmes and Rahe Life Events Scale (24), the Crown-Crisp Experiential Index (10), and the Taylor Manifest Anxiety Scale (75). They found considerably more psychic disturbances in globus patients than in normal controls, with the personalities marked by obsessive traits. They also found two groups of globus patients, one in which psychological disturbances were present, the other in which they were absent. The group with psychological disturbances had often experienced some significant life event prior to the appearance of the globus syndrome. An uncontrolled study of 99 patients (76) used the MMPI to help confirm a diagnosis of globus hystericus. Scores on the depression and hypochondriasis subscales were much higher than normal in 26% of the female and 31% of the male patients. These two subscales were elevated, but not above normal levels, in the remainder of patients. Later, Deary and colleagues (77) compared 96 female and 31 male globus patients with age- and sex-matched ENT patient controls using the Crown-Crisp, the General Hospital Questionnaire, the Hysteroid-Obsessoid Questionnaire, and the Eysenck Personality Inventory. They reported low extraversion scores and high levels of psychoneurotic symptomatology in female globus patients but not in males. They concluded that a substantial minority of globus patients, predominantly female, have significant psychiatric morbidity. Thus, a number of studies have found evidence for the association of psychological symptomatology with the diagnosis of globus.

However, a lack of correlation between globus and psychological symptoms was reported by Moser and colleagues (78) in their study of globus patients using the BDI and the STAI. They concluded that the available data did *not* suggest that personality characteristics and mood states—in particular, anxiety, depression, hypochondriasis, and hysteria—contribute to a significant extent to the exacerbation and maintenance of the globus sensation. It is unclear why the earlier studies of psychological involvement in globus hystericus obtained positive results while this later one did not, but differences in psychometric tests used, diagnostic criteria, and/or types of control groups may have played a part.

E. Functional Esophageal Disorders

These disorders began to be studied intensively beginning in the 1980s. A study by Clouse and Lustman (79) in 1983, using structured psychiatric interviews in patients with contraction abnormalities of the esophagus and matched controls, found that psychiatric diagnoses were made in 84% of patients with certain specific contraction abnormalities but in only 31% of patients with normal esophageal manometric patterns and 33% of a group of patients with other esophageal manometric abnormalities. Later studies, however, obtained different results. A second study by Clouse and Lustman (80) failed to replicate their earlier findings. In this study they used the SCL-90 and found that it did not effectively differentiate patients with esophageal symptoms and contraction abnormalities from patients with other manometric diagnoses. A third study by Clouse and colleagues (81), again using the SCL-90, also failed to find an association between abnormalities in esophageal motility and psychological distress symptoms. Again, differences in psychometric tests used, diagnostic criteria, and/or types of control groups may explain the contradictory results of these studies.

Patients with another esophageal motility disorder, nutcracker esophagus, were compared to IBS patients and three groups of non-GI-disorder patients by Richter and colleagues (82). Nutcracker esophagus is characterized by noncardiac chest pain due to high-amplitude peristaltic contractions in the body of the esophagus. Richter et al. used the Millon Behavioral Health Inventory (MBHI) (83), a comprehensive psychosocial measure designed to aid in the psychological understanding of medically ill patients. Both nutcracker and IBS patients scored significantly higher than controls on scales of GI susceptibility to stress and somatic anxiety, and tended to be hypochondriacal and seek early medical care. Nutcracker esophagus patients, however, did not score above normal on general measures of depression and anxiety, while IBS patients did. This may mean that, at least in the case of nutcracker esophagus, patients with functional esophageal disorders may somaticize stress more than patients with lower functional GI disorders. We could speculate that the reason for the conflicting results in the earlier versus later studies of psychological concomitants of globus hystericus (mentioned above) is that later measures may not have adequately measured somaticized symptoms. If this was the case, then patients with functional esophageal disorders should receive psychometric testing that covers somatic aspects of psychological symptoms, or psychological involvement might be missed.

A 1989 study by Pulliam and colleagues (84) used the SCL-90 and the Millon Behavioral Health Inventory (83) to evaluate patients with gastroesophageal reflex disease (GERD). They found that subjects with higher psychological stress scores reported increased levels of subjective reflux severity across the stress tasks administered, although there was no difference in objective reflux findings based on acidity. They concluded that stress and high psychological-symptom reporting interact to produce increased reports of reflux, and that the commonly reported link between stress and reflux may be due to distorted perceptions rather than to actual increased acid reflux.

III. ASSESSMENT INSTRUMENTS

Given the literature that supports the association between many of the functional GI disorders and personality factors and/or psychiatric symptoms, together with the recent focus on the advantages of treating psychiatric symptoms when they are present in order to optimize clinical outcome, the treating physician may want to integrate psychometric assessment into evaluation procedures. The remainder of this chapter provides brief descriptions and evaluations of the most commonly used assessment devices for personality assessment, scales for evaluation of either single or multiple categories of psychiatric symptoms, and scales for various other psychological constructs that may aid the physician in an understanding of psychological issues in the patient. The Appendix lists commercial sources for many of the measures; others can be found in their references.

A. Measures of Personality

Minnesota Multiphasic Personality Inventory (MMPI)

The MMPI is the most widely used objective personality-assessment instrument and the most widely researched of all psychological tests (12). First published in 1943, the MMPI contains 10 clinical scales and three validity scales. It consists of 550 different items requiring the client to answer either true or false. It can be administered to patients 16 years of age or older with at least 6 years of formal education. It can usually be completed in 1½ to 2 hours. Scoring can be done by hand or by any of several computer services. The raw scores are converted into T scores directly on the scoring sheet. A T score of 70 is considered to indicate some psychopathology in that area. The validity scales take into account the tendency of patients to lie in answering questions or to fake either psychological health or illness. The MMPI can provide information both on mental disorders, such as depression and anxiety, and on variations in personality type. In spite of its length, the MMPI is relatively easy to administer and score, although interpretation of the results requires a good deal of training.

The configuration of the validity scales provides important information regarding test-taking attitudes and biases— for example, whether a patient was defensive and uncooperative in taking the test or trying to look good or bad. In terms of the clinical scales, the meaning of high scores on a particular scale is relative to the entire profile, that is, the scores on all the scales.

Although it was long ago discovered that the scales do not represent that for which they were originally named, each of the scales does represent certain personality characteristics or areas of psychopathology. Scale 1 (Hs) is a measure of the degree of concern regarding bodily functioning, as the items include various somatic complaints. Scale 2 (D) is a trait measure of depression as an ongoing mood. Scale 3 (Hy) reflects patients who are generally immature, egocentric, and demanding, generally denying psychological or emotional problems. Scale 4 (Pd) tends to assess general social maladjustment and a tendency to act out antisocial impulses. Scale 5 (Mf) reflects a dimension of identification with culturally conventional masculine or feminine interest patterns. Scale 6 (Pa) reflects paranoid thinking and can indicate sensitivity to criticism, a basic mistrust of the motives of others, and a tendency to brood and harbor judges. Scale 7 (Pt) reflects chronic or trait anxiety and is a good index of psychological turmoil and discomfort. Scale 8 (Sc) reflects general ego intactness or ego deterioration, and very high scores can reflect psychotic mentation. Scale 9 (Ma) deals with energy level, and the higher scores may be suggestive of a manic disorder. Scale 10 (Si) reflects the social introversion–extroversion dimension.

The important thing to remember about these clinical scales is that usually more than one of them will be high (a T score of over 70), and the *pattern* of high scores is important in interpreting the meaning of the results. This makes a more complete understanding of the patient possible but does require some background in MMPI interpretation to be relatively accurate.

In addition to the clinical scales, a number of special scales have been developed for the MMPI. Welch's Anxiety Scale measures situational anxiety rather than the chronic trait anxiety that is assessed by scale 7. Other special scales include Welch's Depression Scale, an Ego Strength Scale, an Alcoholism Scale, and a Dependency Scale. In 1989 the MMPI was revised significantly, and the revised version is being referred to as the MMPI-2. The MMPI-2 has a much more representative standardization population and much more up-to-date language than the original MMPI. The MMPI-2 contains 704 items, the additional items covering drug abuse, suicide potential, type A behavior patterns, marital adjustment, work attitudes, and treatment amenability. It also includes three new validity scales. In addition, it contains 28 content scales that assess psychological factors such as need for affection, authority problems, and emotional alienation.

In summary, the MMPI is an extremely thorough and well-studied personality test providing information on the personality and psychopathology of an individual. It gives psychological trends but *not* specific psychiatric diagnoses. The main drawbacks are that completion of the test is a lengthy and tedious task for many people (GI patients may be too ill to complete it) and that, while it is easily scored, either by hand or by computerized procedures, its interpretation requires a professional with adequate training.

Eysenck Personality Inventory (EPI)

The EPI (8), developed in England as a further development of the earlier Maudsley Personality Inventory, measures personality in terms of two independent dimensions: extroversion–introversion (E) and neuroticism–stability (N). Each trait is measured by 24 questions, answered yes or no. There is also a distortion-detection (lie) scale. Two parallel forms are available in case retesting is desired, and the test can be completed in about 10 minutes.

High-scoring individuals on the extroversion scale tend to be outgoing, impulsive, uninhibited, optimistic, aggressive, and free with their feelings, and to have many social contacts. A person scoring low on the E scale (an introvert) is typically quiet, retiring, introspective, and much less sociable, does not like excitement, tends to plan ahead, and keeps feelings under control. High scorers on the neuroticism scale tend to be emotionally overresponsive, complain of vague somatic upsets, and report frequent worries and anxieties.

Cutpoints for the EPI are based on percentile norms. These norms for two populations studied are presented in the EPI manual: American college students and British adult industrial workers. Studies have also been done on psychiatric clinical subgroups and subclasses of British reference groups. Cutpoints are the 31st percentile and 70th percentile; individuals scoring above or below these would be considered above or below average in the trait under consideration.

In summary, the EPI is a measure of two personality dimensions. Advantages are its brief administration time, simple scoring procedures, and thorough validation. Disadvantages are the poverty of useful normative data against which to interpret scores; no norms exist for American general medical patients or even normal American adults. The norms for British industrial workers can be used, but the reliability of interpretation based on these is open to question. The authors themselves state that the norms they present should be used with caution, and that it may be desirable for users to develop their own local norms.

NEO Personality Inventory

This personality inventory, developed by Costa and McCrae (50), measures personality in terms of three major domains: Neuroticism, Extroversion–Introversion, and Openness to Experience, which they call second-order dimensions of personality. Within each of these are the more familiar first-order characteristics. Under Neuroticism are scales for anxiety, hostility, depression, self-consciousness, impulsiveness, and vulnerability to stress. In the Extroversion dimension are scales for warmth, gregariousness, assertiveness, activity, excitement-seeking, and cheerfulness, and under the dimension of Openness to Experience are the scales of fantasy, aesthetics, feelings, actions, and ideas and values. In the revised version two more scales have been added: agreeableness and conscientiousness. The NEO inventory–Revised is a 181-item personality measure using a five-point scale, with response options ranging from "strongly agree" to "strongly disagree." Form R is an observer rating scale with two parallel forms, one for male observees and one for females; form S is a self-rating scale, which also comes in an abbreviated version. The NEO-R can be completed in about 25 minutes, the abbreviated version in about 15 minutes. Advantages are its relative brevity, its good reliability and validity, and the inclusion of a full range of adults with regard to age and social class in its normative studies. Also, psychological research supports the five-factor model of personality on which this measure is based. One disadvantage is its assumption of honest answers from respondents and consequent lack of a lie scale. Another is the lack of correspondence to DSM-IV personality-disorder categories.

The Millon Clinical Multiaxial Inventory–III (MCMI-III)

The MCMI is a personality inventory with separate scales constructed in line with the DSM-IV model to distinguish the more enduring personality characteristics of patients from the acute clinical disorders they display (85). The total number of items, 175, is small enough to encourage its use in many types of diagnostic and treatment settings yet large enough to permit the assessment of a wide range of clinically relevant behaviors. most patients can complete the MCMI in 20 to 30 minutes. Personality structure is assessed in scales 1 to 8B and psychopathological functioning in scales A through T, those being for neurotic levels and scales SS, CC, and PP for psychopathology of a more psychotic nature. It is easily computer-scored but, as with the MMPI, interpretation requires training. The interpretive report focuses on a multiaxial framework of assessment as in the DSM-IIIR. It is primarily intended to provide information to clinicians—especially psychologists, psychiatrists, counselors, social workers, physicians, and nurses—who must make assessments and treatment decisions about people with emotional and interpersonal difficulties. However, clinicians working with physically ill patients are advised to use the MCMI's associated inventory, the Millon Behavioral Health Inventory, which is more appropriate to medically ill patients. The MCMI manual can be abstruse and complicated; computer scoring is almost a must.

B. Measures of Multiple Psychiatric Symptoms

Symptom Checklist 90 (SCL-90)

The SCL-90 evolved from the Hopkins Symptom Checklist, a self-report instrument used for measurement of current psychological symptom status in psychiatric and medical outpatients (33). It differs from the psychometric tests discussed above in that it is not a direct personality test but rather focuses on recent psychological symptoms independent of enduring character traits. The SCL-90 is a 90-item self-report symptom inventory, multidimensional in nature. It incorporated the five symptom dimensions of the earlier Hopkins Symptoms Checklist and added four new dimensions. At 90 items, it is much shorter, taking 15 to 20 minutes to complete, and therefore much easier to administer to patients; yet it has high correlations with similar scales of the MMPI.

Each of the 90 items of the SCL-90 is rated on a five-point scale of distress from 0 to 4, which ranges from "not at all" on one pole to "extremely" on the other. The nine symptom dimensions and the problems they reflect are:

- I. Somatization—distress arising from perceptions of bodily dysfunction
- II. Obsessive-Compulsive—the psychiatric disorder of the same name
- III. Interpersonal Sensitivity—feelings of personal inadequacy and inferiority
- IV. Depression—a broad range of the symptoms of depression
- V. Anxiety—symptoms associated with high levels of manifest anxiety
- VI. Hostility—thoughts, feelings, or actions associated with anger
- VII. Phobic Anxiety—persistent fear responses to a specific person, place, object, or situation
- VIII. Paranoid Ideation—a disordered mode of thinking characterized by hostility, suspiciousness, grandiosity, and delusions
- IX. Psychoticism—a withdrawn, isolated lifestyle as well as symptoms of schizophrenia such as hallucinations and thought-broadcasting.

In addition, there are three global indices: the Global Severity Index (GSI), the Positive Symptom Distress Index (PSDI), and the Positive Symptom Total (PST). For scoring and interpretation, these three global raw scores, as well as the individual scale scores, are transformed to standard scores using normative values. Normative values for psychiatric outpatients and inpatients and nonpatients are provided in the manual. A standard score of 63 is suggested as the cutpoint. The SCL-90 is designed to be interpreted in terms of three levels of information: the global, the dimensional, and the discrete symptoms; these are integrated to provide the most meaningful and valid picture of a patient's psychological distress. The SCL-90 has thorough and extensive validation.

In summary, the SCL-90 is a widely used, brief inventory that can provide a reliable multidimensional psychological-symptom profile.

Profile of Mood States (POMS)

The POMS questionnaire is a rapid and economical method of identifying and assessing transient fluctuating mood or affective states (45). The POMS measures six identifiable mood states: tension-anxiety, depression-dejection, anger-hostility, vigor-activity, fatigue-inertia, and confusion-bewilderment. It originally consisted of a set of 55 adjectives describing mood, each of which was rated on a five-point scale from "not at all" to "extremely." The present POMS, representing a refinement of a total of 100 adjectives, consists of 65 adjectives. It is a self-rating questionnaire; patients are told that the list of words describes feeings people have and are asked to rate them according to how they have been feeling during the past week, including that day. The time period is chosen in order to obtain data on the patient's typical and persistent mood reactions and also to assess feelings "in the moment." For scoring the POMS, two profile sheets are available: an outpatient form and a college form. Raw scores are plotted on the profile sheet and can be converted into standard T scores using tables. Abnormally high or low scores are considered to be more than 2 standard deviations from the mean, which would be a score higher than 70 or lower than 30. It takes approximately 3 to 5 minutes for most patients to complete and can easily be administered by technicians or clerical personnel. It may be hand-scored using overlay stencils or computer-scored.

Interpretation of the POMS calls for evaluating each of the six mood-state categories. Factor T (tension-anxiety) includes somatic tension, panic, nervousness, and anxiety, and comprises nine items of the POMS. Factor D (depression-dejection) consists of 15 items of the POMS and represents a mood of depression accompanied by a sense of personal inadequacy, worthlessness, futility, emotional isolation, sadness, and guilt. Factor A (anger-hostility) consists of 12 items and indicates a mood of anger and antipathy toward others. It includes both intense overt anger and mild feelings of hostility. Factor V (vigor-activity), consisting of eight items, depicts a mood of vigorousness, ebullience, and high energy. Factor F (fatigue-inertia) represents a mood of weariness, inertia, and low energy. It consists of seven adjectives: *worn out*, *listless*, *fatigued*, *exhausted*, *sluggish*, *weary*, and *bushed*. Factor C (confusion-bewilderment) consists of seven items: *confused*, *unable to concentrate*, *muddled*, *bewildered*, *inefficient*, *forgetful*, *uncertain about things*. It is not clear from studies whether this represents a mood or a trait of cognitive inefficiency related to anxiety or other such states that might impair cognitive abilities.

The POMS has marginal reliability and validity studies in place at this time. Raw scores are converted to standard T scores on the profile sheet and 2 standard deviations above or below a T score of 50 is considered to be abnormal. Norms for psychiatric outpatients are included in the manual. There are at present no norms for general medical outpatients. A total mood-disturbance score may be obtained by summing scores on the six primary mood factors, with vigor weighted negatively.

In summary, the POMS has been used less in studies of functional GI disorders than some other measures. It is not as yet well validated on outpatient populations and therefore has limited usefulness in medical settings. It can provide potentially useful information about mood states that may need to be considered as part of treatment, but results must be interpreted cautiously. It is quite brief and easy to administer and score.

C. Measures of Depression

Zung Self-Rating Depression Scale

The Zung Depression Scale was published in 1964 in response to a need for a scale that could assess depression simply and specifically as a psychiatric disorder (18,86). Lengthy scales are particularly difficult for depressed patients. The Zung Scale is inclusive with respect to symptoms of depression. It is short and simple, gives a quantitative measure, and is self-administered by the patient. It contains 20 items covering the symptoms of hopelessness, guilt, anxiety, isolation, psychomotor retardation, apathy, hypochondriasis, cognitive disturbances, agitation, clinging, and somatic disturbance. Each of the 20 items is answered on a four-point Likert Scale, with the four points being "a little of the time," "some of the time," "a good part of the time," and "most of the time." The score for the Zung Scale is derived by dividing the sum of the raw score values by the maximum possible score of 80, converting the result to a decimal, and multiplying by 100. The cutpoint for mild depression is 50–60; for moderate depression, 60–70; and for severe depression, 70 and over. Reliability studies indicate that the Zung correlates well with more time-consuming depression-rating scales.

Beck Depression Inventory (BDI)

The BDI is typically administered by a trained interviewer, but can also be self-administered by the patient. It is designed to measure the behavioral manifestations of depression (20). Originally published in 1960, it too was designed in an attempt to create a test that would identify depression specifically. Parenthetically, factor-analytic studies have revealed that the depression scale of the

MMPI contains, among a number of heterogeneous factors, only one that is consistent with the clinical concept of depression. The BDI consists of 21 categories of symptoms and attitudes, each describing a behavioral manifestation of depression, and each consisting of a graded series of four or five self-evaluative statements. These statements are ranked to reflect the range of severity of the symptom from neutral to maximum severity, and numerical scores of 1 to 3 assigned to each statement indicate the degree of severity. The 21 categories are mood, pessimism, sense of failure, lack of satisfaction, guilt feelings, sense of punishment, self-hate, self-accusations, self-punitive wishes, crying spells, irritability, social withdrawal, indecisiveness, poor body image, work inhibition, sleep disturbance, fatigability, loss of appetite, weight loss, somatic preoccupation, and loss of libido. To administer the test, the interviewer reads aloud each statement in the category and asks the patient to select the statement that seems to fit him or her best at the present time (if self-administered, the patient reads and selects). The cutting score is 17 for moderate and 26 for severe depression. In validity studies the BDI showed a highly significant relationship between the scores on the inventory and clinical ratings of depth of depression by experienced psychiatrists. Reliability and validity of the scale have been extensively documented. However, the BDI has been found to underrepresent somatic symptoms of depression.

A short form of the BDI is also available (87). It consists of only 13 questions, taking about 5 minutes for the patient to complete. It was designed for use in a busy medical practice, where most depressed patients are seen but unfortunately rarely detected. The authors used multiple-regression analysis to select items for the short form without loss of reliability and validity.

In summary, the BDI in both standard and short forms provides a standardized, consistent measure of depression. It is economical to use because an interviewer is easily and quickly trained in its use or it can be self-administered by the patient. The inventory provides a quantitative measure of depression and reflects changes in depth of depression over time, thus providing an objective measure for judging improvement resulting from various forms of treatment. However, it tends to underrate somatic symptoms; therefore, the clinician needs to interpret scores with caution in functional GI disorders.

Hamilton Rating Scale for Depression

The Hamilton Depression Scale, developed in 1960, was devised for use only on patients already diagnosed as suffering from depression (14,88). It contains 17 items, which are rated on a five-point scale (from "absent" to "severe"). Four separate items are included (diurnal variation, derealization, paranoid symptoms, obsessional symptoms) in order to classify subtypes of depression; these are rated on a three-point scale (absent, slight or doubtful, clearly present). The rater considers both frequency and intensity when assigning a score for each item. The Hamilton Depression Scale is used to quantify depression and subtypes of depression. It requires a skilled interviewer and therefore has limited value for office use with general medical patients such as those with functional GI disorders.

Center for Epidemiologic Studies Depression Scale (CES-D)

The CES-D Scale was developed for use in studies of the epidemiology of depressive symptomatology in the general population (89). Its purpose differs from that of depression scales that have been used mainly for diagnosis at clinical intake and/or evaluation of severity of illness over the course of treatment. The CES-D scale was designed to measure current level of chronic depressed symptoms, but with an emphasis on mood itself. The CES-D is therefore not comprehensive regarding the spectrum of symptoms of depression. It is a short self-report scale consisting of 20 items to be answered by the respondent in terms of frequency of their occurrence during the past week. The four-point scale ranges from "rarely or none of the time" to "most or all of the time." The items of the scale are symptoms associated with depression that have been used in previously validated longer scales.

The CES-D was tested in household interview surveys and in psychiatric settings and was found to have high internal consistency and adequate test-retest reliability as well as validity, but no attempt has been made to validate it by comparing an individual's score with a psychiatrist's structured clinical rating of depression, as was done, for example, for the BDI. The CES-D is intended only for epidemiological research across population subgroups, not as a clinical diagnostic tool, and interpretations of individual scores should not be made. In its capacity as a tool for epidemiological studies, it is valuable for identifying high-risk groups and studying the relationships between depressive symptoms and other epidemiological variables.

D. Measures of Anxiety

Spielberger State-Trait Anxiety Inventory (STAI)

The STAI, a self-report measure first published in 1970, differentiates anxiety in terms of two very different constructs: one is an unpleasant emotional state, the other is a way of describing relatively stable individual differences in anxiety-proneness as a personality trait (23). An anxiety *state* is characterized by feelings of apprehension, nervousness, and worry, with associated arousal of the autonomic nervous system. *Trait* anxiety is considered the tendency to perceive stressful situations as dangerous or threatening and to respond with increases in state-anxiety reactions. Trait anxiety may also reflect frequency and intensity of anxiety states in an individual, and his or her probability of experiencing them in the future.

The STAI has been used extensively in research and clinically. It contains separate self-report scales for state and trait anxiety, each containing 20 statements that patients rate on a four-point scale. The S-anxiety scale asks how respondents feel "right now" and the T-anxiety scale asks how they feel "generally." The X form of the STAI is the original one; a revised version (the Y form) was published in 1980. Referred to with patients as the Self-Evaluation Questionnaire so as not to bias results, it takes 10 to 15 minutes to complete. Template keys for hand-scoring as well as machine-scoring answer sheets are available.

Scores for both the S- and the T-anxiety scales can vary from a minimum of 20 to a maximum of 80. There are procedures for dealing with unanswered questions. Normative data for form Y are available in the manual for working adults, college students, high-school students, and military recruits, and for form X for male neuropsychiatric patients, general medical and surgical patients, and young prisoners.

Taylor Manifest Anxiety Scale

This longer self-report measure of chronic anxiety states contains 50 items derived from the anxiety scales of the MMPI, together with items from the L, F, and K validity scales of the MMPI and "buffer" items not indicative of anxiety, for a total of 225 items (75). It has the MMPI format of true–false questions. It was originally devised for screening research subjects.

Sheehan Clinician Rated Anxiety Scale (SCRAS) and Sheehan Patient Rated Anxiety Scale (SPRAS)

These scales were designed to provide an overview measure of the severity of anxiety symptoms in panic disorder and phobic disorder (90,91). They are both 35-item scales that elicit the individual symptoms that occur during or as a direct complication of unexpected anxiety attacks or limited symptom attacks. They also reflect improvement in the overall condition and response to treatment.

Part 1 of the SPRAS is a panic-disorder scale; part 2 is an 11-item scale that elicits anxiety symptoms that occur in response to danger, stress, or phobic stimuli. Both scales cover 18 physical symptoms, including chest pain, nausea or other stomach problems, and attacks of diarrhea; eight psychological symptoms, such as fear of dying, anxiety, nervousness, and restlessness; and five behavioral symptoms, such as avoiding situations because they are frightening. In assigning a score to the distress level of each symptom on the SCRAS, the clinician considers the frequency of the symptoms, the severity of the symptom when it occurs, and a description of the last significant occurrences. Symptoms are rated on a five-point scale, from "absent—not at all" (which is 0) to "very severe—extremely" (which is scored 4). Scores above 30 are considered abnormal and scores above 80 are considered severe. Validation studies of this scale are still in progress, the scale being used in several panic disorder multicenter trials.

E. Scales to Measure Obsessive-Compulsive Tendencies

The Leyton Obsessional Inventory (LOI)

The LOI is the most widely used self-rating scale. First published by Cooper in 1970 (92), the 69-question inventory assesses obsessional symptoms and traits. The original form was a card-sorting procedure; paper and pencil forms were developed later (93). It addresses a wide range of obsessive-compulsive symptoms; however, it does not cover unacceptable ideations such as aggression, violence, and blasphemous thoughts. It makes some attempt to assess resistance and subjective distress from obsessional symptoms. Validity and reliability studies are incomplete and inconsistent.

The Maudsley Obsessive-Compulsive Inventory (MOCI)

This is a 30-item true-false self-rated questionnaire that was developed to investigate different types of obsessive-compulsive complaints in patients who had observable rituals (94). It was devised as a research tool to typologize obsessional patients who had already been diagnosed. Reliability and validity studies have been more extensive. One disadvantage of the MOCI is that aggressive and hoarding themes are insufficiently represented whereas checking and cleaning themes are overrepresented. Also, it has no measures that assess the degree of distress or interference of obsessions and compulsions with a patient's daily life.

The Yale-Brown Obsessive-Compulsive Scale (Y-BOCS)

The original version of the Y-BOCS was published in 1986 and the revised version in 1989. This rating scale is designed to rate the severity and type of symptoms in patients with obsessive-compulsive disorder (95,96). The scale is a semistructured interview filled out by the interviewer. The scale contains items that cover aggressive obsessions, contamination obsessions, sexual obsessions, hoarding, saving obsessions, religious obsessions, obsessions with the need for symmetry or exactness, somatic obsessions, cleaning and washing compulsions, checking compulsions, repeating rituals, counting compulsions, ordering and arranging compulsions, hoarding and collecting compulsions, and other obsessions and compulsions.

Another section of the scale asks about the amount of time occupied by obsessive thoughts, obsession-free intervals, how much obsessive thoughts interfere with functioning, how much distress is associated with obsessive thoughts, how much resistance there is against the obsessive thoughts, and how much control the person feels he or she has over obsessive thoughts. The same set of questions is also applied to compulsive behaviors.

Finally, there is a section regarding problems related to obsessions and compulsions, with questions about how much insight into obsessions and compulsions is present, how much avoidance of situations or persons takes place because of them, the degree of indecisiveness, whether there is an over-valued sense of responsibility, whether there is pervasive slowness or inertia, and whether there is pathological doubting. These last two sections are scored on a five-point scale with 0 being none and 4 being extreme. There is a global severity score with 0 equal to "no illness" at one end and 6 to "extremely severe symptoms, completely nonfunctional" at the other end of the spectrum. There is also a place for the interviewer to rate the reliability of the rating scores.

The patient must be provided with readily understood definitions of obsessions and compulsions before the scale is administered. Then the interviewer helps the patient enumerate his or her obsessions and compulsions, list them on the Y-BOCS target-symptom list, determine whether they are bona fide OCD symptoms rather than symptoms of another disorder, and target avoidance behaviors.

In summary, the Y-BOCS is probably the most accurate scale for assessing the range of OCD symptoms and behaviors, and the most sensitive to treatment-induced changes; however, it requires a trained interviewer to administer and interpret it. It has excellent reliability and validity, and good normative data.

A Brief Screening Questionnaire for OCD

This brief screening instrument requires 2 to 5 minutes to complete. It consists of 10 questions to be answered yes or no and can provide a rapid means of detecting whether OCD might be present (97). If present, then a more comprehensive scale such as the Yale-Brown Scale would be indicated.

F. Life Events Scales

A number of questionnaires are available that assess the presence of significant life events. The life events covered are more or less the same for all the commonly used questionnaires and cover such items as death of a family member, major changes in financial status, pregnancy, divorce, sexual difficulties, and retirement.

Holmes and Rahe Schedule of Recent Experiences (SRE)

One of the first life events scales was the SRE, developed in 1967 by Holmes and Rahe (24). It is a self-administered questionnaire containing a list of 43 events. Patients check the events they have experienced in the previous 6 months or 1 year. In creating the questionnaire, each item was "constructed to contain a life event whose advent is either indicative of, or requires a significant change in the ongoing life pattern of the individual" (98). Each broad type of event was given a simple definition and a weighting in terms of its propensity to cause change and disruption. The item *marriage* was used as an anchor and given a score of 500. In this scale the impact of a particular event is assumed to be comparable for all people affected. Another assumption, also later questioned in the literature, is that life changes per se are stressful regardless of their desirability; thus, both positive and negative events re combined in producing a total life-stress score in the SRE. An advantage of the Holmes and Rahe Scale, however, is that it is relatively brief and easy for a patient to fill out. If a physician is mainly interested in qualitative information (e.g., what life events have occurred recently for a particular patient), this would be a useful scale.

Life Experiences Survey (LES)

In an attempt to create an improved questionnaire to measure life changes, Sarason and colleagues (46) created the Life Experiences Survey, a 57-item self-report inventory. Section 1, for all respondents, contains 47 events plus three blank spaces where respondents can add significant events not already covered. Section 2 contains events applicable primarily to students. Many items are similar to items on the SRE, but were made more specific. This questionnaire also asks respondents to rate for each item the positive or negative impact of the event, on a seven-point scale (-3 to +3). Positive and negative change scores are summed separately, and the two can be added together if a total change score is desired. Like the SRE, it asks whether each event happened within the previous 6 months or from 7 months to 1 year previously. Thus, the LES allows for individualized rating of the impact of life events, plus the separate measures of positive and negative change. It requires more time to fill out than the SRE, as patients must decide on a weight for each event; however, it will supply more complete information regarding life events.

Life Events and Difficulties Schedule (LEDS)

A third questionnaire in this area is the LEDS (53). It attempts to avoid distortion due to the patient's mental state by making it interviewer-administered. The interviewer goes through a list of 40 events, giving examples and asking probing questions. Unlike the other two life events scales, it covers ongoing difficulties as well as discrete events. If an event has occurred, further questions are asked regarding nature, severity, and other characteristics to obtain a stress score. As with other interviewer-administered questionnaires, this one requires the presence of an experienced professional for proper use. Its advantage is the relative absence of bias or distortion by the patient.

The question for the physician is the extent to which life events are related to this particular person, at this particular time. So, in addition to life events, information about personality attributes, coping resources, and social support is necessary.

G. Illness Behavior

Illness behavior is a psychological construct designed to reflect variations in psychosocial response to one's state of health.

Illness Behavior Questionnaire (IBQ)

Designed to quantitate abnormal illness behavior, the IBQ was introduced by Pilowsky in 1967 and revised by him in 1983 (47). It consists of 62 items, from which are derived seven scale scores: 1) General Hypochondriasis is characterized by anxious or phobic preoccupation with the possibility of disease; 2) Disease Conviction is characterized by belief in the presence of serious pathology and rejection of reassurances by physicians; 3) Perception of Illness is characterized by items contrasting attribution of illness to either psychological or physical causes, 4) Affective Inhibition is characterized by difficulties in expressing personal feelings, 5) Affective Disturbance is characterized by feelings of anxiety or sadness not attributed to the illness; 6) Denial is characterized by reports of the absence of problems in the patient's life; and 7) Irritability is characterized by hostile reactions, anger, and interpersonal friction.

There is some question as to whether this questionnaire really discriminates normal from abnormal illness behavior, as there is evidence that high scores also occur in patients with clear organic illness when they are distressed by their bodily condition or functioning, or when their lives are disrupted by their illnesses. Therefore, this questionnaire is not recommended, except to assess the degree to which the latter is the case in a particular patient. It might better be called the Illness Impact Scale.

Millon Behavioral Health Inventory (MBHI)

A test that has contributed much to assessment of the psychological concomitants of medical illness is the MBHI. It was developed specifically with physically ill patients and medical-psychosocial issues of treatment in mind (83). It is designed to aid in the psychological understanding of medically ill patients to help the clinician to formulate a comprehensive treatment plan. It can provide information regarding a patient's probable manner of relating to health care personnel, life stressors, attitudes, and possible psychosomatic complications. The inventory is a 150-item self-report questionnaire requiring about 20 minutes to complete. It can be taken by patients 21 years or older with at least eighth-grade-level reading skills.

Four sets of scales make up the MBHI. The Basic Coping Styles Scales assess basic personality or character styles that will influence the way the patient will likely relate to health care personnel. The Psychogenic Attitudes Scales represent the feelings and perceptions of the patint regarding psychological stress, which can increase psychosomatic susceptibility or aggravate the course of a disease. The Psychosomatic Correlates Scales are used only with patients who have previously been medically diagnosed with certain disease syndromes (e.g., gastrointestinal susceptibility). Finally, the Prognostic Indices Scales are aimed at identifying future treatment problems or difficulties (a patient whose illness or treatment could be atypically complicated or unsatisfactory). See Table 2 for a listing of scales in each category.

Computer scoring is recommended, as differential item-weighting and scale overlap complicates scoring by hand. When MBHI sheets are sent for computer scoring, a printed profile is included as part of the interpretative report. The interpretative report provides clinicians with a theoretically and empirically based assessment drawn from an integration of the patient's style of coping, areas of concern, and probable response to treatment. An electronic teleprocessing system is also available to expedite the machine scoring process. Raw scores are transformed into base rate scores rather than to standard scores. Base rate scores utilize estimated class prevalence data. Cutpoints of 75–84 describe "moderate" and 85 or above describe "severe" in each of the subscales of the MBHI. The cutpoints on the psychosomatic correlate scales of the MBHI are based on base rate scores of designated populations. For example, a base rate score of 85 or higher on scale QQ, which is life-threat reactivity, represents a cutpoint above which 11% of a group of patients who have been given diagnosis of illness with

TABLE 2 MBHI Scales

Basic Coping Styles	Psychosomatic Correlates Scales
Scale 1: Introversive style	Scale MM: Allergic inclination
Scale 2: Inhibited style	Scale: NN: Gastrointestinal susceptibility
Scale 3: Cooperative style	Scale OO: Cardiovascular tendency
Scale 4: Sociable style	Prognostic Indices Scales
Scale 5: Confident style	Scale PP: Pain treatment responsivity
Scale 6: Forceful style	Scale QQ: Life threat reactivity
Scale 7: Respectful style	Scale RR: Emotional vulnerability
Scale 8: Sensitive style	
Psychogenic Attitudes Scales	
Scale A: Chronic tension	
Scale B: Recent stress	
Scale C: Premorbid pessimism	
Scale D: Future despair	
Scale E: Social alienation	
Scale F: Somatic anxiety	

potential life-threatening consequences should score. They have no significance for patients who do not fall into this category.

Interpretation of the MBHI is complex enough that special training is necessary if it is to be done in the office. For this reason, clinicians may choose to utilize the automated computer interpretations that are part of the MBHI report. If this automated interpretive report is used, the MBHI authors recommend that the clinician set this information in the context of relevant patient biographical and demographic data. The major limitation of an automated report such as this is that interpretive stereotypes result in a lack of report individualization. This should be taken into account in their use by the clinician. Also, this measure does not provide a diagnosis.

Psychosocial Adjustment to Illness Scale (PAIS)

The PAIS is a relatively new measure, first published in 1985 (99). There is both an interviewer-rated format, which the authors feel is more flexible, and a self-report format. The self-report form contains 46 questions, each with four possible answers from which the patient must choose the one that is most accurate for him or her. There are five to eight questions in each of seven sections: 1) attitude about taking care of health, 2) impact of illness on work life, 3) overview of impact of illness on various aspects of the patient's life, 4) impact on sexual activities, 5) impact on family relationships, 6) impact on leisure activities, and 7) associated psychological symptomatology. Reliability and validity studies to date are promising, and the PAIS has been normed using a number of illness groups (lung cancer, renal dialysis, essential hypertension, acute-burn groups) and for a heterogeneous cancer group and a cardiac-bypass group in the case of the self-report version. Until norms are obtained for patients with functional GI disorders, scores obtained from the use of the PAIS with such patients must be interpreted with caution. The advantage of this scale over the MBHI is its brevity and simpler scoring; however, as noted, it lacks normative data for functional-GI-disorder patients and cannot provide as rich a psychosocial profile as the MBHI.

H. Ego-Strength Scales

The Barron Ego-Strength Scale

The Barron Scale was first published in 1953. It was developed as a construct to predict the response of psychoneurotic patients to psychotherapy, but has since been used in somewhat broader applications (100). It is useful as an assessment device in any situation in which some estimate of adaptability or personal resourcefulness is needed, and it appears to measure the aspects of effective personal functioning that are usually considered under the term ego strength. This scale consists of 68 items from the MMPI selected on the basis of significant correlation with rated improvement in psychoneurotic patients who had been treated for 6 months in psychotherapy. It has adequate validation and reliability. Among the characteristics that are collectively referred to as ego strength in this scale are psysiological stability and good health, a strong sense of reality, feelings of personal adequacy and vitality, permissive morality, lack of ethnic prejudice, emotional outgoingness and spontaneity, and intelligence. The disadvantage of this scale is that physical illness by itself can affect a number of these characteristics.

The Martin-Jacobs Scale of Ego Strength and Ego Weakness

According to Jacobs and colleagues (60), ego strength is defined by capacities to 1) delay discharge of impulse without sacrificing spontaneity, 2) form and sustain interpersonal relationships, 3) function assertively and independently, 4) tolerate affect and frustration, and 5) perceive oneself as esteem-worthy. Jacobs developed this ego-strength scale because he felt that the scales already in use did not relate to what is generally agreed to be ego strength. He felt the Barron scale lacked conceptual relevance to the construct of ego strength. The Jacobs is a self-report scale consisting of 50 items representing 10 aspects of ego strength: obsessiveness, impulsiveness, intrusiveness, isolation, defiance, submissiveness, guardedness, vulnerability, grandiosity, and worthlessness. Each item is rated by the respondent on a five-point scale from "most of the time" to "never." This scale, like the Barron scale, was designed to measure personality changes as a result of psychotherapy, and secondarily to provide a characterological profile of pathology and coping mechanisms. This scale has been subjected to adequate reliability and validity studies.

The cutpoint for the Ego Weakness Scale is 70. A score of 70 or greater is indication of psychopathology; a score below this is associated with mental health and adequate functioning. The cutpoint for the Ego Strength Scale is 25. Those scoring above 25 are considered to have adequate ego strength and those below 25 have significant problems with ego strength. Adequate validation and reliability studies have been performed for this scale, which is useful in delineating those patients with psychopathology as part of the clinical picture who would do well in psychotherapy versus those who would be better treated with medication alone.

I. Miscellaneous Scales

Alexithymia Scale

There is some evidence that patients who suffer from psychosomatic or functional disorders have a relative constriction of their emotional functioning, little in the way of fantasy life, and a relative inability to put their emotions into words. This has been termed *alexithymia* (67). Alexithymia may reflect such difficulty in the use of a psychological idiom of distress in which individuals are compelled to articulate their suffering in exclusively somatic terms.

To assess this construct in patients, Sifneos in 1973 (67) developed the Alexithymia Scale, a 17-item interviewer rating scale containing eight questions aimed at alexithymic characteristics: Does the patient 1) describe endless details rather than feelings? 2) use appropriate words to describe emotion? 3) have a rich fantasy life? 4) use action to express emotion? 5) use action to avoid conflicts? 6) tend to describe circumstances surrounding an event rather than feelings? 7) have difficulty communicating? 8) Is the thought content more concerned with external events than with fantasy or emotion?

This scale is felt to be useful for identifying patients for whom the usual dynamic insight-oriented psychotherapy would not be suitable, and who would do better with psychiatric treatments such as supportive therapy, behavior therapy, or hypnosis. Alexithymia is a useful construct for the clinician to keep in mind when interviewing patients about their symptoms and the impact of their disorder on their lives. Its disadvantages are the need for a trained interviewer to complete the scale and the scale's relative lack of validation in the research literature.

Toronto Alexithymia Scale (TAS)

The TAS, developed by Taylor in 1984 (101), is another self-report measure of alexithymia that canvases all the theoretically positive dimensions of alexithymia. There are good validity and reliability studies on this measure and samples of primary-care patients. The 26-item questionnaire focuses on four components of alexithymia: 1) difficulty identifying feelings and bodily sensations (for example, "I am often puzzled by sensations in my body" or "I have feelings that I can't quite identify"), 2) externally oriented thinking ("I prefer to analyze problems rather than just describe them"), 3) difficulty expressing feelings ("people tell me to describe my feelings more"), 4) reduced daydreaming ("I daydream rarely").

Despite the good reliability and validity studies on the TAS, some critics (102) point out how different the various factors subsumed under alexithymia are. They point to studies that show different correlations between sociodemographic and illness cognition variables and these various factors, and note that they may reflect other personality variables, such as neuroticism, introversion, and openness to experience as measured on the Eysenck Personality Questionnaire. They also point out that there are reasons other than alexithymia for patients' tendency to amplify somatic distress.

Rotter Internal-External Locus of Control Scale

A good deal of research literature supports the notion that the perception that control over one's life lies outside oneself is associated with a greater likelihood of developing stress-related physical ailments and psychopathology. If a person perceives an event as the result of luck, chance, or fate, or as being under the control of powerful others or unpredictable because of the great complexity of the forces surrounding him or her, this is labeled as a belief in external control. If a person perceives that the event is contingent on his or her own behavior or his or her own relatively permanent characteristics, this belief is termed internal control (103).

The Locus of Control Scale (34) was developed to measure the degree to which a person perceives one has control over one's life versus perceiving control as lying somewhere outside oneself. It is a forced-choice, 29-item scale that includes six filler items. For each item, one sentence depicts a belief in external control and one a belief in internal control regarding an event or circumstance. The respondents are asked to choose one or the other item. Adequate reliability and validity studies have been done on the Rotter Scale. Studies have shown that an individual who scores high on internal control is likely to 1) be more alert to those aspects of the environment that provide useful information for steps to take to improve his or her environmental condition, 2) place greater value on skill or achievement, and be generally more concerned with ability, and 3) be resistant to subtle attempts to influence him or her. The Rotter Scale is scored such that the total score is the total number of external choices, so that the higher the score, the greater the person's belief in external control.

J. British Questionnaires

A number of studies of functional GI disorders appearing in British medical and psychiatric journals have used questionnaires developed in England. They are included here to provide the reader with information for comparison with studies using American measures.

General Health Questionnaire

This is a self-administered screening questionnaire designed for use in outpatient settings and aimed at detecting patients with a diagnosable psychiatric disorder (16). It focuses on two major kinds of phenomena: the inability to carry out once normal "healthy" functions and the appearance of new phenomena of a distressing nature. It focuses on symptoms that the authors felt best differentiate psychiatric patients as a general class from those who consider themselves well. The 28 items all start with "Have you recently . . ." Each is rated on a four-point rating scale, ranging from "better than usual" to "much worse than usual." A global score indicates the likelihood of some psychiatric disorder being present, and six factors within the questionnaire provide information on how a patient scores in several diagnostic categories: severity of illness, psychic versus somatic depression, social dysfunction, suicidal depression, sleep disturbance, and head pains. The cutpoint score for defining a patient as having a diagnosable psychiatric disorder is 5 or above. The subscale division is recommended more for research, but it does given an indication of which category of psychiatric illness the patient may suffer from primarily.

Crown-Crisp Experiential Index (CCEI)

This instrument, formerly known as the Middlesex Hospital Questionnaire, was designed in 1966 by Crown and Crisp to provide a means of rapidly quantifying a broad range of common symptoms and traits relevant to diagnostic categories of psychoneurotic illness (10). The 48-item self-report inventory, which requires 5 to 10 minutes to complete, asks patients a series of questions about how they feel and act. Some require a yes-or-no response; some have a three-point graded response, with the most psychopathological answer having the greatest score. The inventory contains five subscales: free-floating anxiety, phobic, somatic, depressive, hysteric, and obsessive scales. Some studies have questioned the discriminate validity of the scales of the CCEI.

Hospital Anxiety and Depression (HAD) Questionnaire

The HAD is a more recent and more restricted self-report questionnaire that measures only anxiety and depression, the scores on the two subscales also validly measuring severity of these two emotional disorders (72). It was designed to help physicians in busy nonpsychiatric hospital practices to sort out whether these two most prevalent emotional disorders are complicating the clinical picture. It is brief, so it can easily be filled out while a patient is waiting to see the physician. There are eight items on each subscale. To lessen the effect of physical illness on scores, items relating to physical symptoms are excluded; the items in the HAD are based solely on psychic symptoms associated with depression and anxiety. A score of 8–10 on a subscale indicates marginal symptom levels; a score of 11 or greater indicates definite psychopathology in that area.

Delusions-Symptoms-States Inventory

This is a self-report inventory intended to measure a range of psychiatric syndromes in psychiatric patients. First published in 1975 by Foulds and Bedford (26), it consists of 84 items in 12 sets of seven items each. The 12 sets of items are categorized into four classes: dysthymic states (anxiety, depression, hypomania), neurotic symptoms (conversion, dissociative, phobic, obsessive, compulsive), integrated delusions (paranoid disorder, mania, psychotic depression), and nonintegrated delusions (psychosis).

TABLE 3 Characteristics of Personality Tests Used in Functional GI Disorder Research

	Skill req. for interp.?	Self-report?	Copy-righted?	How scored	Admin. time	Comments
MMPI	Yes	Yes	Yes	Computer	1–2 hr	Thorough but very long and requires professional interpretation
EPI	No	Yes	Yes	Hand or service	10 min	Measures only two personality dimensions
NEO-R	No	Yes	Yes	Hand	40 min	Measures five personality dimensions
MCMI-III	Yes	Yes	Yes	Computer	30 min	Aligned with DSM-IV, focus is on medically healthy

TABLE 4 Characteristics of Illness Behavior Scales Used in Functional GI Disorder Research

	Skill req. for interp.?	Self-report?	Copy-righted?	How scored	Admin. time (min)	Comments
IBQ	No	Yes	No	Hand	10	May not discriminate normal from abnormal illness behavior
MBHI	Yes	Yes	Yes	Computer or teleprocessing	30	Thorough but automated reports are stereotyped
PAIS	No	Yes, and interviewer	Yes	Hand	20	Less comprehensive but good general psychosocial information

TABLE 5 Characteristics of Multiple Psychiatric Symptoms and Ego-Strength Scales Used in Functional GI Disorder Research

	Skill req. for interp.?	Self-report?	Copy-righted?	How scored	Admin. time (min)	Comments
Multiple psychiatric symptoms						
SCL-90	No	Yes	Yes	Hand or computer	15	Brief; provides reliable multi-dimensional psychological profile.
POMS	No	Yes	Yes	Hand	5	Currently no norms for medical outpatients
Ego strength						
Barron	Yes	Yes	No	Hand	20	Scale is affected by physical illness itself
Martin-Jacobs	No	Yes	No	Hand or machine	15	Measures both ego strength and ego weakness

Table 6 Characteristics of Depression and Anxiety Scales Used in Functional GI Disorder Research

	Skill req. for interp.?	Self-report	Copy-righted?	How scored	Admin. time (min)	Comments
Depression scales						
Zung	No	Yes	No	Hand	5	Excellent short scale
BDI	No	Yes, and interviewer	Yes	Hand	10-15	Underrepresents somatic symptoms
BDI (short)	No	Yes	Yes	Hand	5	Underrepresents somatic symptoms
Hamilton	Yes	No	No	Hand	10-20	For quantifying depression and discriminating subtypes
CES-D	No	Yes	No	Hand	5	Not intended as clinical diagnostic tool
Anxiety scales						
STAI	No	Yes	Yes	Hand or machine	10-15	Measures both situational and more enduring anxiety
Taylor Manifest Anxiety	No	Yes	No	Machine	30-40	Uses items from the MMPI, including validity scales
SCRAS	No	No	No	Hand	10	Specific for panic disorder
SPRAS	No	Yes	No	Hand	10	Specific for panic disorder

Table 7 Characteristics of Obsessive-Compulsive Symptom Scales Used in Functional GI Disorder Research

	Skill req. for interp.?	Self-report?	Copy-righted?	How scored	Admin. time (min)	Comments
LOI	No	Yes	Yes	Hand	20	Does not cover unacceptable ideation; has poor reliability studies
MOCI	No	Yes	Yes	Hand	10	Aggressive and hoarding underrepresented, checking and cleaning overrepresented
Y-BOCS	Yes	No	Yes	Hand	30	Most thorough; asks about insight, avoidance, indecisiveness
OCD Screen	No	Yes	Yes	Hand	3–5	Only for screening; if positive, follow with longer scale

Table 8 Characteristics of Miscellaneous Psychometric Tests Used in Functional GI Disorder Research

	Skill req. for interp.?	Self-report?	Copy-righted?	How scored	Admin. time (min)	Comments
Alexithymia						
Alexithymia Scale	Yes	No	Yes	Hand	20–30	Good screen for suitability for psychotherapy but little validation currently
TAS	No	Yes	Yes	Hand	10	Better validated; focuses on four components
Locus of control						
Rotter	No	Yes	Yes	Hand	10	Forced-choice format makes comparison to other patients problematic

TABLE 9 Characteristics of Life Events Scales Used in Functional GI Disorder Research

	Skill req. for interp.?	Self-report?	Copy righted?	How scored	Admin. time (min)	Comments
Holmes and Rahe (SRE)	No	Yes	Yes	Machine	10	Combines positive and negative events to compute score, scale rates impact of event
LES	No	Yes	No	Hand	20	Positive and negative scores are separate, patient rates impact
LEDS	Yes	No	No	Hand	30	Interviewer administration is attempt to avoid distortion by patient

TABLE 10 Characteristics of British Psychometric Tests Used in Functional GI Disorders Research

	Type of test	Skill req. for interp.?	Self report?	Copy righted?	How scored	Admin. time (min)	Comments
GHQ	Psychiatric symptoms	No	Yes	Yes	Hand	10	Outpatient setting; used to detect psychiatric disorder but not for specific diagnosis
CCEI	Psychiatric symptoms	No	Yes	Yes	Hand or machine	5–10	Discriminant validity has been questioned
HADQ	Anxiety and depression	No	No	No	Hand	5	Physical symptoms are excluded
DSSI	Psychiatric symptoms	Yes	No	No	Machine	20–30	Complicated hierarchical exclusion criteria for arriving at psychiatric diagnosis

APPENDIX: COMMERCIAL SOURCES

Beck Depression Inventory: The Psychological Corporation, 555 Academic Court, San Antonio, TX 78204-2498

Crown-Crisp Experiential Index: Hodder & Stoughton Educational, Hodder Headline PLC, 338 Euston Road, London NW1 3BH, England

Eysenck Personality Inventory: EdITS/Educational & Industrial Testing Service, P.O. Box 7234, San Diego, CA 92167

General Health Questionnaire: NFER-Nelso Publishing Company, Ltd., Darville House, 2 Oxford Road East, Windsor, Berkshire SL4 1DF, England

Holmes and Rahe Schedule of Recent Experiences: University of Washington Press, P.O. Box 50096, 4045 Brooklyn Avenue N.E., Seattle, WA 98145-5096

Millon Clinical Multiaxial Inventory III: NCS Assessments, P.O. Box 1416, Minneapolis, MN 55440

Minnesota Multiphasic Inventory-2: NCS Assessments, P.O. Box 1416, Minneapolis, MN 55440

NEO Personality Inventory: Psychological Assessment Resources, Inc., P.O. Box 998, Odessa, FL 33556-0998

PAIS: Clinical Psychometric Research, Inc., P.O. Box 619, Riderwood, MD 21139

Profile of Mood States: Renesis Likert Associates Inc., Suite 401, Wolverine Tower, 3001 S.E. State Street, Ann Arbor, MI 48104-7352

SCL-90: NCS Assessments, P.O. Box 1416, Minneapolis, MN 55440

Spielberger State-Trait Anxiety Inventory: Consulting Psychologists Press, Inc., 3803 E. Bayshore Road, Box 10096, Palo Alto, CA 94303

REFERENCES

1. Almy TP, Tulin M. Alterations in colonic function in man under stress: experimental production of changes simulating "the irritable colon." Gastroenterology 1957; 8:616–626.
2. Chaudhary N, Truelove SC. The irritable colon syndrome. Q J Med New Series XXXI 1962; 123:307–322.
3. Hislop IG. Psychological significance of the irritable colon syndrome. Gut 1971; 12:452–457.
4. Liss J, Alpers D, Woodruff R. The irritable colon syndrome and psychiatric illness. Dis Nerv System 1973; 34:151–157.
5. Young S, Alpers D, Norland C, Woodruff R. Psychiatric illness and the irritable bowel syndrome: practical implications for the primary physician. Gastroenterology 1976; 70:162–166.
6. Feighner JP, Robins E, Guze SB, et al. Diagnostic criteria for use in psychiatric research. Arch Gen Psychiatry 1972; 26:57–63.
7. Hill O, Blendis L. Physical and psychological evaluation of "non-organic" abdominal pain. Gut 1967; 8:221–229.
8. Eysenck HJ, Eysenck S. Eysenck personality inventory. Educational and Industrial Testing Service, 1963.

9. Palmer RL, Crisp AH, Stonehill E, Waller S, Misiewicz JJ. Psychological characteristics of patients with the irritable bowel syndrome. Postgrad Med J 1974; 50:416–419.
10. Crown S, Crisp AH. A short clinical diagnostic self-rating scale for psychoneurotic patients, the Middlesex Hospital questionnaire (M.H.Q.). Br J Psychiatry 1966; 112:917–923.
11. Welgan P, Meshkinpour H, Beeler M. Effect of anger on colon motor and myoelectric activity in irritable bowel syndrome. Gastroenterology 1988; 94:1150–1156.
12. Hathaway SR, McKinley JC. Minnesota Multiphasic Personality Inventory-2, Manual for Administration and Scoring. Minneapolis, MN: University of Minnesota Press, 1989.
13. Gomez J, Dally P. Psychologically mediated abdominal pain in surgical and medical outpatient clinics. Br Med J 1977; 1:1451–1453.
14. Hamilton M. A rating scale for depression. J Neurol 1960; 23:4–62.
15. MacDonald A, Bouchier I. Non-organic gastrointestinal illness: a medical and psychiatric study. Br J Psychiatry 1980; 13:276–283.
16. Goldberg DP, Hillier VF. A scaled version of the General Health Questionnaire. Psychol Med 1979; 9:139–145.
17. Welch GW, Stace NH, Pomare EW. Specificity of psychological profiles of irritable bowel syndrome patients. Aust NZ J Med 1984; 14:101–104.
18. Zung WWK. A self-rating depression scale. Arch Gen Psychiatr 1965; 12:63–70.
19. Rose JDR, Throughton AH, Harvey JS, Smith PM. Depression and functional bowel disorders in gastrointestinal outpatients. Gut 1986; 27:1025–1028.
20. Beck AT, Ward CH, Mendelson M, Mock J, Erbaugh J. An inventory for measuring depression. Arch Gen Psychiatry 1960; 4:561–571.
21. Kumar D, Pfeffer J, Wingate DL. Role of psychological factors in the irritable bowel syndrome. Digestion 1990; 45:80–87.
22. Schwarz SP, Blanchard EB, Berreman CF, Scharff L, Taylor AE, Greene BR, Suls JM, Malamood HS. Psychological aspects of irritable bowel syndrome: comparisons with inflammatory bowel disease and nonpatient controls. Behav Res Ther 1993; 31(3):297–304.
23. STAI: Self-rating questionnaire, item booklet (form HS). Psychological Assessment Resources 1979, 1986, 1988.
24. Holmes TH, Rahe RH. The Social Readjustment Rating Scale. J Psychosom Res 1967; 11:213–218.
25. Fowlie S, Eastwood MA, Prescott R. Irritable bowel syndrome: assessment of psychological disturbance and its influence on the response to fiber supplementation. J Psychosom Res 1992; 36(2):175–180.
26. Bedford A, Foulds GA. Validation of the Delusions-Symptoms States Inventory. Br J Med Psychol 1977; 50:163–171.
27. Longstreth GF, Wolde-Tsadik G. Irritable bowel-type symptoms in HMO examinees: prevalence, demographics, and clinical correlates. Dig Dis Sci 1993; 38(9):1581–1589.
28. Helzer JE, Stillings WA, Chammas S, Norland CC, Alpers DH. A controlled study

of the association between ulcerative colitis and psychiatric diagnoses. Dig Dis Sci 1982; 27(6):513–518.

29. Bergeron CM, Monto GL. Personality patterns seen in irritable bowel syndrome patients. Am J Gastroenterol 1985; 80(6):448–451.
30. Heefner J, Wilder R, Wilson ID. Irritable colon and depression. Psychosomatics 1978; 19(9):540–547.
31. Lancaster-Smith MJ, Prout BJ, Pinto T, Anderson JA, Schiff AA. Influence of drug treatment on the irritable bowel syndrome and its interaction with psychoneurotic morbidity. Acta Psychiatr Scand 1982; 66:33–41.
32. Wise TN, Cooper JN, Ahmed S. The efficacy of group therapy for patients with irritable bowel syndrome. Psychosomatics 1982; 23(5):465–469.
33. Derogatis L, Rickels K, Rock A. The SCL-90 and the MMPI: a step in the validation of a new self-report scale. Br J Psychiatry 1976; 128:280–289.
34. Rotter J. Generalized expectancies for internal versus external control of reinforcement. Psychol Monographs: Gen Appl 1966; 80(1):1–10.
35. Whitehead W, Engel B, Schuster M. Irritable bowel syndrome: physiological and psychological differences between diarrhea-predominant and constipation-predominant patients. Dig Dis Sci 1980; 25(6):404–413.
36. Latimer P. Psychophysiologic disorders: a critical appraisal of concept and theory illustrated with reference to the irritable bowel syndrome. Psychol Med 1979; 9:71–80.
37. Latimer P, Sarna S, Campbell D, Latimer M, Waterfall W, Daniel EE. Colonic motor and myoelectrical activity: a comparative study of normal subjects, psychoneurotic patients, and patients with irritable bowel syndrome. Gastroenterology 1981; 80:893–901.
38. Campbell D, Shannon S, Collins S. Colonic motility and personality. Dig Dis Sci 1984; 29(6):554.
39. Kingham JGC, Dawson AM. Origin of chronic right upper quadrant pain. Gut 1985; 26:783–788.
40. Hamilton M. Development of a rating scale for primary depressive illness. Br J Soc Clin Psychol 1967; 6:278–296.
41. Whitehead WE, Holtkotter B, Enck P, Hoelzl R, Homes KD, Anthony J, Shagsin HS, Schuster MM. Tolerance for rectosigmoid distention in irritable bowel syndrome. Gastroenterology 1990; 98:1187–1192.
42. Cook IJ, VanEeden A, Collins SM. Patients with irritable syndrome have a greater pain tolerance than normal subjects. Gastroenterology 1987; 93:272–733.
43. Welch GW, Hillman LC, Pomare EW. Psychoneurotic symptomatology in the irritable bowel syndrome: a study of reporters and non-reporters. Br Med J 1985; 291:1328–1384.
44. Drossman DA, McKee DC, Sandler RS, Mitchell CM, Cramer EM, Lowman BC, Burger AL. Psychosocial factors in the irritable bowel syndrome: a multivariate study of patients and nonpatients with irritable bowel syndrome. Gastroenterology 1988; 95:701–708.
45. McNair DM, Lorr M, Doppleman LF. Profile of Mood States Instruction Manual. San Diego: Educational & Industrial Testing Service, 1971.

46. Sarason IG, Johnson JH, Siegel JM. Assessing the impact of life changes: development of the life experiences survey. J Consult Clin Psychol 1978; 45(5):932–946.
47. Pilowsky I, Spence ND. Manual for the Illness Behavior Questionnaire. 2nd ed. 1983. Available from the authors, Department of Psychiatry, Royal Adelaide Hospital, University of Adelaide, Adelaide, South Australia.
48. Greenbaum D, Abitz L, VanEgeren L, Mayle J, Greenbaum R. Irritable bowel symptom prevalence, rectosigmoid motility and psychometrics in symptomatic subjects not seeing physicians. Gastroenterology 1983; 84(5–2):1174.
49. Whitehead WE, Bosmajian L, Zonderman AB, Costa PT, Schuster NM. Symptoms of psychologica distress associated with irritable bowel syndrome. Gastroenterology 1988; 95:709–714.
50. McCrae R, Costa P. Joint factors in self-reports and ratings: neuroticism, extraversion and openness to experience. Person Individ Diff 1983; 4(3):245–255.
51. Craig TKJ, Brown CW. Life events, meaning and physical illness: a review. Health Care Hum Behav 1984; 7:39.
52. Craig TKJ, Brown GW. Goal frustration and life events in the aetiology of painful gastrointestinal disorder. J Psychosom Res 1984; 28(5):411–421.
53. Brown GW. Life events, psychiatric disorder, and physical illness. J Psychosom Res 1981; 25(5):461–473.
54. Blanchard EB, Radnitz, CL, Evans DD, Schwarz SP, Neff DF, Gerardi MA. Psychological comparisons of irritable bowel syndrome to chronic tension and migraine headache and nonpatient controls. Biofeedback Self-Reg 1986; 11(3):221–230.
55. Creed F, Guthrie E. Psychological factors in the irritable bowel syndrome. Gut 1987; 28:1307–1318.
56. Engle GL. Studies of ulcerative colitis. III. The nature of the psychologic processes. Am J Med 1955; 19:231–256.
57. Alexander F. Psychosomatic medicine: Its Principles and Applications. New York: WW Norton, 1950.
58. Olden KW. Inflammatory bowel disease: a biopsychosocial perspective. Psychiatr Ann 1992; 22:619–623.
59. McMahon AW, Schmitt P, Patterson JF, Rothman E. Personality differences between inflammatory bowel disease patients and their healthy siblings. Psychosom Med 1973; 35(2):91–103.
60. Jacobs M, Pugatch D, Spilken A. Ego strength and ego weakness, comparison of psychiatric patients and functioning normals. J Nerv Ment Dis 1968; 147(3):297–307.
61. West KL. MMPI correlates of ulcerative colitis. J Clin Psychol 1988; 26:214–219.
62. Helzer JE, Stillings WA, Chammas S, Norland CC, Alpers DH. A controlled study of the association between ulcerative colitis and psychiatric diagnoses. Dig Dis Sci 1982; 27(6):513–518.
63. Helzer JE, Chammas S, Norland CC, et al. A study of the association between Crohn's disesae and psychiatric illness. Gastroenterology 1984; 86:324–330.
64. Esler M, Goulston K. Levels of anxiety in colonic disorders. N Engl J Med 1973; 288(1):16–20.

65. Cattell RB, Scheier IH, Handbook for the IPAT Anxiety Scale Questionnaire. Champaign, IL: Institute for Personality & Ability Testing, 1963.
66. Fava GA, Pavan L. Large bowel disorders II: psychopathology and alexithymia. Psychother Psychosom 1976/77; 27:100–105.
67. Sifneos PE. The prevalence of "alexithymic" characteristics in psychosomatic patients. Psychother Psychosom 1973; 22:255–262.
68. Tucker D, Sandstead H, Logan G, Klevay L, Mahalko J, Johsonn L, Inman L, Englett G. Dietary fiber and personality factors as determinants of stool output. Gastroenterology 1981; 81:879–883.
69. Devroede G, Girard G, Bouchoucha M, Roy T, Black R, Camerlain M, Pinard G, Schang J, Arhan P. Idiopathic constipation by colonic dysfunction, relationship with personality and anxiety. Dig Dis Sci 1989; 34(9):1428–1433.
70. Wald A, Hinds J, Caruana B. Psychological and physiological characteristics of patients with severe idiopathic constipation. Gastroenterology 1989; 97:932–937.
71. Fisher SE, Breckon K, Andrews HA, Keighley MRB. Psychiatric screening for patients with faecal incontinence or chronic constipation referred for surgical treatment. Br J Surg 1989; 76:352–355.
72. Zigmond AS, Snaith RP. The hospital anxiety and depression scale. Acta Psychiatr Scand 1983; 67:361–370.
73. Whitehead WE, Burgio KL, Engel BT. Biofeedback treatment of fecal incontinence in geriatric patients. J Am Geriatr Soc 1985; 33:320–325.
74. Lehtinen V, Puhakka H. A psychosomatic approach to the globus hystericus syndrome. Acta Psychiatr Scand 1976; 53:21–28.
75. Taylor J. A personality scale of manifest anxiety. J Abnorm Soc Psychol 1953; 48(2):285–290.
76. Pratt LW, Tobin WH, Gallagher RA. Globus hystericus—office evaluation by psychological testing with the MMPI. Laryngological Office (Waterville, ME) 1976; 1540–1551.
77. Deary I, Wilson J, Mitchell L, Marshall T. Covert psychiatric disturbance in patients with globus pharyngis. Br J Med Psychol 1989; 62:381–389.
78. Moser G, Vacariu-Granser G, Schneider C, Abatzi T, Pokieser P, Stacher-Janotta G, Gaupmann G, Weber U, Wenzel T, Roden M, Stacher G. High incidence of esophageal motor disorders in consecutive patients with globus sensation. Gastroenterology 1991; 101:1512–1521.
79. Clouse R, Lustman P. Psychiatric illness and contraction abnormalities of the esophagus. N Engl J Med 1983; 30(22):1337–1342.
80. Clouse R, Lustman P. Value of recent psychological symptoms in identifying patients with esophageal contraction abnormalities. Psychosom Med 1989; 51:570–576.
81. Clouse R, McCord G, Lustman P, Edmundowicz S. Clinical correlates of abnormal sensitivity to intraesophageal balloon distension. Dig Dis Sci 1991; 36(8):1040–1045.
82. Richter J, Obrecht WF, Bradley L, Young L, Anderson K. Psychological comparison of patients with nutcracker eophagus and irritable bowel syndrome. Dig Dis Sci 1986; 31(2):131–138.

83. Millon T, Green C, Meagher R Jr. Millon Behavioral Health Inventory. Minneapolis: National Computer Systems, 1987.
84. Pulliam TJ, Bradley LA, Dalton CB, Salley AN, Richter JE. Role of psychological stress in gastroesophageal reflux disease (GERD). Gastroenterology 1989; 96:A401.
85. Millon T. Millon Clinical Multiaxial Inventory II. 2nd ed. Minneapolis: National Computer Systems, 1987.
86. Zung WWK. Factors influencing the Self-Rating Depression Scale. Arch Gen Psychiatry 1967; 16:543–547.
87. Beck AT, Beck RW. Screening depressed patients in family practice—a rapid technic. Postgrad Med Dec 1972; 81–85.
88. Hamilton M. Development of a rating scale for primary depressive illness. Br J Soc Clin Psychol 1967; 6:278–296.
89. Radloff L. The CES-D scale: a self-report depression scale for research in the general population. Applied Psychol Measurement 1977; 1(3):385–401.
90. Sheehan Clinician Rated Anxiety Scale. Copyright 1980, D. V. Sheehan.
91. Sheehan DV. Sheehan Patient Rated Anxiety Scale: The Anxiety Disease. New York: Charles Scribner & Sons, 1983:126–128.
92. Cooper J. The Leyton Obsessional Inventory. Psychol Med 1970; 1:48–64.
93. Snowdon J. A comparison of written and postbox forms of the Leyton Obsessional Inventory. Psychol Med 1980; 10:165–170.
94. Hodgson RJ, Rachman S. Obsessional-compulsive complaints. Behav Res 1977; 15:389–395.
95. Goodman WK, Price LA, Rasmussen LH, et al. The Yale-Brown Obsessive Compulsive Scale (Y-BOCS). Part I: Development, use and reliability. Arch Gen Psychiatry 1989; 46:1006–1011.
96. Goodman Wk, Price LA, Rasmussen LH, et al. The Yale-Brown Obsessive Compulsive Scale (Y-BOCS). Part II: Validity. Arch Gen Psychiatry 1989; 46:1012–1016.
97. Griest JH. Screening for OCD During Routine Mental Health Examinations. Ciba-Geigy, 1992.
98. Rahe RH. Life crisis and health changes. In: May PRA, Wittenbourn JR, eds. Psychotropic Drug Response: Advances in Prediction. Springfield, MO: CC Thomas, 1969.
99. Derogatis LR. The psychosocial adjustment to illness scale. J Psychosom Res 1986; 30(1):79–81.
100. Barron F. An ego-strength scale which predicts response to psychotherapy. J Consult Psychol 1953; 17(5):327–333.
101. Taylor GJ. Alexithymia: concept, measurement, and implications for treatment. Am J Psychiatry 1984; 141:725–732.
102. Kirmayer L, Robbins J. Cognitive and social correlates of the Toronto alexithymia scale. Psychosomatics 1993; 34(1):41–52.
103. Lefcourt HM. Locus of Control: Current Trends in Theory and Research. 2nd ed. London: Lawrence Erlbaum Associates, 1982.

6

Survey Research Methods in Functional GI Disorders

Sylvia S. Hom
St. Mary's Medical Center
San Francisco, California

I. INTRODUCTION

Survey research methods are used increasingly to study the functional gastrointestinal (GI) disorders. The nature and characteristics of these disorders make them especially amenable to study with survey research methodologies. First and foremost, the diagnosis of functional GI disorders is currently made based on symptom criteria, not by structural or biochemical abnormalities that can be empirically observed (1,2). Standardized criteria for diagnosing patients with specific functional GI disorders have recently been developed. One set of diagnostic criteria are referred to as the "Rome criteria," after the international working teams that developed them (3,4). In clinical research, the Rome criteria are now often used as a means of classifying patients. It is particularly important to ensure that patients entered into research studies be properly classified using common criteria. In the past, variable inclusion criteria made assessment of the accuracy of results difficult and prohibited comparability across investigators. While the Rome criteria have not been completely validated, they at least provide a common reference point for use in survey research in the functional GI disorders. Provisions for ongoing modification of the Rome diagnostic criteria make them a living document subject to continuous scrutiny and refinement.

Second, the biopsychosocial model employed to understand these disorders implies that GI symptoms are caused by a multitude of factors, incorporating biological, psychological, and sociocultural factors. It is important to recognize these interactions when studying the functional GI disorders. Survey questionnaires can be effectively used to delineate the impact of each of these dimensions in the development of a functional GI symptom. In research studies, questionnaires can be employed to identify a wide spectrum of both intestinal and extraintestinal symptoms, including psychological and demographic factors that are often difficult to assess by other methods.

II. DESIGN OF SURVEY RESEARCH

Epidemiological or *population surveys* are studies aimed at identifying the characteristics and illness experience of a specific population. Epidemiological surveys are conducted to determine the prevalence of functional GI disorders in large populations based on specific demographic characteristics (e.g., geography, age, and occupation). In addition to sociodemographic characteristics, the health-related attitudes and beliefs of patients with functional GI disorders and the impact of their illness experience can be established through surveys. This information gives valuable insight into how patients cope with their illness and their overall state of health. In addition to providing descriptive information about a population, surveys can be used to describe the relationship between the characteristics of a population and the specific disorder under study. In the functional GI disorders, GI symptoms have been associated with a number of sociodemographic factors, including female gender, younger age, and lower household income (1,2).

The two primary designs for epidemiological surveys are retrospective (case–control) or prospective (cohort). In a *retrospective*, or case–control, study, two groups of individuals are compared to identify the prevalence of a medical condition or disease and the factors associated with it. Both cases and controls are selected retrospectively—as of a given time that has already occurred. These two groups should be similar in all respects except for classification of the condition or disease, e.g., individuals diagnosed with irritable bowel syndrome and those who are not.

In a *prospective*, or cohort, study, a group of individuals representative of a specified population is selected based on sociodemographic characteristics, which frequently include geographical, occupational, or other criteria. The cohort is then studied prospectively over a period of time to determine the rates of occurrence (incidence) of the medical condition or disease. Characteristics of the members of the cohort who develop the condition are then compared to those who do not. These characteristics can then be evaluated as specific risk factors for developing the condition or disease. In summary, Table 1 illustrates the kinds of information sought through both prospective and retrospective surveys.

III. PREVALENCE OF FUNCTIONAL GI DISORDERS

Many earlier studies that sought to establish estimates of the prevalence of the functional GI disorders were limited in scope. These surveys incorporated samples that were often lacking in demographic range (5–7). Recently, however, investigators have striven to overcome sampling limitations to provide national estimates. Estimates of the national prevalence of a variety of functional GI disorders from a survey of U.S. households were recently established (1). The proportion of individuals having at least one functional symptom of any kind was extremely high (69%). The prevalence of specific disorders was also established, including functional abdominal bloating (32%), functional heartburn (29%), and irritable bowel syndrome (9%). In addition, important associations with sociodemographic and other factors, such as health-care seeking, were also identified. These findings were obtained from a sample of over 8000 households in the United States. Quotas based on geographic region and sociodemographic characteristics (age, gender, household size, and income) were established to ensure that the resulting sample was representative of the entire U.S. householder population.

A. Random Sampling

As the U.S. Householder Survey illustrates, it is important to ensure that appropriate sampling is undertaken in population surveys. Since the primary goal is to estimate the prevalence of a medical condition in a specified population, a representative sample of healthy individuals is imperative to make the proper infer-

TABLE 1 Uses of Survey Research

Information sought	Retrospective study (case-control)	Prospective study (cohort)
Prevalence of functional GI disorder	×	
Incidence of functional GI disorder		×
GI symptomatology	×	×
Extraintestinal symptomatology	×	×
Health-related attitudes and beliefs	×	×
Health-care-seeking behavior	×	×
Health-related quality of life	×	×
Sociodemographic characteristics	×	×

ence. To ensure the representation of the sample, a method of *random sampling* should be employed, in which each member of the specified population has an equal chance of being selected for the sample. A basic method of selecting a random sample is to number the individuals sequentially in a list and then select individuals based on their corresponding numbers from a random number table.

Systematic sampling, another method often used in population surveys, has been found to be as precise as random sampling (8). In a systematic sample, every *n*th (e.g., fifth) individual is chosen from a list ordered sequentially. The starting number is determined randomly. The major pitfall of systematic sampling is the existence of a bias that may be hidden from the investigator in the ordered list of individuals from which the sample will be drawn. For example, in a list of HMO members, every fifth individual may have been hospitalized in the last year. One way of checking for possible biases is to select several systematic samples using different starting points and then analyze the composition of the sample to rule out nonrandom selection.

B. Stratified Sampling

Care should also be taken to ensure that all identifiable subgoups within a population are sufficiently represented in the sample. *Stratified sampling* is employed when subgroups (or strata) can be identified, and sufficient numbers are needed to ensure representation within the sample. In population surveys, strata are often identified by geography or sociodemographic characteristics such as age, gender, ethnicity, and employment or educational status. Individuals within these strata are then randomly selected for the sample. If certain strata are known to be "underrepresented" in the sample, care should be taken to oversample members within these strata to ensure that proper inferences can be made from them (often call *quota sampling*).

IV. IRRITABLE BOWEL SYNDROME

In the investigation of irritable bowel syndrome (IBS), the development of standard diagnostic criteria was a key to improving research methodologies. Prior to development of standard criteria, problems of definition made it virtually impossible to assess the validity of results, especially in clinical treatment trials (9). It is crucial to ensure that individuals entered into research studies on IBS be classified using standard criteria. Moreover, consistency of diagnostic criteria enables comparability of research results across different study populations.

Standardizing the criteria also eliminated the use of loosely described terms for disturbed bowel patterns, such as functional "diarrhea" and "constipation," that were not subject to consistent definition in the past. Both terms are commonly used by health practitioners and patients alike, but they may have different meanings depending on who is using them (10). Instead of employing such ambiguous terms, the Rome diagnostic criteria describe patterns of bowel symptoms that are actually being experienced, e.g., the sensation of incomplete evacuation and the actual frequency or infrequency of stools. The prevalence of IBS is often estimated in populations whose members were classified using variable diagnostic criteria. It is difficult to assess the accuracy of these estimates if the questions used to determine a diagnosis are vague or differ remarkably from one another. The Rome criteria have become a standard method of determining the diagnosis of IBS in research studies. Moreover, they are easily incorporated into survey questionnaires on IBS (4).

A population survey of HMO members who underwent routine health assessment to determine the prevalence of symptoms indicative of IBS demonstrated a number of important associations (11). The sample of HMO members was used to represent a population of healthy individuals from which prevalence estimates could be obtained. The primary method of data collection was a questionnaire that was self-administered to HMO members. The questionnaire elicited information on demographic characteristics, bowel-function symptoms, and extraintestinal complaints. Past health and social history was also obtained. Finally, two psychological tests for depression and anxiety were included to evaluate the prevalence of psychological symptoms in this population. In addition to describing the characteristics of HMO members with IBS, the survey findings revealed a number of clinical correlates to IBS. Several of these correlates were found to be independent markers for IBS (incontinence, laxative use, sexual abuse, and physician visits).

V. NON-ULCER DYSPEPSIA

Non-ulcer dyspepsia (NUD) is another functional GI disorder that has benefited from epidemiological investigation with survey research methodologies. However, like that of IBS, the study of NUD has been considerably hampered by the lack of consistent definition among investigators. This deficiency is due to fact that the diagnosis of NUD is currently made based on symptom criteria, and only after organic disease is ruled out. The Rome criteria have made the distinction of subdividing categories of functional dyspepsia by symptom location and pattern (3,12,13). *Ulcer-like dyspepsia* refers to the presence of epigastric pain associated with characteristics suggestive of classic ulcer complaints. *Dysmotility-like dyspepsia* refers to symptoms suggestive of an underlying abnormality in motility, including symptoms of early satiety, postprandial fullness, nausea, vomiting, and bloating in the upper abdomen. Finally, *unspecified dyspepsia* includes all other symptoms that do not fall clearly into the other two categories. In studying

NUD, it is particularly important to distinguish among the individual symptoms that comprise the disorder and to apply a consistent description of these symptoms for both investigators and respondents alike (14).

A considerable symptom overlap with IBS also exists (13,15,16). Symptoms characterized as being compatible with IBS frequently appear in patients with NUD, and the opposite has also been found. While patients with IBS report disturbed bowel patterns, it has been documented that two-thirds of patients with dyspepsia without ulcer or other organic disease report a normal bowel habit (16). In research studies, it is this difference in bowel patterns that distinguishes patients as having IBS while those with unaltered bowel patterns are classified as having NUD.

The significant problem created by the lack of standard diagnostic criteria for NUD was illustrated in a recent prospective study undertaken to describe the symptoms and clinical features of the common causes of dyspepsia. A detailed questionnaire was used to elicit symptom information from a sample of mostly outpatients referred for dyspepsia over a 15-year period in Glasgow, Scotland. The investigators found that the certainty of diagnosis among physicians was much lower in the functional GI disorders, particularly IBS and functional dyspepsia, than in organic disease. In fact, the diagnosis of functional dyspepsia was made based on physicians' clinical opinion, and no attempt was made to apply a consensus definition (17).

Population studies of the prevalence of NUD have been difficult to obtain because of the necessity to rule out organic disease in respondents that report NUD symptoms. In the U.S. Householder Survey, the national prevalence of functional dyspepsia was estimated to be 2–3%, after self-reports of structural diagnoses were excluded (1,2). Moreover, most of the epidemiological surveys done in the past have yielded estimates of the prevalence of dyspepsia that range from 20 to 40% of the adult population in the United States and parts of Europe, including the United Kingdom, Denmark, Sweden, and Norway (13). The variation in prevalence rates has been attributed to the problem of inconsistent definition.

Research into the associations that may give clues to the etiology of NUD have focused on the role of psychological factors, including major life event stress and sociodemographic characteristics. The psychological distress associated with NUD does not appear to be one of etiology, but may affect a patient's coping style with the disorder; i.e., psychological distress may influence an individual's desire to seek health care for his or her symptoms (13). Few studies have evaluated relationships with sociodemographic characteristics. One study found no differences among study participants and controls in various measures of socioeconomic status and other factors, including family environment, structure, and migration (18).

VI. HOW TO USE SURVEY RESEARCH IN THE FUNCTIONAL GI DISORDERS

For the clinical investigator who desires to study the functional GI disorders, survey research can be an extremely useful tool. The relative ease and low cost of developing and conducting a survey give it advantages over other forms of investigation. Moreover, a survey can address the full range of behavioral, psychological, and sociocultural dimensions that are specific to the functional GI disorders.

The first step in designing a survey is to determine the exact purpose of the investigation. As described above, the kind of information that the investigator wishes to uncover should guide the investigator in selecting the appropriate research design. The information desired will identify the population and sampling method that will best elicit the anticipated results. For example, to estimate the incidence of a functional GI disorder in a community, a cohort study must be undertaken of a group of healthy individuals rather than patients admitted to a hospital. Obviously, a sample chosen from a list of hospital patients will overstate the incidence of the medical condition under study because, by definition, hospital patients are seeking care for their condition.

A. Constructing Questionnaires

The next vital step in designing a survey is the construction of the questionnaire, the primary tool for data collection. The items or measures that an investigator includes in a questionnaire must be valid. Validity ensures that proper conclusions can be drawn from these measurements. The validity of a questionnaire incorporates the following two concepts: whether an instrument actually assesses what it seeks to measure (*face validity*) and whether the instrument includes all the relevant areas or content under study (*content validity*). To yield valid information, the instrument must be well designed and tested with respondents before actual full-scale implementation.

To make this step easier, standard questionnaires that can be used for specific research purposes have been validated by a number of other investigators. An examination of the literature can identify the validated questionnaires that have been used effectively in a number of settings (see Table 2). One example is the bowel-symptom questionnaire developed by Talley et al. (19), which was used to study a population of healthy individuals to estimate the prevalence of specific functional GI disorders. Questions differentiate symptomatic from asymptomatic individuals and identify specific disorders, both functional and organic (including NUD, IBS, and organic GI disease).

If the investigator has constructed a unique questionnaire, validation can be accomplished in pilot studies. In a pilot study, the questionnaire is adminis-

TABLE 2 Validated Questionnaires with Applicability to the Functional GI Disorders

Purpose	Investigator	Date
Diagnostic criteria		
Rome diagnostic criteria for classifying functional GI disorders	Drossman et al. (4)	1994
Non-ulcer dyspepsia, IBS, organic GI disease	Talley et al. (19)	1989
Bowel symptoms		
Functional bowel complaints	Talley et al. (19)	1989
Physical and sexual abuse	Drossman et al. (35)	1990
Health-related quality of life (HRQL)		
Sickness Impact Profile	Bergner et al. (38)	1981
Generic HRQL in gastroenterology setting	McGee et al. (46)	1991
HRQL in inflammatory bowel disease	Guyatt et al. (43)	1993
Other		
Patient knowledge questionnaire in inflammatory bowel disease	Jones et al. (47)	1993

tered to a small group of individuals selected for the study whose responses are not included in the final analysis of the results. The questionnaire is scrutinized to evaluate both face and content validity. Problems with the wording of questions and in determining consistency of responses and getting precise answers to what you are seeking to measure can all be resolved in pilot studies. Further, succeeding revisions to a questionnaire can be tested during a pilot study. Questionnaires are almost always improved from pilot studies (20).

Using validated questionnaires is imperative for investigators to compare their findings to the results of other researchers (*reliability*). The reliability of a measure or instrument ensures that the results obtained are reproducible in a consistent manner across respondents, observers, and investigators. A simple method of testing the reliability of a unique questionnaire is to administer both the study questionnaire and a previously validated one to a sample of individuals and then compare the results (21). The results from the unique questionnaire should be similar to those obtained from the validated one. In addition to enabling replication by other investigators, results from validated questionnaires are used to compare findings from different populations.

However useful, there are a number of pitfalls in constructing survey questionnaires, especially in studying the functional GI disorders. The specific wording of questions is extremely important. "Leading" questions may overstate results; vague questions may underestimate them. The need to avoid the use of vague and imprecise definitions or descriptions of symptomatology cannot be overemphasized. Another important obstacle in using survey questionnaires is the problem of poor retrospective recall. It is often difficult for people to evaluate their experiences as precisely as the investigator wishes when these experiences and the factors associated with them occurred long ago. Questionnaires are especially prone to this problem. To minimize the impact of vague recall, specific time frames should be used for questions, especially those about symptoms. For example, a question can be phrased "For the past 3 weeks, indicate whether you have experienced the following symptoms" rather than "Have you ever experienced these symptoms?" Other methods of collecting symptom information that rely on contemporaneous recall, e.g. diary cards, have been used with results that are judged to be more accurate than questionnaires (22).

B. Rating Scales

Rating scales are useful devices that are often employed to elicit information about symptomatology, both GI and extraintestinal. Various rating scales have been used in studying the functional GI disorders, especially to measure the intensity or frequency of symptoms. The construct of rating scales and their pitfalls have been described extensively (21–23). In *ordinal* (or *adjectival*) *scales*, both categorical and numerical constructs have been used (Figure 1). In categorical constructs, intervals are described using verbal phrases that approximate the intensity of experience. For example, to describe the physical distress that accompanies a specific symptom, a scale can typically be constructed as follows: "not at all distressing," "a little distressing," "moderately distressing," "quite a bit distressing," and "extremely distressing." The major deficiency of these categorical constructs is the inconsistency of meaning between the intervals among study subjects. What is "a little distressing" to one individual may be "moderately distressing" to another.

Instead of verbal phrases, another method of describing the intervals is to use numbers. In the example above, physical distress would be described using a scale of 1 to 5, with 1 being "not at all distressed" and 5 "extremely distressed." Respondents can select any number within the scale to describe their experience. Studies have shown that the optimal number of intervals is either 7 or 10 (21). However, intersubject variation also exists with numerical constructs. Therefore, care must be taken to construct intervals that are sensitive enough to describe the experience but not so specifically that the respondent is overwhelmed by the number of possible ratings.

The *visual analog scale* (VAS) was devised to eliminate the inconsistency of meaning among study subjects responding to exclusively verbal or numerical descriptions of the intervals. One of the most useful applications has been in the assessment of pain (24). The simplicity of the VAS is apparent because the scale consists of a straight line of fixed length, usually 10 cm, with the extremes corresponding to the minimum and maximum intensity of the experience (Figure 1).

Ordinal Scales

Categorical Responses:

How much have you been distressed by abdominal bloating during the last 7 days?

Not at all	A little bit	Moderately	Quite a bit	Extremely
☐	☐	☐	☐	☐

Numerical Responses:

Please describe the distress you have experienced from abdominal bloating during the last 7 days, using a scale of 1-7, with 1 being "Not at all distressed" and 7 being "Extremely distressed."

Not at all distressed...Extremely Distressed

1 2 3 4 5 6 7

Visual Analog Scale

How much have you been distressed by abdominal bloating during the last seven days?

No distress whatsoever ———————————————— Distress as bad as it can be

FIGURE 1 Rating scales.

Respondents place a mark along the line corresponding to their perceived experience. Although the VAS is a popular scaling method because of its apparent simplicity, studies have shown that the results obtained from VAS and ordinal scales are similar (25,26). It has been argued that the problem with the VAS is not in the construct of the scale itself but in its application in health-care research (21). For example, the VAS uses only a single scale to assess pain although pain may be influenced by a number of factors. Using multiple visual analog scales to assess all aspects of the condition under study would eliminate this shortcoming.

C. Statistical Analysis

Analysis of results from survey research in the area of functional GI disorders has focused on identifying associations. To properly determine associations, it is imperative that a sample of individuals not classified with the disorder but similar to the study group in all other respects be used as controls. Statistical methods used to assess associations constitute single and multivariate techniques, including contingency tables, multiple regression, and odds ratios. Another technique with particular application in the functional GI disorders is analysis of variance, which is used to assess the different sources of variability in a measure or value.

Frequently, the proportion of a group of individuals with a specified characteristic is compared to the proportion of individuals without it to determine if the characteristic is associated to the outcome measurement. The data can be arranged in a *contingency table*, of which the 2 × 2 table is a common design (see Table 3). In a 2 × 2 table, a characteristic or variable is divided into two mutually exclusive categories, e.g., male or female gender, age over 65 or age 65 and under. The outcome measure is similarly divided into two mutually exclusive categories, e.g., high or low score on functional status. The proportions within the groups are then statistically compared to determine if the characteristic is indeed associated with the outcome measurement. In a study of IBS in patients infected with HIV, analysis with 2 × 2 contingency tables was used to demonstrate the prevalence of IBS in this population (27).

Multiple regression plays an important role in analyzing data in studies on the functional GI disorders. As described earlier, many dimensions of a biological, psychological, and sociocultural nature can influence the illness experience of individuals with a functional GI disorder. Multiple regression seeks to assess the effects of a set of characteristics on a single dependent variable to determine whether the factors are indeed interrelated. For example, in the functional GI disorders, multiple regression has been used to determine the factors that contribute to illness severity and health-related quality of life (28).

In prospective surveys, a measure of the *relative risk* of contracting the medical condition or disease under study is of primary interest. Relative risk is the increased risk of incurring the condition or disease in those who possess certain characteristics or who are exposed to certain factors compared to those who are not. The characteristics are determined to be risk factors for developing the condition or disease. Relative risk can be determined only from prospective studies because the risk is determined from the incidence rates of contracting the medical condition or disease. In retrospective surveys, relative risk is approxi-

TABLE 3 2 × 2 Contingency Table

	Abdominal Bloating		
Age	Yes	No	Total
65 or older	9	12	21
Under 65	10	7	17
Total	19	19	38

mated with the *odds ratio*: the proportionate difference of the prevalence rates of the group of individuals possessing or exposed to the suspected risk factors and the rates of those who are not. In the functional GI disorders, odds ratios have been used to evaluate the relationship between sociodemographic characteristics and health-care-seeking behavior of individuals with IBS (2,11) and psychosocial factors in NUD (29).

Analysis of variance (ANOVA) is a technique used to assess the reliability of a measure or value. The variability in the answers given by different respondents and in evaluations given by different observers, as well as the variability that exists randomly, are all assessed by ANOVA. An analysis of variance can quantify how each source of variability contributes to the overall variability of a measurement. In the functional GI disorders, ANOVA has been used extensively to test for reliability of symptom measures. In one study to develop a numerical index of illness severity, ANOVA was used to compare physicians' ratings of illness severity across several study sites to assess variability in observers (28). Another application of ANOVA techniques in the functional GI disorders is the comparison of the composition of a sample by demographic or other characteristics in order to assess the comparability of results from different study sites (28).

Controlling for covariates—characteristics that are closely allied with each other (e.g., age and height)—can be done statistically, and is necessary to identify confounding associations. For example, an important dimension to recognize in studying the functional GI disorders is the influence of psychological distress. Psychosocial factors play a key role in the perception of health and illness in the functional GI disorders. Since psychiatric distress can affect symptom recall and reporting, care should be taken to establish psychological status and analyze its impact (22). For example, individuals may have a lower threshold to pain when feeling anxious. In reporting the intensity or frequency of symptoms, individuals with psychological distress may also magnify them (30,31).

The role of psychological factors also becomes an important consideration when drawing samples for population surveys. For example, individuals with IBS who seek treatment are more likely to have psychological distress than those who do not see physicians (32,33) or who are seen in primary-care practice (34). Therefore, the investigator must be careful in considering the effect of psychological status, both in selecting a sample of individuals for study and as a confounding variable.

D. Clinical Inference

The investigator who embarks on a survey using appropriate sampling methods and analysis techniques can be reasonably assured that the findings will have some statistical meaning. After all, the application of proper techniques will allow the investigator to draw the conclusion as to whether a particular result was due merely to chance. However, not all statistically significant results will have relevance clinically. Thus, research findings must be evaluated within the context of the clinical setting to determine whether the finding has any wider clinical application. In the functional GI disorders, determining clinical significance can be especially challenging because of the many biological and psychosocial variables that play a role in their etiology and expression.

VII. SPECIAL CONSIDERATIONS

A. Physical and Sexual Abuse

In the study of functional GI disorders, two specific areas of investigation have recently been undertaken that deserve special mention. First, research has demonstrated a strong relationship between the functional GI disorders and a patient's social history of abuse, especially physical and sexual abuse (35). Physical or sexual abuse is a form of life stress that can increase the magnitude of the illness experience of patients with functional GI disorders. The increased severity of GI symptoms has resulted in more frequent usage of health care services and results in poorer response to standard treatment (35). Moreover, the prevalence of psychological disorders is high in patients with an abuse history (36). Current research in the area of abuse and its effects in patients with functional GI disorders has focused on its impact on a patient's health status.

Inquiry into an individual's history of sexual abuse is particularly sensitive because of the nature of the information being asked. Many people are unwilling to reveal such information, even to a health professional. A survey questionnaire that can be completed anonymously is advantageous for such an intimate area of inquiry. In designing such questionnaires, it is especially important to avoid ill-constructed questions that may overstate or miss the abuse entirely. However, the problem of nondisclosure cannot be totally avoided with self-administered questionnaires. One method to avoid these pitfalls is to use or modify questions from validated instruments (35). Structured psychiatric and sexual trauma interviews have also been shown to be effective in eliciting sensitive information. These methods were used in a study of patients with IBS and inflammatory bowel disease to determine the prevalence rates of sexual victimization in the two groups (36).

B. Health-Related Quality of Life

A second area of special interest in the functional GI disorders that is particularly amenable to the use of survey research methods is *health-related quality of life* (HRQL). The terms *health status* and *functional status* have been used interchangeably with HRQL, which has been defined as the aspects of life experience that impact directly on an individual's perception of health and well-being.

These factors usually determine how well individuals believe they are coping with their illness in their daily lives—physically, mentally, and emotionally. Despite the absence of structural defects or significant metabolic deficiencies, the functional GI disorders can produce significant distress that negatively affects an individual's perception of his or her daily functioning and overall well-being. Disease activity and its impact on the individual often cannot be measured by laboratory or imagery studies alone, and the physical examination can give few clues to the severity of a functional GI complaint.

To better determine how patients cope in the context of a functional GI disorder, it is extremely important to identify the individual factors specific to the disorder that comprise the patient's health status. The key factors include the nature and severity of GI symptoms, functional status in physical and social contexts (e.g., mobility and the ability to take care of oneself), and psychological distress and other extraintestinal complaints. HRQL measures that encompass the multidimensional realms of the functional GI disorders—physical, psychological and sociocultural—are the most relevant and can lead to meaningful assessment of overall health.

The two primary types of HRQL measurements are generic instruments and disease-specific instruments. *Generic instruments* evaluate the overall aspects of health status or functioning. They are most often used in population surveys to document the range of disability in a specified population or group of patients (37). One of the most widely used is the Sickness Impact Profile (SIP), a comprehensive, 136-item instrument that assesses health-related dysfunction in 12 areas of activity, including work, sleep, eating, mobility, and social interaction (38). The SIP was developed in the early 1970s based on input from patients, healthy individuals, care-givers, and health professionals into the factors comprising health and well-being. Subsequent testing and revision of the instrument took place in both pilot and large-scale field studies from which validity and reliability were determined. Another generic instrument frequently used in assessing HRQL in patients with functional GI disorders is the Health Status Questionnaire (SF36), a more concise battery of 36 items that evaluate eight areas of functioning, primarily physical and psychosocial aspects. Wider application of both the SIP and the SF36 in the functional GI disorders is still being investigated; few studies have been undertaken to date.

Disease-specific HRQL instruments evaluate the factors impacting functional status and well-being that are associated with a single medical condition or disease. HRQL measures have been developed for a variety of chronic diseases, including cancer (39), rheumatoid arthritis (40), heart disease (41), and inflammatory bowel disease (42,43). Most of the previous studies in the functional GI disorders have relied on generic instruments. For example, Whitehead and colleagues (44) found that individuals with IBS report lower HRQL than do those who did not have bowel symptoms. In the U.S. Householder Study (1,2), individuals with functional GI disorders reported higher levels of absenteeism from work and higher rates of physician visits than did individuals without GI symptoms.

HRQL measures that are specific to the functional GI disorders have recently been proposed and validated (28). The obvious advantage of using disease-specific measures is that they more accurately characterize how a particular functional GI disorder can affect functionality in daily life. They can also help to better identify the degree of illness severity and lead to better identification of subgroups of patients based on severity of illness. The primary consideration in selecting validated HRQL measures or developing new ones is the application of the items to the specific functional GI disorder under study. A recent critique of HRQL instruments found that the major deficiency was that the measures had poor face validity (45). Frequently, investigators neglected to define exactly what they conceptualized as quality of life, nor did they solicit input from the patients. In the functional GI disorders, it is particularly important to assess the relevance of the HRQL measures to the patients themselves because there are no universal determinants of symptom severity. The development of effective instruments will significantly improve our assessment of how the functional GI disorders are impacting our patients' perception of their health and well-being.

REFERENCES

1. Drossman DA, Li Z, Andruzzi E, et al. U.S. Householder Survey of functional gastrointestinal disorders: prevalence, sociodemography and health impact. Dig Dis Sci 1993; 38:1569–1580.
2. Drossman DA. U.S. national prevalences of functional gastrointestinal disorders. In: Drossman DA, ed. The Functional Gastrointestinal Disorders: Diagnosis, Pathophysiology and Treatment. Boston: Little, Brown, 1994:311–328.
3. Drossman DA, Thompson WG, Talley NJ, et al. Identification of sub-groups of functional gastrointestinal disorders. Gastroenterol Int 1990; 3:159–172.
4. Drossman DA. The functional gastrointestinal disorders and their diagnosis: a coming of age. In: Drossman DA, ed. The Functional Gastrointestinal Disorders: Diagnosis, Pathophysiology and Treatment. Boston: Little, Brown, 1994:1–23.
5. Heaton KW, O'Donnell LJD, Braddon FEM, et al. Symptoms of irritable bowel syndrome in a British urban community: Consulters and nonconsulters. Gastroenterology 1992; 102:1962–1967.
6. Jones R, Lydeard S. Irritable bowel syndrome in the general population. Br Med J 1992; 304:87–90.
7. Talley NJ, O'Keefe EA, Zinsmeister AR, et al. Prevalence of gastrointestinal symptons in the elderly: a population-based study. Gastroenterology 1992; 102:895–901.
8. Armitage P, Berry G. Statistical Methods in Medical Research. Oxford: Blackwell Scientific Publications, 1994.
9. Klein KB. Controlled treatment trials in the irritable bowel syndrome: a critique. Gastroenterology 1988, 95:232–240.

10. Talley NJ, Weaver A, Zinsmeister A, et al. Self-reported diarrhea: what does it mean? Am J Gastroenterol 1994; 89:1160–1164.
11. Longstreth GF, Wolde-Tsadik G. Irritable bowel-type symptoms in HMO examinees: prevalence, demographics and clinical correlates. Dig Dis Sci 1993; 38:1581–1589.
12. Talley NJ. Non-ulcer dyspepsia: myths and realities. Aliment Pharmacol Therap 1991; 5:145–162.
13. Talley NJ. Functional gastroduodenal disorders. In: Drossman DA, ed. The Functional Gastrointestinal Disorders: Diagnosis, Pathophysiology and Treatment. Boston: Little, Brown, 1994:311–328.
14. Nyren O. The epidemiology of non-ulcer dyspepsia. In: Galmiche JP, Jian R, Mignon M, Ruszniewski PH, eds. Non-Ulcer Dyspepsia: Pathophysiological and Therapeutic Approaches. Paris: John Libbey Eurotext, 1991:7–13.
15. Talley NJ, Piper DW. The association between non-ulcer dyspepsia and other gastrointestinal disorders. Scand J Gastroenterol 1985; 20:896–900.
16. Talley NJ, Phillips SF. Non-ulcer dyspepsia: potential causes and pathophysiology. Ann Intern Med 1988; 108:865–879.
17. Crean GP, Holden RJ, Knill-Jones RP, et al. A database on dyspepsia. Gut 1994; 35:191–202.
18. Drossman DA. Psychosocial factors in functional dyspepsia. Eur J Gastroenterol Hepatol 1992; 4:602–607.
19. Talley NJ, Phillips SF, Melton J III, et al. A patient questionnaire to identify bowel disease. Ann Intern Med 1989; 111:671–674.
20. Hulley SB, Cummings SR, eds. Designing Clinical Research: An Epidemiologic Approach. Baltimore: Williams & Wilkins, 1988.
21. Streiner DL, Norman GR. Health Measurement Scales: A Practical Guide to their Development and Use. Oxford: Oxford University Press, 1994.
22. Talley NJ. Optimal design of treatment trials. In: Drossman DA, ed. The Functional Gastrointestinal Disorders: Diagnosis, Pathophysiology and Treatment. Boston: Little, Brown, 1994:265–310.
23. Dunn-Rankin P. Scaling Methods. Hillsdale NJ: Erlbaum, 1983.
24. Huskisson EC. Measurement of pain. Lancet 1974; ii:1127–1131.
25. Downie WW, Leatham PA, Rhind VM, et al. Studies with pain rating scales. Ann Rheum Dis 1978; 37:378–381.
26. Jaeschke R, Singer J, Guyatt GH. A comparison of seven point and visual analogue scales: data from a randomized trial. Controlled Clin Trials 1990; 11:43–51.
27. Desta T, Olden KW, Hom SS. Irritable bowel syndrome: a common cause of GI symptoms in HIV infection (abstr). Gastroenterology 1995; 108:A10.
28. Drossman DA, Li Z, Toner BB, et al. Functional bowel disorders: a multicenter comparison of health status and development of illness severity index. Dig Dis Sci 1995; 40:986–995.
29. Talley NJ, Jones M, Piper DW. Psychosocial and childhood factors in essential dyspepsia: a case-control study. Scand J Gastroenterol 1988; 23:341–346.
30. Barsky AJ. Investigating the psychological aspects of irritable bowel syndrome. Gastroenterology 1987; 93:902–904.

31. Guthrie E, Creed FH, Dawson D, et al. A controlled trial of psychological treatment for the irritable bowel syndrome. Gastroenterology 1991; 100:450–457.
32. Whitehead WE, Bosmajian L, Zonderman AB, et al. Symptoms of psychological distress associated with irritable bowel syndrome: comparison of community and medical clinic samples. Gastroenterology 1988; 95:709–714.
33. Drossman DA, McKee D, Sandler R, et al. Psychosocial factors in the irritable bowel syndrome. Gastroenterology 1988; 95:701–708.
34. Drossman DA. Illness behavior in the irritable bowel syndrome. Gastroenterol Int 1991; 4:77–81.
35. Drossman DA, Leserman J, Nachman G, et al. Sexual and physical abuse in women with functional or organic gastrointestinal disorders. Ann Intern Med 1990; 113:828–833.
36. Walker EA, Katon WJ, Roy-Byrne PP, et al. Histories of sexual victimization in patients with irritable bowel syndrome or inflammatory bowel disease. Am J Psychiatry 1993; 150:1502–1506.
37. Guyatt GH, Feeny DH, Patrick DL. Measuring health-related quality of life. Ann Intern Med 1993; 118:622–629.
38. Bergner M, Bobbitt, RA, Carter WB, et al. The Sickness Impact Profile: development and final revision of a health status measure. Med Care 1981; 19:787–805.
39. Spitzer W, Dobson A, Hall J. Measuring the quality of life in cancer patients: a concise QL index for use by physicians. J Chron Dis 1981; 34:585–597.
40. Bombardier C, Ware J, Russell IJ, et al. Auranofin therapy and quality of life in patients with rheumatoid arthritis. Am J Med 1986; 81:565–578.
41. Wiklund I, Comerford MB, Dimenas E. The relationship between exercise tolerance and quality of life in angina pectoris. Clin Cardiol 1991; 14:204–208.
42. Drossman DA, Patrick DL, Mitchell CM, et al. Health related quality of life in inflammatory bowel disease. Dig Dis Sci 1989; 34:1379–1386.
43. Guyatt GH, Mitchell A, Irvine EJ, et al. A new measure of health status for clinical trials in inflammatory bowel disease. Gastroenterology 1989; 96:804–810.
44. Whitehead WE, Burnett CK, Cook E, et al. Health related quality of life in IBS: patients compared to IBS non-consulters and asymptomatic individuals (abstr). Am J Gastroenterol 1994; 89:1700.
45. Gill TM, Feinstein AR. A critical appraisal of the quality of quality of life measurements. JAMA 1994; 619–626.
46. McGee H, O'Boyle C, Hickey A, et al. Assessing the quality of life of the individual: The SEIQOL with a healthy and a gastroenterology unit population. Psychol Med 1991; 3:749–759.
47. Jones SC, Gallacher B, Lobo AJ, et al. A patient knowledge questionnaire in inflammatory bowel disease. J Clin Gastroenterol 1993; 17:21–24.

7

Esophageal Disorders and Their Relationship to Psychiatric Disease

Laurence A. Bradley
University of Alabama at Birmingham
Birmingham, Alabama

Joel E. Richter
The Cleveland Clinic Foundation
Cleveland, Ohio

I. INTRODUCTION

It has long been recognized that psychiatric disease and other psychosocial factors may interact with and influence the onset or course of esophageal disorders. Indeed, Kronecker and Meltzer (1) observed in 1883 that "psychic upset" could induce esophageal contractions. Since the early 1980s, investigators have shown marked interest in studying relationships between psychosocial factors and motility disorders. This renewed and sustained emphasis on the "biopsychosocial" (2) dimensions of esophageal disease may be attributed to new collaborative relationships that have developed among behavioral and biomedical scientists, improvements in the measurement of esophageal function and psychosocial variables, the formation of active patient advocacy groups (e.g., the International Foundation for Bowel Dysfunction), and the dedication of funds for biobehavioral research by the National Institutes of Health and private organizations.

This chapter reviews the evidence concerning the relationships between the major esophageal disorders and psychiatric diseases or psychosocial factors. The esophageal disorders include gastroesophageal reflux disease, achalasia, globus sensation, hypertensive lower-esophageal sphincter, spasmodic disorders, and chest pain of unknown etiology. Our discussion of each disorder includes an examination of its a) biological and psychophysiological components, b) psychiatric and psychosocial dimensions, and c) appropriate medical and behavioral treatment interventions.

II. GASTROESOPHAGEAL REFLUX DISEASE

Gastroesophageal reflux disease (GERD) is the most common disorder of the esophagus and the major indication for antacid consumption (3). A recent Gallup survey showed that 20% of 800 randomly sampled adults reported heartburn more than three times in the previous month, and an additional 25% complained of heartburn at least once in the preceding month. In addition to the common complaint of heartburn, many patients with GERD will report such symptoms as dysphagia, sour regurgitation, waterbrash (bland liquid secreted by the salivary glands), nausea, vomiting, hiccups, or belching. Other, more atypical symptoms of GERD include chest pain, hoarseness, frequent coughing, asthma, and recurrent pneumonia.

A. Biological and Psychophysiological Components

Multiple factors contribute to GERD, including a) the competence of the lower-esophageal sphincter (LES) in serving as a barrier to gastric reflux, b) the effectiveness of the esophagus in clearing refluxed material by gravity, peristalsis, and acid neutralization by saliva, c) the potential of reflux material, e.g., acid and pepsin, to damage the esophageal mucosa, d) the intrinsic resistance of the esophageal mucosa to potentially damaging reflux material, e) delayed gastric emptying and acid hypersecretion, and f) hiatal hernia. An important biological factor that may initiate or aggravate GERD is pregnancy. Indeed, 15% of pregnant women suffer daily heartburn (4). The relationship between pregnancy and heartburn is probably mediated both by increased abdominal pressure and by the reduction in LES pressure produced by estrogens and progesterone (5).

The LES is considered the major barrier to acid reflux. The circular smooth muscle of the LES maintains tonic closure predominantly due to intrinsic muscular activity. However, there is also some cholinergic contribution as atropine can decrease resting LES pressure (6). The LES tone is dynamic and frequently changes throughout the day as a result of eating, smoking, gastric distension, increased abdominal pressure, and the interaction of various hormones and peptides. Contrary to common belief, fewer than 25% of reflux episodes are associated with free reflux across an atonic sphincter or a low LES overwhelmed by transient increases in intra-abdominal pressure. Instead, reflux more frequently occurs in association with transient LES relaxations that are not related to swallowing (7). This appears to be the primary mechanism of postprandial reflux brought about by gastric distension and perhaps by vagal properties (8).

The development of prolonged esophageal pH monitoring has produced several interesting findings about GERD. Although acid reflux can cause heartburn, the relationship between reflux and symptoms is often poor. Postprandial reflux, for example, commonly occurs in healthy persons but symptoms of heartburn are rare (8). In patients with esophagitis, intraesophageal pH monitoring frequently shows excessive reflux; patients, however, usually experience heartburn during fewer than 20% of these reflux episodes (9). Indeed, it has been shown that patients with GERD do not report symptoms during reflux episodes unless they are quite certain that symptoms have occurred (10).

Patterns of reflux episodes may be important in the development of symptoms and esophagitis. Patients who reflux acid at night tend to have low symptom levels but more severe evidence of esophagitis. In contrast, patients who reflux during the day tend to exhibit minimal mucosal damage but frequently report heartburn, aerophagia, and belching (11). There is evidence that these individuals may habitually swallow air, which can produce belching and subsequent reflux (12). Alternatively, acid reflux may trigger multiple dry swallows in an attempt to enhance acid clearance, which can lead to belching because each dry swallow contains 1 to 2 ml of air (11). Other biological factors that may influence reflux-induced symptoms include the hydrogen ion concentrations of the reflux material, total volume of reflux material contributing to esophageal distension, the acid clearance mechanisms, the interaction of pepsin with acid in the esophageal mucosa, and the patient's overall sensitivity to physiological and pathological stimuli.

B. Psychiatric and Psychosocial Dimensions

It is well known that certain behaviors tend to aggravate GERD. These include overeating, bending over, lying down soon after meals, smoking, ingestion of alcohol and spicy or acidic foods, and the use of certain medications such as theophylline and progesterones (4).

Many reflux patients and physicians believe that environmental stressors increase the likelihood of GERD symptoms in predisposed individuals. The Gallup survey described earlier reported that 64% of the respondents believed that stress exacerbated their reflux symptoms. Indeed, one can imagine many instances in which stress might interact with behavioral and physiological factors to produce GERD symptoms. For example, an individual with posttraumatic stress disorder may perceive many events as threatening and possess few adaptive strategies for coping with rapid anxiety reactions to these events. Moreover, his or her repertoire of coping strategies may include several behaviors that aggravate GERD, such as smoking or drinking alcohol. This individual may also frequently swallow air involuntarily during anxiety episodes (12,13). Swallowed air tends to elicit a peristaltic wave that helps clear the esophagus; this wave, however, may also relax the LES and further increase the probability of GERD symptoms.

Laboratory studies of the effects of stress on reflux episodes have tended to produce negative results. Cook and Collins (14), for example, reported that stressful dichotic listening tasks failed to influence either the number or the duration of objectively determined reflux episodes in healthy volunteers. Moreover, we found that three prolonged stressors (e.g., rapid presentation of difficult mental arithmetic problems), relative to neutral events (e.g., listening to acoustic guitar music presented on audiotape), produced significant increases in physiological stress measures such as blood pressure but did not influence intraesophageal acid exposure in patients with GERD. We also found, however, that patients' reports of the severity of their reflux symptoms during stress and neutral conditions varied as a function of psychological distress. Patients with low anxiety levels, as measured by the Millon Behavioral Health Inventory (16), reported similar levels of reflux symptoms during stress and neutral conditions. These reflux ratings were consistent with patients' intraesophageal acid exposure levels. In contrast, highly anxious patients reported significantly greater reflux symptom activity during stress compared to neutral conditions despite the fact that intraesophageal acid exposure did not vary with stress. These findings suggest that the common belief in a relationship between stress and increased reflux symptoms may be due to the experiences of a subgroup of persons who are characterized by high levels of anxiety.

One might question what factors may account for the reflux symptoms of highly anxious patients during stress. It is possible that the experience of anxiety during stressful situations contributes to a psychologically mediated response bias for symptom reporting. That is, anxious patients may devote excessive attention to a wide variety of esophageal events and label them as painful (17). There is also evidence, however, that anxiety influences neural input during stressful situations (17). It may be that when chronically anxious patients with GERD are exposed to prolonged stress, afferent somatovisceral information from the esophagus is modulated by cortical or subcortical (e.g., thalamus) activity so that low-intensity esophageal events are perceived as reflux symptoms (18).

C. Medical and Behavioral Treatment Interventions

Conservative medical treatment of GERD usually entails frequent doses of antacids, histamine H_2 blocking drugs (e.g., cimetidine, ranitidine, famotidine), or prokinetic agents (bethanechol, metoclopramide). Omeprazole may also be used to control acid secretion, especially in patients with erosive esophagitis (19).

In addition to the medications noted above, several behavioral changes are usually recommended to patients. These include a) elevating the head of the bed 6 inches to decrease reflux episodes during sleep, b) reducing the amount of food eaten during meals, and c) abstaining from eating for 2 or 3 hours prior to going to bed (4).

A few investigators have examined the efficacy of behavioral therapies for GERD. Schuster and colleagues (20) were the first to describe the effectiveness of a biofeedback procedure for increasing LES pressures in GERD patients. They reported that three healthy individuals and six patients learned to double their resting pressures after approximately 90 minutes of practice with visual LES pressure feedback. It was reported later that seven of 10 patients treated with the biofeedback method learned to double their resting LES pressures (21). Moreover, two of the patients with severe GERD who had not responded to traditional medical treatment showed "excellent" levels of symptom reduction.

Two other investigators have reported that biofeedback reduces patients' GERD symptoms. Gordon and colleagues (22) administered LES pressure biofeedback to an individual with an 8-year history of GERD. The patient learned to raise mean resting LES pressure from 2.7 to 8.9 mm Hg. Consistent with this improvement in LES pressure, macroscopic esophagitis was eliminated and the patient reported a decrease in heartburn episodes from at least three times daily to once every two weeks.

Shay and colleagues (23) used electromyographic (EMG) biofeedback from the rectus abdominal muscle to treat a patient with a 20-year history of rumination and a 1-year history of heartburn. The EMG biofeedback allowed the patient to reduce abdominal muscle tone and thus reduce intra-abdominal pressure. This was followed by an 80% improvement in the patient's symptom reports that was maintained for 6 months after treatment without additional physican visits.

Two drawbacks are associated with the use of biofeedback interventions for GERD. First, persons with exceptionally low resting LES pressure (<4 mm Hg) might not respond well to treatment given that maximum improvement appears to be limited to twice their baseline pressures. In addition, successful biofeedback training requires special equipment and experience in designing treatment protocols.

In light of these drawbacks, we recently performed a controlled trial of the effects of progressive muscle relaxation on symptom perception and intraesophageal acid exposure in patients with GERD and high levels of anxiety (24). Progressive muscle-relaxation training is an effective pain-management procedure that requires no equipment and only a small amount of specialized training. It is easily taught to patients, produces a deep state of relaxation, and is usually quite acceptable to medical patients. We found that patients who received relaxation training, relative to those who received a credible attention-placebo, were characterized by lower heart rates and total esophageal acid exposure (Table 1). The relaxation-training patients also reported lower levels of anxiety and fewer reflux symptoms than the attention-placebo patients.

These results suggest that progressive muscle-relaxation training can be a useful adjunct to traditional antireflux therapy in patients with GERD who have anxiety as a component of their illness presentation. In contrast to LES pressure biofeedback, the mechanisms underlying the effectiveness of relaxation training are not clear. It is possible that the diaphragmatic breathing associated with relaxation training increases the pressure of the crural diaphragm, thereby increasing overall LES pressure, which in turn reduces the number of episodes of gastric contents refluxing into the esophagus. However, it is also possible that relaxation training activates central mechanisms similar to those involved in hypnosis that decrease gastric-acid secretion, thereby reducing the amount of material that might be refluxed (24). Additional research is necessary to better identify the mechanisms that mediate the

Table 1 Effects of Relaxation Training Versus Attention-Placebo on Measures of Stress, Reflux Symptom Ratings, and Percentage Total Acid Exposure

Posttreatment variable	Treatment Group		
	Relaxation	Attention-placebo	*p*-value
Heart rate	81.1 ± 2.3	89.9 ± 2.4	<0.03
Anxiety rating	23.9 ± 6.0	60.6 ± 6.3	<0.03
Percentage total acid exposure	6.9 ± 4.2	28.1 ± 10.6	<0.05
Reflux symptom rating	1.3 ± 0.3	2.6 ± 0.3	<0.006

Values are expressed as mean ± SEM
Source: Ref. 24.

effects of relaxation training on esophageal acid reflux and patients' symptom perceptions.

III. GLOBUS SENSATION

Globus sensation and globus "hystericus" are terms used to describe the common symptom of cervical fullness, or a "lump in the throat" (4). It is a constant symptom that usually does not interfere with swallowing and, in fact, may be relieved by deglutition. Globus appears to be a common symptom although it is rarely brought to the attention of physicians. It is not known what factors cause some individuals with globus to seek health care and others to cope with the symptom using their own resources, although health-care-seeking behavior generally is associated with symptom severity and psychological distress (25–27). Nevertheless, Watson and colleagues (28) found that 18% of a group of women attending a gynecological clinic reported the presence of globus and that 34% of patients with irritable bowel syndrome also described globus symptoms. Thompson and Heaton (29) studied 147 healthy individuals and found that 45% experienced globus sensation, including 35% of the men and 53% of the women. Finally, Moloy and Charter (30) surveyed 4330 consecutive new patients at a general otolaryngology clinic and found that 4.1% identified globus sensation as their primary health problem. These investigators also reported that, among patients below the age of 50 years, globus was three times more prevalent in women than in men. However, there was no difference in the prevalence of globus between men and women over the age of 50.

A. Biological and Psychophysiological Components

The physiological mechanisms underlying globus sensation are unknown. It has been suggested that spasm of the upper-esophageal sphincter (UES) might account for globus, but empirical studies have produced conflicting results (31,32). It also has been suggested that globus is associated with hiatal hernia or reflux esophagitis. Wilson and colleagues (33) reported that abnormal gastroesophageal reflux occurred in 37 of 142 (23%) of globus patients. This indicates that, although reflux may be associated with globus sensation, it probably does not contribute to globus sensation in most patients with this symptom.

B. Psychiatric and Psychological Dimensions

It is widely believed that stress and anxiety contribute to the perception of globus symptoms. However, the term "globus hystericus" appears to be a misnomer. Lehtinen and Puhakka (34), for example, reported that during psychiatric interviews globus patients were more likely to display obsessive personality traits and depression than hysterical personality traits. Similarly, Cook and colleagues

(35) found that globus patients, relative to healthy controls, produced significantly higher scores on self-report measures of neuroticism, introversion, anxiety, and depression.

A series of British investigations have suggested that psychological distress may vary as a function of gender in globus patients (36–38). Wilson and colleagues (36,37) demonstrated that, compared to matched otolaryngology patients and healthy controls, only women with globus produced elevated scores on self-report measures of neuroticism, anxiety, depression, somatic concern, and general psychological distress. The women's high levels of somatic concern led Wilson et al. to speculate that these patients might be unusually sensitive to esophageal stimuli. The investigators attempted to test this hypothesis using forearm immersion in cold water as a noxious stimulus (38). It was found that globus patients and matched healthy controls did not differ in pain threshold for this stimulus. However, this procedure failed to provide an adequate test of the hypothesis concerning esophageal sensitivity since the noxious stimulus did not produce visceral stimulation. Thus, it currently is not known whether globus sensation may be related to abnormal neurosensory processing of esophageal stimuli.

Cook and colleagues (35) have examined the role of stress in UES pressures and symptom reports in globus patients. They reported that stress induced by a dichotic listening task produced nearly equivalent increases in UES pressure in both globus patients (31%) and healthy controls (25%). In contrast to the pattern found in anxious patients with GERD (15), the stressor did not produce globus sensation in any of the patients or controls. Thus, it was not possible to conclude that stress is associated with the production of globus sensation. It should be noted, however, that, unlike the study of stress in GERD patients, this investigation used a relatively brief environmental stressor and did not evaluate whether anxiety might interact with stress to produce unpleasant symptoms or influence UES pressure.

C. Medical and Behavioral Treatment Interventions

Globus sensation frequently recurs in patients despite the treatment efforts of physicians (39). This is probably due to the fact that the etiopathogenesis of the disorder, which may involve multiple factors, is unknown. We have recommended that physicians evaluate patients for underlying esophageal motility disorders or GERD (4). The high levels of somatic concern, depression, and anxiety associated with globus suggest that a psychological evaluation should be obtained for all patients. A few case studies have shown that antidepressant therapy (e.g., imipramine) can produce substantial and rapid improvement in globus patients with psychiatric disorders such as panic disorder, somatization, major depression, and agoraphobia (40). It should be noted that imipramine and other tricyclic medications reduce pain independently of their antidepressant effects (41). Thus, effective treatment of globus with psychotropic medication may not be mediated entirely by reduction of psychological distress.

Few studies have examined the efficacy of behavioral interventions for globus sensation. However, one case study (42) described the use of EMG biofeedback to treat constricted throat muscles and globus symptoms in a young woman. The patient was taught to reduce forehead EMG levels during 20 training sessions, which produced complete symptom relief. This report is typical of the behavioral literature regarding globus sensation in that there is no known causal pathway between the relaxation of frontal muscles and relief of globus symptoms. It may be that forehead EMG biofeedback training and other behavioral treatments shown to be effective for globus (e.g., relaxation training, desensitization of swallowing fear) (43) are successful because they provide patients with an adaptive coping strategy that they can successfully employ in situations that tend to evoke their symptoms (44).

IV. ESOPHAGEAL MOTILITY DISORDERS

Esophageal motility disorders are produced by a variety of abnormalities in the coordinated neuromuscular components responsible for orderly peristalsis in the esophagus. The primary symptoms of esophageal motility disorders are dysphagia (difficulty with food transport down the esophagus) and chest pain. The underlying motor abnormalities are most readily diagnosed by careful esophageal manometric studies. It should be noted that, until the mid-1980s, our manometric techniques allowed us only to define achalasia and markedly diminished LES pressure. However, recent advances in technology now permit accurate recording of pressures generated in the esophageal body as well as in the upper and lower sphincters. Several laboratories have established criteria for normal esophageal contractile activity in studies of large numbers of healthy adults (45,46). In addition, newer esophageal motility disorders have been recognized, particularly in patients with chest pain of unknown etiology (see Table 2).

A. Achalasia

The most thoroughly studied and best understood esophageal motility disorder is achalasia (4). First described in the 17th century by Willis, achalasia is associated with a loss of smooth-muscle ganglion cells that produces two major defects in esophageal function: an obstruction in the esophagogastric junction associated with incomplete relaxation of the LES and an absence of normal peristalsis in the distal smooth-muscle segment of the esophagus. The resulting symptoms include chronic dysphagia, regurgitation of bland material, and weight loss. In addition,

TABLE 2 Manometric Criteria Proposed for Primary Esophageal Motility Disorder

- Achalasia
  - Aperistalsis of esophageal body
  - Incomplete LES relaxation
  - Elevated LES pressure (>45 mm Hg)
  - Elevated intraesophageal baseline
- Diffuse esophageal spasm
  - Simultaneous contraction (>10%)
  - Intermittent normal peristalsis
  - May also find:
    - Repetitive contractions (more than two peaks)
    - Spontaneous contractions
    - Incomplete LES relaxation
    - Increased duration and/or amplitude
- Nutcracker esophagus
  - Increased distal amplitude (>180 mm Hg)
  - Normal peristalsis
  - May have increased duration (>6 sec)
- Hypertensive LES
  - Elevated LES pressure (>45 mm Hg)
  - Normal peristalsis and LES relaxation
- Nonspecific esophageal motility disorder
  - Any combination of:
    - Increased nontransmitted waves (>20%)
    - Prolonged contractions (>6 sec)
    - Triple-peak contractions
    - Retrograde contractions
    - Low-amplitude waves (<30 mm Hg)
    - Absent peristalsis with normal LES

Based on values exceeding mean + 2 SD in 95 healthy normal volunteers (Ref. 46).
Source: Ref. 4.

young patients may have severe substernal chest pain. Nevertheless, barium esophagrams and radionuclide studies of esophageal transit will confirm the absence of peristalsis and marked delay in esophageal emptying in these patients.

Given the straightforward relationships between the biological components and the symptoms of achalasia, little attention has been devoted to the psychiatric and psychosocial dimensions of this disorder. Accordingly, the preferred initial treatment for achalasia is pneumatic dilatation (47). This procedure produces long-term relief of dysphagia and chest pain in 75 to 80% of patients; however, it reduces pain in only 50% of patients with vigorous achalasia (48).

Esophageal myotomy also relieves dysphagia in 80 to 90% of achalasia patients. Unfortunately, it may produce esophageal reflux as a side effect that requires treatment on a continual basis (49).

One case study has been published regarding the efficacy of a behavioral treatment protocol for a woman with vigorous achalasia (50). This patient's symptoms had been present for 12 years and had been unresponsive to myotomy, pneumatic dilatations, and multiple medications, including diazepam, nitroglycerin, ranitidine, and nifedipine. The behavioral treatment protocol consisted of progressive muscle relaxation, frontal electromyographic and finger-temperature biofeedback, and cognitive-behavioral therapy directed toward increases in social activities as well as decreases in pain behaviors. It was found that the 16-week behavioral treatment protocol eliminated all chest-pain episodes; this effect was maintained for 1 year following treatment termination. However, there were no changes in her esophageal manometry studies between baseline and follow-up. The patient showed simultaneous contractions and loss of peristalsis in both manometric studies. It was suggested that behavioral treatment reduced psychological distress, which in turn eliminated the patient's tendency to interpret GI sensations as pain.

B. Diffuse Esophageal Spasm and Related Motility Disorders

In contrast to achalasia, diffuse esophageal spasm and related motility disorders are characterized by variable manometric patterns and symptoms. The motility patterns displayed by patients with these disorders are distinct from those of patients with achalasia. The former, however, frequently fluctuate between normal and abnormal, with contractile activity featuring periods of normal peristalsis interrupted by simultaneous repetitive contractions, high-amplitude or long-duration waves, and occasional dysfunction of the LES. The accepted criteria for these motility disorders are shown in Table 2. Intermittently, patients with diffuse esophageal spasm may have striking changes in their barium esophagram, described by such colorful terms as "rosary bead esophagus" and "corkscrew esophagus." The related motility disorders, especially nutcracker esophagus and hypertensive LES, usually are characterized by normal motility and esophageal emptying on barium esophagrams and radionuclide studies. In nutcracker esophagus, the peristaltic waves may last longer and are higher distally. The symptoms that accompany all these disorders involve intermittent chest pain or dysphagia that is usually progressive and does not show consistent relationships with variations in motility.

It should be noted that the proliferation of manometric classifications shown in Table 2 has raised questions as to whether each set of criteria corresponds to a distinct motility disorder that may vary with respect to pathophysiology and appropriate intervention. We believe that there are not sufficient data to support this "splitter" approach. Indeed, each set of manometric criteria appears to be associated with similar symptoms that do not require diverse management approaches. Thus, we recommend a "lumper" approach in which these manometric criteria are clustered under the general term "spastic motility disorders of the distal esophagus."

1. Biological and Psychophysiological Components

The pathophysiology of the spastic motility disorders is poorly understood. Since these disorders rarely require surgery or lead to death, little biological material has been available for examination. Nevertheless, three biological abnormalities have been found in some patients with spastic motility disorders. First, thickening of esophageal muscle has been observed in some patients (51), although the esophageal muscle and neural plexus have been normal in the majority of patients studied to date. Second, early physiological studies suggested that there may be neural dysfunction in many patients with spastic motility disorders. The esophagus appears to be especially sensitive to cholinergic stimulation, which produces an exaggeration of abnormal manometric findings (52). These responses, however, are not sensitive or specific for the spastic disorders and may be observed in persons with achalasia as well as healthy individuals (53). Finally, electromyographic studies in patients with diffuse esophageal spasm have revealed spike-independent contractions of the esophageal body and increased excitability of spontaneous spike activity (54). These findings may represent impaired noncholinergic, nonadrenegic, inhibitory neural mechanisms. Indeed, an imbalance between excitatory and inhibitory innervation could produce the motility changes associated with the spastic disorders. However, some of these abnormalities are also observed in healthy persons in response to normal physiological stimuli such as dry swallows (46) and ingestion of very cold liquids (55).

2. Psychiatric and Psychosocial Dimensions

Several studies have shown that the spastic motility disorders are associated with high levels of psychological distress. For example, Clouse and Lustman (56) found that 21 of 25 (84%) patients with spastic esophageal motility disorders met criteria for psychiatric disorders based on structured interview criteria. However, only four of 13 (31%) patients with normal manometry and four of 12 (33%) patients with other manometric abnormalities met criteria for psychiatric diagnoses. The most common diagnoses among the patients with spastic motility disorders were depression, anxiety disorder, and somatization disorder. These are similar to the psychiatric diagnoses frequently associated with irritable bowel syndrome (57). However, they also are consistent with psychiatric disturbances frequently found in patients with musculoskeletal pain syndromes (58,59). Thus, frequent depression, anxiety, and somatization are not unique to patients with painful GI disorders.

It has also been found that patients with spastic motility disorders tend to produce elevated scores on some self-report measures of psychological distress. For example, we have found that patients with nutcracker esophagus produce significantly higher scores on the Gastrointestinal Susceptibility and Somatic Anxiety scales of the Millon Behavioral Health Inventory (MBHI) than do healthy controls and patients with benign structural abnormalities of the esophagus. Similar to the results reported by Clouse and Lustman, the scores of the nutcracker esophagus patients did not differ from those of patients with irritable bowel syndrome. Thus, both of these groups produced responses to the MBHI that are similar to those of medical patients who react to psychological stress with severe GI symptoms and who exhibit unusually high levels of concern regarding bodily functions as well as depression.

We also have found elevated Gastrointestinal Susceptibility scores in a small group of patients with hypertensive LES (60). It is possible, then, that patients with spastic motility disorders are characterized by enhanced tertiary contraction responses to stress that in turn are associated with increased symptomatology. However, we have shown that few abnormal tertiary contractions occur in response to stress when relatively stringent criteria (≥10 mm Hg increase in pressure) are used to differentiate tertiary contractions from normal respiratory changes of the esophageal baseline (61). We have also shown that increased peristaltic-wave amplitudes represent the primary response to stress in both healthy individuals and patients with the nutcracker esophagus (62). Furthermore, after adjusting for baseline differences among the subject groups, the increases displayed by the nutcracker esophagus patients were significantly greater than those of the healthy controls, and were substantially larger than those of patients with chest pain and normal motility. Nevertheless, stress did not induce pain in any of the nutcracker esophagus patients. Indeed, 24-hour ambulatory pH monitoring has shown that contraction abnormalities occur as frequently after the onset of chest pain as before (63). This evidence suggests, then, that the nutcracker esophagus, and perhaps the other spastic motility disorders, may be markers for chest pain but do not represent the causes of the pain.

3. Medical and Behavioral Treatment Interventions

The first-line treatments for diffuse esophageal spasm and related motility disorders include: 1) antireflux therapy, 2) nitrate, anticholinergic, or calcium channel blocking agents, and 3) anxiolytic or antidepressant medications such as alprazolam, buspirone, amitriptyline, or trazodone (64). However, it may be necessary for physicians to perform trials of all these treatments in a serial fashion, as most of these therapies have not been shown to be superior to placebo in controlled studies (4).

Esophageal pneumatic dilation and myotomy have been used in some patients with diffuse esophageal spasm and other motility disorders (65,66). However, the potential risks and limited benefits of these procedures for patients with spastic motility disorders suggest that great care must be taken in their usage. We have previously suggested that pneumatic dilation be performed only with patients with documented delays in esophageal emptying and that myotomy is appropriate only for patients with significant chest pain, dysphagia, and disability who do not respond to first-line treatments (4). Physicians may also consider referring unresponsive patients for behavioral therapies before recommending pneumatic dilatation or surgery. These therapies have not been tested in controlled clinical trials, but case studies suggest that they may be effective, especially for patients with diffuse esophageal spasm (67).

Finally, we have shown that an essential treatment component is confident reassurance, based on careful diagnostic studies, that the patient's symptoms are due to an esophageal motility disorder rather than cardiac disease or some other life-threatening or progressive disease (68). Reassurance helps patients to accept their symptoms, reduces their emotional distress, and thus leads to reductions in chest pain as well as pain-related, functional impairments.

V. CHEST PAIN OF UNKNOWN ETIOLOGY

Approximately 500,000 coronary angiograms are performed in the United States each year. It is estimated that 15 to 30% of these angiograms are normal, resulting in 75,000 to 150,000 patients with chest pain and normal coronary arteries (69). It has been shown that, even though these patients do not suffer from a life-threatening disease, many do not return to work, continue to have restricted lifestyles, and persist in believing that they have coronary artery disease that has not yet been detected (69). As a result, patients frequently continue to take cardiac medications, visit emergency rooms, and use other health care resources, resulting in costs of approximately $315 million per year (4,69).

A. Biological and Psychophysiologic Components

Many studies have shown that esophageal motility disorders are frequently found in patients with chest pain and normal coronary arteries. For example, we reported that motility disorders were present in 255 of 910 (28%) patients (70). The most common motility disorder was nutcracker esophagus (48%); diffuse esophageal spasm was found relatively infrequently (10%). However, the presence of these motility disorders was generally independent of chest-pain episodes.

Given the lack of association between the presence of motility disorders and chest pain, some investigators have used provocative testing in an effort to reproduce patients' chest pains. The provocative agents used in this testing have included ice-water swallows, intraesophageal acid perfusion, and systemic injections of bethanechol, edrophonium, ergonovine, and pentagastrin (4,69). Edrophonium, the most frequently used provocative agent, provokes chest pain in 18 to 34% of patients but does not induce pain in healthy volunteers (53,71). However, provocative testing has not clarified the cause of patients' chest pain since motility changes do not distinguish those who respond to testing from nonresponders (4).

The development of ambulatory monitoring devices for 24-hour esophageal pH monitoring has made an important contribution to our understanding of the biological components of chest pain in patients with normal coronary arteries. Studies using this measurement system have shown that GERD is the most common cause of the chest pain. For example, we found that 50 of 100 patients with chest pain and normal coronary arteries showed definite evidence that acid reflux contributed to their pain episodes (72). In contrast, ambulatory esophageal-pressure monitoring studies have suggested that fewer than 30% of chest pain episodes are associated with abnormal motility (73). However, motility changes are often associated with periods of reflux activity, suggesting that multiple biological processes may underlie many of the patients' chest pain symptoms.

Our ability to identify GERD in about 50% of patients with chest pain and normal coronary arteries has enhanced our understanding of this disabling pain syndrome. However, despite the development of sophisticated ambulatory monitoring devices, we still cannot identify biological abnormalities in approximately one-half of the patients who seek medical treatment for their chest pain. These patients, who are labeled as suffering from chest pain of unknown etiology (CPUE), are the focus of the remainder of this discussion.

B. Psychiatric and Psychosocial Dimensions

It has been found consistently that high levels of neuroticism and psychological distress tend to be associated with CPUE. This distress is manifested by somatic preoccupation, anxiety, depression, and perceived vulnerability to serious heart disease (74–76). High levels of neuroticism in patients with CPUE are associated with poor prognosis for improvement (75), high levels of pain and breathlessness (77), and the use of maladaptive pain coping strategies (78).

Clouse (79) has suggested that it is most appropriate to evaluate the psychological features of medical patients using structured psychiatric interviews. A large number of psychiatric interview studies have found a high prevalence of panic disorder among patients with CPUE. These prevalence rates, which range between 34 and 59%, are substantially higher than those found among patients with other chronic pain syndromes (80–83). It has been shown that patients with panic disorder show greater awareness of cardiac symptoms (e.g., rapid heartbeat) and more accurate perception of heart rate than patients with simple phobias and healthy controls (84). This might help account for the high prevalence of panic disorder among chest pain patients. Indeed, some investigators have suggested that panic disorder and related psychiatric variables may represent one cause of CPUE (85).

It should be noted that high frequencies of panic disorder may not be specific to patients with CPUE. For example, it has been found that there is a 40% prevalence rate of panic disorder among patients with chest pain and abnormalities in the smaller endocardial vasculature without fixed lesions or spasm of the epicardial vessels, i.e., microvascular angina (86). In addition, we have found similar frequencies of panic disorder among patients with CPUE and GERD (87). Thus, although panic disorder may enhance patients' perceptions of chest pain, it is unlikely that it represents a unique cause of CPUE (88).

During the past several years, we have examined the hypothesis that patients with CPUE are characterized by abnormal pain perception and responsiveness to noxious esophageal stimulation. We have performed two studies that demonstrated that patients with CPUE display lower pain thresholds than healthy controls during intraesophageal balloon distension (89,90). Moreover, we have used sensory decision theory (SDT) methods to increase our understanding of the perceptual factors that account for these differences in pain threshold (91). Our SDT methods require subjects to rate the intensity levels of a large series of stimuli presented in random order. The ratings then are used to derive two statistically independent parameters: the accuracy with which subjects differentiate stimuli of relatively high and low intensity levels (i.e., discrimination ability) and subjects' characteristic tendencies to report pain at either high or low intensity levels (i.e., response bias). Variations in discrimination ability are determined primarily by changes in neurosensory processing of afferent stimuli at either the peripheral or the central levels. Thus, high discrimination ability reflects high levels of neural input that may be produced by hyperresponsiveness of peripheral receptors or altered central processing of afferent stimuli. Low discrimination ability reflects relatively diminished neural input levels that may be produced by medications. In contrast, variations in response bias are determined largely by changes in central factors involved in pain perception. These factors may be physiological or they may represent the influence of psychosocial factors such as culturally based values regarding the expression of pain. Thus, low response bias reflects a characteristic tendency to report pain in response to numerous stimuli. High response bias represents a tendency to adopt a stoic response pattern during exposure to potentially painful stimuli. It has been shown, for example, that the administration of imipramine, which tends to reduce serotonin reuptake at central levels, produces increases in pain threshold levels and response bias (92). This suggests that the increase in pain threshold may be mediated by the inhibition of nociceptive transmission or by mood alteration associated with altered serotonin levels.

TABLE 3 Mean (±SEM) Pain Threshold Levels as a Function of Stimulus and Subject Group

	Subject group			
Stimulus	Chest pain	Irritable bowel	Reflux disease	Healthy control
Intraesophageal balloon distension (ml)[a]	10.6 ± 0.7	11.8 ± 1.0	13.2 ± 0.7	12.2 ± 0.7
Mechanical finger pressure (kg)[b]	84.5 ± 5.1	81.3 ± 7.3	94.5 ± 5.6	90.3 ± 5.7

[a] $p = 0.05$. Patients with chest pain of unknown etiology exhibited significantly lower pain threshold levels than patients with gastroesophageal reflux disease and healthy controls ($p \leq 0.05$ for both).
[b] $p = 0.28$. There were no significant differences in pain threshold levels among the subject groups.

We compared pain threshold levels and SDT parameters in patients with CPUE and three groups of control subjects. The control groups were composed of healthy individuals as well as patients with either GERD or irritable bowel syndrome (IBS). We evaluated the pain threshold and SDT parameters in response to two forms of noxious stimuli: esophageal balloon distension and mechanical finger pressure. Table 3 shows that patients with CPUE exhibited significantly lower pain threshold levels than healthy controls and patients with GERD only in response to esophageal balloon distension. In addition, Table 4 shows that the CPUE patients produced significantly lower response bias values than the healthy controls and GERD patients during esophageal stimulation. There were no group differences in discrimination ability (93).

These findings indicate that CPUE patients' low pain thresholds are specific to esophageal balloon distension. Moreover, the difference between the CPUE patients and those with GERD suggests that the CPUE patients' low pain thresholds cannot be attributed to altered function of peripheral receptors related to acid exposure. Finally, the response bias values provide evidence that central factors are involved in the CPUE patients' low pain threshold levels. This is consistent with the results reported by Castell (94), Lenz et al. (95), and McDonald-Haile (96).

C. Medical and Behavioral Treatment Interventions

We have emphasized that the medical treatment of patients with chest pain must begin with the evaluation of cardiac disease as the cause of their pain (4). Once cardiac disease has been ruled out, it is necessary to determine whether the pain

TABLE 4 Mean (±SEM) SDT Discrimination Ability and Response Bias Values During Intraesophageal Balloon Distension as a Function of Subject Group

	Subject group			
STD value	Chest pain	Irritable bowel	Reflux disease	Healthy control
Discrimination ability[a]	29.7 ± 0.9	27.7 ± 1.3	28.5 ± 1.0	28.1 ± 1.0
Response bias[b]	9.0 ± 0.2	9.5 ± 0.3	9.8 ± 0.2	9.9 ± 0.2

SDT = Sensory Decision Theory
[a] $p = 0.20$. There were no significant differences in discrimination ability among the subject groups
[b] $p = 0.002$. Patients with chest pain of unknown etiology exhibited significantly lower response bias values than patients with gastroesophageal reflux disease and healthy controls ($p \leq 0.004$ for both).

may be associated with musculoskeletal causes, GERD, or the motility disorders described earlier. At the same time, it is quite helpful to have the patients undergo a thorough psychological evaluation, including the administration of a structured psychiatric interview or psychometric tests (97). This assessment should also include an interview concerning early learning experiences such as episodes of childhood chest pain or frequent health care usage, family histories of cardiac or other forms of recurrent pain, and sexual or physical abuse (98,99). We have provided a detailed description of our psychological assessment procedures elsewhere (97).

After the psychological evaluation has been completed, it is very useful to provide patients and their referring physicians with a preliminary verbal report followed by a written report that integrates the results of the medical and psychological evaluations. The integration of the medical and psychological evaluations greatly reduces patients' resistance to psychological or behavioral treatments and reassures them that all possible causes of their pain have been investigated.

The treatment of patients with chest pain and normal coronary arteries is an empirical endeavor. First, patients must be reassured that cardiac disease has been ruled out as a cause of their pain. Second, for patients with chest pain and evidence of acid reflux, a vigorous 1- to 2-month trial of antireflux therapy should be initiated. Similarly, nitrate, anticholinergic, and calcium channel blocking agents may be used if motility disorders are found during esophageal manometry. It should be noted, however, that these medications may not effectively relieve the patients of their chest pain. Therefore, we treat the nonresponders in the same manner as those patients with CPUE and no other physiological abnormalities.

The third treatment approach for chest pain involves the use of psychotropic medications. Gupta and colleagues (100) recently reported that imipramine significantly reduces the frequency of chest pain episodes relative to placebo and clonidine. It has been shown that other tricyclic medications have analgesic effects, although none of these medications has been tested in controlled trials in patients with CPUE (41). Similarly, none of the selective serotonin reuptake inhibitors has been evaluated for use with these patients. A small uncontrolled study has shown that patients with CPUE and panic disorder respond well to alprazolam (101). It should be noted, however, that alprazolam and other benzodiazepines are most appropriate for short-term use since patients have difficulty in discontinuing these medications (102). Thus, we tend to prescribe alprazolam for appropriate patients using 6-month trial periods and planned withdrawal schedules to minimize drug dependency. Alternatively, we will use buspirone; this medication has not been subjected to clinical trials with CPUE patients, but it frequently is helpful to patients and it may be discontinued without adverse side effects.

The fourth approach to treatment is the use of psychological therapy. One review has indicated that psychological therapies are as effective in treating panic disorder as are the anxiolytic and antidepressant medications (103). The psychological therapies also appear to prevent relapse more effectively than do the pharmacological treatments. However, only one controlled trial of psychological therapy has been performed with CPUE patients. Klimes and colleagues (104) evaluated the efficacy of a cognitive-behavioral intervention relative to a waiting-list control condition in reducing pain in 35 patients with CPUE who also suffered symptoms of panic or generalized anxiety. It was found that the intervention, relative to the control condition, produced significant improvements in chest pain, mood, and performance of daily activities. These effects were maintained over a 3-month follow-up period. Nevertheless, persons who administer cognitive-behavioral or other psychological therapies for CPUE patients must provide relapse prevention training that will help patients cope effectively with new stressors or other events that may exacerbate pain after treatment termination. Keefe and Van Horn (105) have provided a detailed description of these relapse-prevention procedures. Briefly, relapse-prevention training requires patients to identify events that are likely to lead to pain episodes or increased pain levels. The patients are then encouraged to develop plans for coping with these events and to practice their coping strategies. Keefe and Van Horn have suggested that relapse-prevention training be provided during all phases of psychological therapies for chronic pain.

VI. SUMMARY

This review has shown that psychosocial factors, including psychiatric illnesses, contribute to the onset or course of all the esophageal disorders, with the possible exception of achalasia. For example, high levels of psychological distress are associated with globus sensation, diffuse esophageal spasm and related motility disorders, and chest pain of unknown etiology. Indeed, psychological factors such as panic disorder may contribute to symptom perception in some patients in the absence of esophageal dysfunction.

The role of environmental stress in esophageal disorder, however, is less clear. It has been established that stress alters esophageal functioning in both normal individuals and patients. Nevertheless, few patients display symptoms of globus sensation or chest pain when they are exposed to laboratory stressors. In contrast, high levels of stress in GERD patients with chronic anxiety produce increases in reflux symptoms, even when low levels of acid are present in the esophagus.

Investigators are also beginning to devote attention to differences in pain perception between patients and healthy controls. Most of the research on pain perception has been performed with patients with CPUE. These patients exhibit lower pain thresholds than healthy persons and GERD patients in response to intraesophageal balloon distension. Moreover, analyses based on sensory decision theory suggest that these differences in pain threshold levels are mediated by central rather than peripheral factors. In contrast, CPUE patients do not differ from GERD patients or healthy controls in pain threshold levels during exposure to mechanical finger pressure. It appears, then, that it is important to study patients' responses to organ-specific as well as more general noxious stimulation.

Finally, treatment of the esophageal disorders reviewed in this chapter is largely empirical. That is, trials of several classes of pharmacological agents may be used for globus sensation, most of the motility disorders, and chest pain with normal coronary arteries. These agents include antireflux therapies, nitrates, anticholinergics, and calcium channel blocking drugs. However, none of these medications has been shown to be consistently effective in controlled clinical trials. There is also some evidence that various psychotropic medications are helpful with some patients with globus sensation, motility disorders, and CPUE. The only controlled trials, however, have been performed with trazodone and imipramine. Both of those trials produced positive results in patients with chest pain and normal coronary arteries.

Most of our knowledge regarding the effects of behavioral or psychological therapies on esophageal symptoms has been derived from case reports. As a consequence, it is not possible to determine the factors that may mediate the beneficial effects of most of these therapies. It is clear, however, that the effects of lower-esophageal-sphincter biofeedback for reflux disease are mediated by increases in LES pressure changes. Cognitive-behavioral therapy has produced positive results in one controlled trial using patients with CPUE. Thus, the reductions in chest pain produced by this therapy cannot be attributed to nonspecific factors such as patients' expectations for improvement. Nevertheless, it is not possible to determine at present which components of this treatment intervention are the most effective in producing improvement. Moreover, greater attention should be devoted to helping patients prevent relapse following termination of psychological and behavioral therapies.

In conclusion, a great deal of progress has been made in understanding the relationships between the esophageal disorders and psychiatric disease and other psychosocial factors. As we continue to learn about the interactions of physiological events with stress, psychological distress, psychiatric illness, and symptom perceptions, it will be possible to develop pharmacological, behavioral, and psychological therapies that are targeted for specific esophageal disorders. We look forward to contributing to these developments.

ACKNOWLEDGMENT

Preparation of this chapter was supported by NIDDK R01 42428.

REFERENCES

1. Kronecker H, Meltzer SJ. Der schluckmechanismus, sein erreging und seine Hemmung. Arch Anat Physiol 1883; 7(suppl):328–362.
2. Engel GL. The need for a new medical model: a challenge to biomedicine. Science 1977; 196:129–136.
3. Henderson RD. Motor Disorders of the Esophagus. 2nd ed. Baltimore: Williams & Wilkins, 1980.
4. Bradley LA, McDonald JE, Richter JE. Psychophysiological interactions in the esophageal diseases: implications for assessment and treatment. Sem Gastrointest Dis 1990; 1:5–22.
5. Schuster MM. Disorders of the esophagus: applications of psychophysiological methods to treatment. In: Hözl R, Whitehead WE, eds. Psychophysiology of the Gastrointestinal Tract. New York: Plenum, 1983:33–42.
6. Dodds WJ, Dent J, Hogan WJ, et al. Effect of atropine on esophageal motor function in humans. Am J Physiol 1978; 235:392–396.
7. Dodds WJ, Dent J, Hogan WJ, et al. Mechanisms of gastroesophageal reflux in patients with reflux esophagitis. N Engl J Med 1982; 307:1547–1552.
8. Holloway RH, Hongo M, Berger K, et al. Gastric distention: a mechanism for postprandial gastroesophageal reflux. Gastroenterology 1985; 89:779–784.
9. Peters LJ, Maas LC, Petty D, et al. Spontaneous noncardiac chest pain: evaluation by 24-hour ambulatory esophageal motility and pH monitoring. Gastroenterology 1988; 94:878–886.

10. Clark WC, Bennett Clark S. Application of the medical decision making model to esophageal reflux disease: commentary on a study by Breumelhof and Smout. Am J Gastroenterol 1992; 87:924–926.
11. Johnson LF, De Meester TR. 24-hour pH monitoring of the distal esophagus—a quantitative measure of gastroesophageal reflux. Am J Gastroenterol 1974; 62:325–332.
12. Cuevas JL, Cook EW, Richter JE, McCutcheon M, Taub E. Spontaneous swallowing rate and emotional state: possible mechanism for stress-related gastrointestinal disorders. Dig Dis Sci 1995; 40:282–286.
13. Fonagy P, Calloway SP. The effect of emotional arousal on spontaneous swallowing rates. J Psychosom Res 1986; 30:183–188.
14. Cook IJ, Collins SM. Does acute emotional stress influence frequency or duration of gastroesophageal reflux in human subjects? (abstr). Gastroenterology 1986; 90:1380.
15. Bradley LA, Richter JE, Pulliam TJ, Haile JM, Scarinci IC, Schan CA, Dalton CB, Salley AN. The relationship between stress and symptoms of gastroesophageal reflux: the influence of psychological factors: Am J Gastroenterol 1993; 88:11–19.
16. Millon T, Green CJ, Meagher RB. Million Behavioral Health Inventory. Minneapolis: Interpretive Scoring Symptoms, 1983.
17. Malow RM, West JA, Sutker PB. Anxiety and pain response changes across treatment: sensory decision analysis. Pain 1989; 38:35–44.
18. Mayer EA, Raybould HE. Role of visceral afferent mechanisms in functional bowel disorders. Gastroenterology 1990; 99:1688–1704.
19. Hetzel DJ, Dent J, Reed WD, et al. Healing and relapse of severe peptic esophagitis after treatment with omeprazole. Gastroenterology 1988; 95:903–912.
20. Schuster MM, Nikoomanesh P, Wells P. Biofeedback control of lower esophageal sphincter contraction. Rendiconti di Gastroenterol 1973; 5:14–18.
21. Schuster MM. Disorders of the esophagus: applications of psychophysiological methods to treatment. In: Hözl R, Whitehead WE, eds. Psychophysiology of the Gastrointestinal Tract. New York: Plenum, 1983:33–42.
22. Gordon A, Gordon E, Berelowitz M, et al. Biofeedback improvement of lower esophageal sphincter pressures and reflux symptoms. J Clin Gastroenterol 1983; 5:235–237.
23. Shay SS, Johnson LF, Wong RKH, et al. Rumination, heartburn, and daytime gastroesophageal reflux: a case study with mechanisms defined and successfully treated with biofeedback therapy. J Clin Gastroenterol 1986; 8:115–126.
24. McDonald-Haile J, Bradley LA, Bailey MA, Schan CA, Richter JE. Relaxation training reduces symptoms and acid exposure in patients with gastroesophageal reflux disease. Gastroenterology 1994; 107:61–69.
25. Drossman DA, McKee DC, Sandler RS, Mitchell Cm, Cramer EM, Lowman BC, Burger AL. Psychosocial factors in the irritable bowel syndrome: a multivariate study of patients and non-patients with irritable bowel syndrome. Gastroenterology 1988; 95:701–708.
26. Bradley LA, Alarcón GS, Triana M, Aaron LA, Alexander RW, Stewart KE, Martin M, Alberts K. Health care seeking behavior in fibromyalgia: associations with pain

thresholds, symptom severity, and psychiatric morbidity. J Musculoskel Pain 1994; 2:79–87.
27. Cameron L, Leventhal EA, Leventhal H. Symptom representations and affect as determinants of care seeking in a community-dwelling, adult sample population. Health Psychol 1993; 12:171–179.
28. Watson WC, Sullivan SN, Corke M, et al. Globus and headache: common symptoms of the irritable bowel syndrome. Can Med Assoc J 1978; 118:387–388.
29. Thompson WG, Heaton KW. Heartburn and globus in apparently healthy people. Can Med Assoc J 1892; 126:46–48.
30. Moloy PJ, Charter R. The globus symptom. Arch Otolaryngol 1982; 108:740–744.
31. Caldarelli DD, Andrews AH, Derbyshire AJ. Esophageal motility studies in globus sensation. Ann Otol Rhinol Laryngol 1970; 79:1098–1100.
32. Watson WC, Sullivan SN. Hypertoxicity of the cricopharyngeal sphincter: a cause of globus sensation. Lancet 1974; ii:1417–1419.
33. Wilson JA, Maran AGD, Pryde A, et al. Globus sensation is not due to gastroesophageal reflux. Clin Otolaryngol 1987; 12:271–275.
34. Lehtinen V, Puhakka H. A psychosomatic approach to the globus hystericus syndrome. Acta Psychiatr Scand 1976; 53:21–28.
35. Cook IJ, Dent J, Collins SM. Upper esophageal sphincter tone and reactivity to stress in patients with a history of globus sensation. Dig Dis Sci 1989; 34:672–676.
36. Wilson JA, Deary IJ, Maran AGD. Is globus hystericus? Br J Psychiatry 1988; 153:335–339.
37. Deary IJ, Wilson JA, Mitchell L, et al. Covert psychiatric disturbance in patients with globus pharyngis. Br J Med Psychol 1989; 62:381–389.
38. Wilson JA, Deary IJ, Mardon SL. Globus. Lancet 1989; ii:780.
39. A lump in the throat (editorial). Lancet 1989; i:534.
40. Brown SR, Schwartz JM, Summergrad P, et al. Globus hystericus syndrome responsive to antidepressants. Am J Psychiatry 1986; 143:917–918.
41. Onghena P, Van Houdenhove B. Antidepressant-induced analgesia in chronic nonmalignant pain: a meta-analysis of 39 placebo-controlled studies. Pain 1992; 49:205–219.
42. Haynes SN. Electromyographic biofeedback treatment of a woman with chronic dysphagia. Biofeedback Self-Reg 1976; 1:121–126.
43. Solzom L, Sookman D. Fear of choking and its treatment. Can J Psychiatry 1980; 25:30–34.
44. Holroyd KA, Andrasik F, Noble J. Comparison of EMG biofeedback and a credible pseudotherapy in treating tension headache. J Behav Med 1980; 3:29–39.
45. Clouse RE, Staiano A. Contraction abnormalities of the esophageal body in patients referred for manometry: a new approach to manometric classification. Dig Dis Sci 1983; 28:784–791.
46. Richter JE, Wu WC, Johns DN, et al. Esophageal manometry in 95 healthy adult volunteers: variability of pressures with age and frequency of "abnormal" contractions. Diag Dis Sci 1987; 35:583–592.
47. Richter JE, Bradley LA, Castell DO. Esophageal chest pain: current controversies in pathogenesis, diagnosis, and therapy. Ann Intern Med 1989; 110:66–78.

48. Vantrappen G, Hellemans J. Treatment of achalasia and related motor disorders. Gastroenterology 1980; 79:144–154.
49. Pope CE. Motor disorders. In: Sleisenger MH, Fordtran JS, eds. Gastrointestinal Disease: Pathophysiology Diagnosis, and Management. Philadelphia: Saundesr, 1983:424–448.
50. Shabsin HS, Katz PO, Schuster MM. Behavioral treatment of intractable chest pain in a patient with vigorous achalsia. Am J Gastroenterol 1988; 83:970–973.
51. Gillies M, Nicks R, Shyring A. Clinical, manometric and pathologic studies in diffuse esophageal spasm. Br Med J 1967; 2:527–530.
52. Kramer P, Fleshler B, McNally E, et al. Oesophageal sensitivity to mecholyl in symptomatic diffuse spasm. Gut 1967; 8:120–125.
53. Richter JE, Hackshaw BT, We WC, et al. Edrophonium: a useful provocative test for esophageal chest pain. Ann Intern Med 1985; 103:14–21.
54. Ouyang A, Reynold JC, Cohen S. Spike-associated and spike-independent esophageal contractions in patients with diffuse esophageal spasm. Gastroenterology 1983; 84:907–914.
55. Meyer GW, Castell DO. Human esophageal response during chest pain induced by swallowing cold liquids. JAMA 1981; 246:2057–2060.
56. Clouse RE, Lustman PJ. Psychiatric illness and contraction abnormalities of the esophagus. N Engl J Med 1983; 309:1337–1342.
57. Latimer P, Sarna S, Campbell D, et al. Colonic motor and myoelectrical activity: a comparative study of normal subjects, psychoneurotic patients, and patients with irritable bowel syndrome. Gastroenterology 1981; 80:893–901.
58. Magni G, Marchetti M, Moreschi C, Merskey H, Luchini SR. Chronic musculoskeletal pain and depressive symptoms in the National Health and Nutrition Examination. I. Epidemiologic follow-up study. Pain 1993; 53:163–168.
59. Aaron LA, Bradley LA, Alarcón GS, Alexander RW, Triana-Alexander M, Martin MY, Alberts KR. Psychiatric diagnoses are related to health care seeking behavior rather than illness in fibromyalgia. Arthritis Rheum 1995. In press.
60. Waterman DC, Dalton CB, Ott DJ, et al. Hypertensive lower esophageal sphincter: what does it mean? J Clin Gastroenterol 1989; 11:139–146.
61. Young LD, Richter JE, Anderson KO, et al. The effects of psychological and environmental stressors on peristaltic esophageal contractions in healthy volunteers. Psychophysiology 1987; 24:132–140.
62. Anderson KO, Dalton CB, Bradley LA, et al. Stress induces alteration of esophageal pressures in healthy volunteers and noncardiac chest pain patients. Dig Dis Sci 1989; 34:83–91.
63. Peters LJ, Maos LC, Petty D, et al. Spontaneous noncardiac chest pain: evaluation by 24-hour ambulatory esophageal motility and pH monitoring. Gastroenterology 1988; 94:878–886.
64. Clouse RE, Lustman PJ, Eckert TC, et al. Low-dose trazadone for symptomatic patients with esophageal contraction abnormalities: a double-blind, placebo-controlled trial. Gastroenterology 1987; 92:1027–1036.
65. Horton ML, Goff JS. Surgical treatment of nutcracker esophagus. Dig Dis Sci 1986; 31:878–883.

66. Traube M, Tummala V, Baue AE, et al. Surgical myotomy in patients with high-amplitude peristaltic esophageal contractions: manometric and clinical effects. Dig Dis Sci 1987; 32:16–21.
67. Latimer PR. Biofeedback and self-regulation in the treatment of diffuse esophageal spasm: a single-case study. Biofeedback Self-Reg 1981; 6:181–189.
68. Ward BW, Wu WC, Richter JE, et al. Long-term follow-up of symptomatic status of patients with non-cardiac chest pain: is diagnosis of esophageal etiology helpful? Am J Gastroenterol 1987; 82:215–218.
69. Richter JE, Bradley LA, Castell DO. Esophageal chest pain: current controversies in pathogenesis, diagnosis, and therapy. Ann Intern Med 1989; 110:66–78.
70. Katz PO, Dalton CB, Richter JE, et al. Esophageal testing in patients with non-cardiac chest pain or dysphagia: results of three years' experience with 1161 patients. Ann Intern Med 1987; 106:593–597.
71. Lee CA, Reynolds JC, Ouyang A, et al. Esophageal chest pain: value of high-dose provocative testing with ediophonium chloride in patients with normal esophageal manometries. Dig Dis Sci 1987; 32:682–688.
72. Hewson EG, Sinclair JW, Dalton CB, et al. Evaluation of 100 non-cardiac chest pain patients finds 24-hour pH study to be most useful diagnostic test. Gastroenterology 1990; 98:58A.
73. Janssens J, Vantrappen G, Ghillebert G. 24-hour recording of esophageal pressure and pH in patients with non-cardiac chest pain. Gastroenterology 1986; 90:1978–1984.
74. Barefoot JC, Beckham JC, Peterson BL, Haney TL, Williams RB. Measures of neuroticism and disease status in coronary angiography patients. J Consult Clin Psychol 1992; 60:127–132.
75. Bass C, Wade C. Chest pain with normal coronary arteries: a comparative study of psychiatric and social morbidity. Psychol Med 1984; 14:51–61.
76. Wielgosz AT, Earp J. Perceived vulnerability to serious heart disease and persistent pain in patients with minimal or no coronary disease. Psychosom Med 1986; 48:118–24.
77. Costa PT, Fleg JL, McCrae RR, et al. Neuroticism, coronary artery disease, and chest pain complaints: cross-sectional and longitudinal studies. Exp Aging Res 1982; 8:37–44.
78. Vitaliano PP, Katon W, Maiuro RD, et al. Coping in chest pain patients with and without psychiatric disorders. J Consult Clin Psychol 1989; 57:338–343.
79. Clouse RE. Psychiatric disorders in patients with esophageal disease. Med Clin North Am 1991; 75:1081–1096.
80. Beitman BD, Mukerji V, Lamberti JW, et al. Panic disorder in patients with chest pain and angiographically normal coronary arteries. Am J Cardiol 1989; 63:1399–1403.
81. Beitman BD, Basha I, Flaker G, et al. Atypical or nonanginal chest pain: panic disorder or coronary artery disease? Arch Intern Med 1987; 147:1548–1552.
82. Katon W, Hall ML, Russo J, et al. Chest pain: relationship of psychiatric illness to coronary arteriographic results. Am J Med 1988; 84:1–9.
83. Katon W, Egan K, Miller D. Chronic pain: lifetime psychiatric diagnoses and family history. Am J Psychiatry 1989; 142:1156–1160.

84. Ehlers A, Breuer P. Increased cardiac awareness in panic disorder. J Abnorm Psychol 1992; 101:371–382.
85. Beitman BD, Mukerji V, Kushner M, et al. Validating studies for panic disorder in patients with angiographically normal coronary arteries. Med Clin North Am 1991; 75:1143–1155.
86. Roy-Brynne PP, Schmidt P, Cannon RO, et al. Microvascular angina and panic disorder. Int J Psychiatry Med 1989; 19:315–325.
87. Bradley LA, Scarinci I, McDonald JE, Schan CA, Richter JE. Choice of psychiatric criteria affects relationship between non-cardiac chest pain (NCCP) and panic disorder (PD). Gastroenterology 1991; 100:A425.
88. Harford WV. Southwestern internal medicine conference. The syndrome of angina pectoris: role of visceral pain perception. Am J Med Sci 1994; 307:305–315.
89. Barish CF, Castell DO, Richter JE. Graded esophageal balloon distention: a new provocative test for noncardiac chest pain. Dig Dis Sci 1986; 31:1292–1298.
90. Richter JE, Barish CF, Castell DO. Abnormal sensory perception in patients with esophageal chest pain. Gastroenterology 1986; 91:845–852.
91. Clark WC. Pain sensitivity and the report of pain: an introduction to sensory decision theory. Anesthesiology 1974; 40:272–282.
92. Kvinesdal B, Molin J, Froland A, Gram LF. Imipramine treatment of painful diabetic neuropathy. JAMA 1984; 251:1727–1730.
93. Bradley LA, Richter JE, Sconici IC, Haile JE, Schon CA. Mechanisms of altered pain perception in non-cardiac chest pain patients. Gastroenterology 1993; 104:A482.
94. Castell DO. Evoked potentials and the irritable esophagus. In: Mayer EA, Raybould HE, eds. Basic and Clinical Aspects of Chronic Abdominal Pain. Amsterdam: Elsevier, 1993; 283–291.
95. Lenz FA, Gracely RH, Hope EJ, Baker FH, Rowland LH, Dougherty PM, Richardson RT. The sensation of angina can be evoked by stimulation of the human thalamus. Pain 1994; 59:119–125.
96. McDonald-Haile J, Bradley LA, Bailey MA, Mountz J, Deutsch G, Inampudi C, Richter JE. Low regional cerebral blood flow (rCBF) to caudate nuclei is associated with chest pain of undetermined etiology (CPUE). Gastroenterology 1994; 106:A1038.
97. Bradley LA, Haile JM, Jaworski TM. Assessment of psychological status by interviews and self-report instruments. In: Turk DC, Melzack R, eds. Handbook of Pain Assessment. New York: Guilford, 1992: 193–213.
98. Scarinci IC, Haile JM, Bradley LA, Richter JE. Altered pain perception and psychosocial features among women with gastrointestinal disorders and history of abuse: a preliminary model. Am J Med 1994, 97:108–118.
99. Drossman DA, Leserman J, Nachman G, Li ZM, Gluck H, Toomey TC. Sexual and physical abuse in women with functional or organic gastrointestinal disorders. Ann Intern Med 1990; 113:828–833.
100. Gupta PK, Stark MT, Maher KA, Cannon RO. Imipramine is superior to clonidine and placebo for amelioration of chest pain symptoms in patients enrolled in a double-blinded, two-drug, placebo controlled study in chest pain of undetermined etiology. Am J Gastroenterology 1992; 87:1248.
101. Beitman BD, Basha IM, Trombka LH, et al. Alprazolam in the treatment of cardiology patients with atypical chest pain and panic disorder. J Clin Psychopharmacol 1988; 8:127–130.
102. Committee on the Review of Medicines. Systematic review of the benzodiazepines. Br Med J 1980; 280:910–912.

103. Clum GA. Psychological interventions vs. drugs in the treatment of panic. Behav Ther 1989; 20:429–457.
104. Klimes I, Mayou RA, Pearce MJ, et al. Psychological treatment for atypical non-cardiac chest pain: a controlled evaluation. Psychol Med 1990; 20:605–611.
105. Keefe FJ, Van Horn Y. Cognitive-behavioral treatment of rheumatoid arthritis pain. Arthritis Care Res 1993; 6:213–222.

8

Functional Disorders of the Stomach and Duodenum

Kevin W. Olden
University of California, San Francisco
and St. Mary's Medical Center
San Francisco, California

I. INTRODUCTION

In the popular literature, the stomach is considered the "heart" of the gastrointestinal (GI) tract. Irrespective of where patients may actually have pathology, they are most likely to refer to a problem with "their stomach." Likewise, gastroenterologists are often referred to informally as "stomach specialists." The stomach is indeed a key organ of the GI tract, with a number of features that make it unique. First, it serves as a reservoir of ingested food. Second, it serves as a powerful crushing tool, using the high-amplitude contractions of the antrum to grind ingested food particles to less than 2 millimeters, thus creating chyme for processing in the small bowel. Third, the process of digestion begins with the stomach introducing hydrochloric acid and pepsinogen into the chyme.

Beyond these obvious physiological processes, the stomach has a number of more subtle but important functions. It has significant decision-making responsibility for ensuring the integrity of the digestive process. It is the stomach that initially assesses whether a substance is toxic and initiates a process to expel it, i.e., vomiting. Likewise, overindulgence, defined by the stomach as oral intake too great for the GI tract to handle safely, will also result in a decision to reject excess volume, again by the mechanism of vomiting. Finally, the sensation of hunger is mediated by a complex communication between the hypothalamus and the cerebral cortex of the brain. The enteric nervous system in turn influences the stomach through the action of a variety of excitatory and inhibitory neuropeptides in combination with input from the vagus nerve, which results in a pattern of gastric motility commonly referred to as "hunger pains."

The significant physiological responsibilities delegated to the stomach require that it have a sophisticated neurological capability to integrate input from the cerebral cortex, the thalamus and hypothalamus, and the chemoreceptor trigger zone. Utilizing this neurological division of labor, communication takes place via the enteric nervous system to influence gastric motility. The actual motility of the stomach is influenced by a complex interaction among a large number of inhibitory and prokinetic peptides (Table 1). The ability of the stomach to differentiate solids from liquids, large from small particles, and foods of high viscosity (e.g., fats) from those of low viscosity (e.g., sugars) requires significant afferent input to communicate to higher centers the volume, osmolality, and other characteristics of the ingested gastric contents. This interaction of input from the stomach to the brain results in a pattern of motility appropriate to gastric intraluminal conditions. Given the wide spectrum of nutrients presented to the stomach for digestion on a daily basis, the stomach and antroduodenum are required to possess an ever-changing pattern of motility. The stomach is well adapted to this task.

II. FUNCTIONAL ANATOMY

The stomach is divided into four distinct anatomical regions. First is the gastroesophageal junction, containing the lower esophageal sphincter and the gastric cardia. The proximal stomach tends not to display propulsive patterns of contrac-

Table 1 Neuropeptides Affecting Gastroduodenal Motility

Peptide	Effect
Cholecystokinin	Inhibitory; activates gastric sensory neurons
Gastrin	Trophic
Motilin	Trophic
Secretin	Inhibits gastric emptying
Somatostatin	Inhibits ACh release
Vasoactive inhibitory peptide	Reduces lower-esophageal-sphincter pressure

tion and serves mainly as a reservoir for ingested contents. Distally, this is followed by the fundus and body of the stomach. The division between the distal body and the beginning of the antrum is demarcated at the incisura angularis on the lesser curvature. Finally, there is the distal antrum and pylorus and proximal duodenum. This latter area functions in such a coordinated manner that the three components are collectively referred to as the "antroduodenal segment." To coordinate its complex physiological functions, the stomach has its own pacemaker. It is located in the midbody of the stomach along the greater curvature. This area generates action potentials, which in turn result in symmetrical anterograde contractions that mainly influence the distal portions of the stomach. Antral pacemaker action potentials are superimposed on the normal resting "slow-wave" (three cycles per minute) contractions of the gastric myocytes. The slow-wave depolarizations themselves are not associated with significant propulsive activity of the gastric musculature. However, in the distal antrum, slow-wave action potentials interact with the pacemaker-generated contractions to produce powerful sustained muscular contraction of the antroduodenum. These antral pacemaker potentials are generated three to four times per minute, and they propagate distally at approximately 4 centimers/second. This effect is not seen in the more proximal regions of the stomach, i.e., the body or fundus, consistent with the storate role of those parts of the stomach.

Normal antral motility is characterized by a three- to four-cycle-per-minute pattern of contractions. However, the pattern of contraction is cyclic, with intense bursts of activity occurring approximately every 90 to 120 minutes. These cycles of intense electrical activity resulting in high-amplitude contractions are termed the interdigestive migrating motor complex (MMC). The MMC consists of four phases, from a period of quiescence (phase I) to periods of increasing intense activity (phases II and III), followed by a transitional period of reorganization (phase IV) (Table 2). The MMC, although initiated in the stomach, moves transpylorically to migrate down the entire length of the small bowel. The MMC is extinguished by feeding. This process is induced partly by the presence of fats and carbohydrates in the bowel lumen itself. In addition, nutrients, as they enter the stomach, initiate the secretion of a variety of prokinetic peptides, including glucagon, cholecystokinin, and gastrin. These peptides, in turn, stimulate gastric and intraduodenal motility and also extinguish the MMC. Fi-

TABLE 2 Phases of the Migrating Motor Complex

Phase I	Slow-wave resting potentials; no muscular contraction
Phase II	Increasing frequency of irregular muscular contractions
Phase III	Maximal frequency of contractions
Phase IV	Decreasing frequency of contractions toward a phase I pattern

nally, the vagus nerve is stimulated by the presence of food in the stomach to increase cholinergic tone to the stomach and small bowel. The net result of the combined efforts of these multiple trophic stimuli is to produce a pattern of intense contraction and propulsive activity (1).

Disruptions in the basic physiology of the stomach can occur as a result of abnormalities of the gastric pacemaker or from the presence of ectopic pacemakers. Abnormalities in gastric pacemaker activity can result in antral slow waves occurring in as many as five to 10 cycles per minute. These hyperactive patterns of contraction are called *tachygastrias*. Likewise, decreased activity of the gastric pacemaker can result in fewer than three cycles of contractions per minute, or *bradygastrias*. Finally, discoordinated electrical activity of the gastric pacemaker can produce chaotic patterns of contraction (2).

Pacemaker-generated electrical activity can be measured by a variety of means, but the most common one uses silver/silver-chloride external recording electrodes on the abdominal wall over the stomach, resulting in an electrogastrogram (EGG). Disturbances of gastric rhythm have been associated with the nausea and vomiting of pregnancy (3) and non-ulcer dyspepsia (4,5). However, a large percentage of the patients who complain of chronic nausea, bloating, and dyspepsia do not have observable abnormalities of gastric motility (6). The inability to detect gastric motility disturbances in many patients presenting with functional GI complaints has led investigators to explore the epidemiological and psychosocial aspects of chronic nausea and vomiting of unclear etiology, non-ulcer dyspepsia, and upper-abdominal bloating. The best studied of these disorders, non-ulcer dyspepsia, can serve as a model for discussion.

III. NON-ULCER DYSPEPSIA

Dyspepsia is extremely common. Surveys done in both the United States and Europe show that, at any given time, 20–40% of the population meet the Rome diagnostic criteria for non-ulcer dyspepsia (NUD) (7,8). The highest prevalence rates, ranging from 16 to 54% of the population, have been reported in Europe (9,10). Lower rates, from 10 to 36%, have been reported in the United States. Dyspepsia complaints tend to decrease with age (9). Gender association is unclear, with some studies showing no gender differences while others show a greater prevalence in women (10).

Endoscopic studies have shown that more than 80% of patients who present with ulcer-like symptoms of abdominal pain, nausea, and food intolerance do not haev evidence of gastric or duodenal ulcers (11). This large group of patients can logically be labeled as having NUD. The nomenclature associated with NUD is not without its difficulties. Vague upper-abdominal symptoms such as chronic belching, abdominal pain, food intolerance, early satiety, and chronic nausea and vomiting, as well as symptoms of pyrosis and occasional regurgitation of food, all fall under the umbrella of NUD. NUD is defined as a pattern of upper-abdominal discomfort above the umbilicus and below the xiphisternum that appears in the absence of known peptic ulcer disease. Dyspepsia has been classified as follows: *ulcer-like dyspepsia*, consisting of symptoms extremely suggestive of peptic ulcer disease but in the absence of ulcers; *dysmotility-like dyspepsia*, which is commonly associated with bloating, belching, postprandial fullness, nausea, vomiting, and early satiety; and *reflux-like dyspepsia*, the sensation of pyrosis and other symptoms of gastroesophageal reflux in patients who do not have endoscopic or other evidence of esophagitis, often accompanied by a predominant complaint of upper-abdominal discomfort.

However, the clinical utility of these dyspepsia subgroups has yet to be demonstrated. Talley et al. (12) evaluated 820 consecutive patients presenting for endoscopy. Forty-six GI symptoms were measured. Seventeen percent of patients had ulcer-like dyspepsia; 9%, dysmotility-like dyspepsia; and 16%, reflux-like dyspepsia. However, 31% fell into two or more symptom groups, and 27% had symptoms that were nonspecific. When patients with and without functional dyspepsia were compared, lower age, female gender, frequent upper-abdominal pain, lack of symptom relief with antacids, and infrequent vomiting were predictors of functional dyspepsia. Dyspepsia subgroups were poor discriminators of functional disorders compared to other GI diagnoses.

The vague nature of these symptoms presents a significant diagnostic as well as nomenclatural challenge. An attempt at developing a rational system to categorize these symptom complexes, for both clinicians and investigators, has been undertaken by the international working teams of the World Congress of Gastroenterology (13). The proposed classifications have not been fully validated. However, even in their preliminary form, they serve a valuable role in providing a common point of reference for studying patients in clinical trials.

Crean and coworkers (14) studied 1540 patients who were evaluated for complaints of dyspepsia in a regional hospital in Glasgow, Scotland. Patients were screened for the presence of duodenal ulcer, functional dyspepsia, and irritable bowel syndrome. Duodenal ulcer was identified as the most common source of pain in 26% of the patients, followed by functional dyspepsia (22%). Fifteen percent of the patients were found to suffer from irritable bowel syndrome. The study also found that 31% of patients met the criteria for two of the three possible diagnoses, and 6% met the criteria for all three. Where multiple diagnoses were found together, functional disorders, including functional dyspepsia and irritable bowel syndrome, together accounted for 39% of all diagnoses. However, the lack of a consensus definition of functional disorders may have overstated their prevalence. NUD has commonly been associated with a variety of other functional and organic conditions separate from peptic ulcer disease. These disorders include gastroesophageal reflux disease, aerophagy (swallowing air out of proportion to what is considered normal swallowing), biliary tract disease, including gallstones and sphincter of Oddi dysfunction, and chronic pancreatitis (15).

The workup for dyspepsia is straightforward. The American College of Physicians Committee on Health and Public Policy has recommended that, in the absence of cardinal symptoms of GI malignancy or complicated ulcer disease, patients should be empirically treated with antacids or H_2 blockers. Patients who fail to improve within 4 to 6 weeks on this regimen should undergo upper endoscopy (11). Studies have shown that evaluations beyond endoscopy are not likely to lead to other diagnostic possibilities (16).

A. NUD, Gastritis, and *Helicobacter pylori*

One of the most recent developments in gastroenterology has been the discovery of the strong association between *Helicobacter pylori* and the development of chronic gastritis and peptic ulcer disease. Contemporary classifications of gastritis include type A gastritis, associated with autoimmune conditions such as pernicious anemia, and type B gastritis, associated with an environmental factor such as *H. pylori* infection. Type A gastritis involves the fundus and body of the stomach but not the antrum. It is associated with a histamine-fast achlorhydria, hypergastrinemia, and vitamin B_{12} malabsorption. This autoimmune disease is also associated with parietal cell antibodies along with antibodies to intrinsic factor in 90% of patients. Type B gastritis, on the other hand, usually involves the antrum without extension in the body and fundus. It is associated with normal acid secretion, normal serum gastrin levels, and normal absorption of vitamin B_{12}. It is not associated with antibodies to intrinsic factor or parietal cells. It is type B gastritis that is often seen with *H. pylori* infection (17). Rates of *H. pylori* infection are extremely high in Western countries; about 10% to 20% of people in their 20s are infected, gradually increasing to 50% at age 60. The incidence is higher in people with lower socioeconomic backgrounds, particularly in the developing world. Studies from South America have demonstrated an incidence of *H. pylori* antibodies in 70–87% of patients who are 20 years old (18). The high prevalence of *H. pylori* infection and its role in the etiology of chronic type B gastritis have led to investigation of *H. pylori* as a possible cause of the symptoms of NUD.

Tucci and colleagues (19) evaluated 45 consecutive patients with chronic idiopathic dyspepsia in whom gastroduodenoscopy showed no evidence of any focal lesions. Symptoms included postprandial fullness, nausea, vomiting, and epigastric pain or burning. *H. pylori* was found in 60% of the dyspeptic group and 30% of controls. Among those infected with *H. pylori*, 89% of the dyspeptic patients and 80% of controls had histological evidence of chronic gastritis, almost exclusively in the antrum. Gastric acid output, both basally and maximally stimulated, was normal in both groups, with no significant differences. Gastric-emptying studies revealed significantly longer emptying times in dyspeptic patients. The proportion of infected patients with delayed gastric emptying (33%) was the same as that among nondyspeptic controls (33%) but significantly lower among patients with normal gastric emptying (78%). Tucci concluded that there were two main subtypes of dyspeptic patients. Patients with one type had *H. pylori* infection with no gender specificity and generally normal gastric emptying, and their main symptom was epigastric pain or burning. The second type included patients with delayed gastric emptying and was associated with female gender and lower age. In this group, *H. pylori* infection was relatively uncommon, and postprandial fullness was the major symptom of dyspepsia.

Frazzoni et al. (20) investigated 53 patients with dyspeptic complaints who had normal upper endoscopies. Patients were randomized in a placebo-controlled double-blind manner to either anti–*H. pylori* therapy consisting of colloidal bismuth subscitrate plus metronidazole or placebo (20 patients). Patients who had normal antral mucosa and who were *H. pylori*–negative were randomized to receive either cisapride or placebo (28 patients). There was no significant difference in the mean symptom scores between *H. pylori*–positive and –negative patients prior to the treatment intervention. Both treatment groups achieved significant improvement of symptoms. Mean symptom scores after treatment did not differ significantly between the *H. pylori*–positive and –negative groups.

A significant eradication rate of *H. pylori* and reduction in the gastritis score compared to that in the pretreatment biopsy were documented. However, symptom improvement, judged by patients' self-reports, was equivalent to that obtained by placebo, despite the fact that the placebo regimen clearly did not affect *H. pylori*–infection status. One patient in the treatment group and all 12 *H. pylori*–positive patients in the placebo group experienced symptom remission. Frazzoni and colleagues concluded that duodenal bulb and antral biopsies did not prove useful in the management of dyspeptic patients with normal endoscopic findings. They did not find any correlation between *H. pylori* eradication and symptom improvement.

The possibility that *H. pylori* infection could induce GI motility disorders and subsequently contribute to NUD-like symptoms was investigated by Pieramico and colleagues (21). In a study of 46 patients with endoscopy-negative dyspepsia symptoms, no difference, either qualitative or quantitative, in symptom scores between *H. pylori*–positive and negative subgroups was found. Eighteen patients (39%) had chronic gastritis and were *H. pylori*–positive. Analysis of motility tracings showed impaired antral motility in the postprandial state in approximately half the patients with NUD. Antral hypomotility was observed in two-thirds of the patients who were *H. pylori*–negative and in one-third of the patients who were positive. Neither duration nor the individual phases of the migrating motor complex were changed in the NUD patients. Postprandial antral hypomotility was probably present in a subset of patients with NUD. Antral motility was impaired in NUD without regard to the presence of *H. pylori* infection. Chronic active gastritis resulting from *H. pylori* infection played no causal role in either the postprandial antral motility disorders or symptoms of NUD.

Subsequent studies have also found that dyspepsia was equally common among both *H. pylori*–positive and –negative patients (22). In a comprehensive review of the literature from 1983 to 1992 on *H. pylori* and its relationship to duodenal ulcer, gastric ulcer, and NUD, Veldhuyzen van Zanten and Sherman (23) found that the literature was unequivocal in establishing a strong causal relationship between *H. pylori* infection and gastritis and duodenal ulcer, but only a moderate association with gastric ulcer. There was no evidence to support a causal relationship between *H. pylori* infection and NUD.

Some of the supporting evidence for *H. pylori* as a possible cause of functional dyspepsia has come from treatment trials. A number of trials have been performed over the years in which patients treated for *H. pylori* subsequently "improved." However, in an extensive review of 16 trials published between 1984 and 1993, Talley (24) noted that, of studies that reported positive results from *H. pylori* eradication, eight failed to detect a statistically significant benefit from treatment. Moreover, Talley noted that numerous design flaws existed in these studies, including failure to randomize patients, absence of a placebo control arm, lack of an adequate definition of dyspepsia, and inclusion of patients whose only symptoms were of gastroesophageal reflux. Studies also failed to accurately assess the effects of patient compliance, lack of posttherapy follow-up, and inadequate study power. Therefore, no one type of pharmacological intervention for NUD can be recommended as having benefits over others.

B. Psychosocial Correlates of NUD

Given the lack of correlation with structurally based GI disorders, a number of investigators have explored the biopsychosocial correlates of NUD-like symptoms. Talley and Jones (25) compared 109 consecutive patients who presented to a university endoscopy service with NUD-like symptoms to the same number of randomly selected, sociodemographically matched controls from th e general community who had no GI complaint. Study patients had a mean of 8 years of dyspepsia, and none reported the onset of dyspepsia prior to 15 years of age. The dyspeptic patients had a significantly lower occupational status, and they were more apt to report an unhappy childhood, as assessed by a simple but validated measure in which patients were asked directly, "Did you have a happy childhood?" However, there were no significant differences between dyspeptics and controls in marital status, family stability, age at separation of parent, number of siblings, or migration. The investigators concluded that developmental history—

specifically, events in early childhood—played only a small role in the development of "essential dyspepsia."

However, recent studies have suggested a correlation between sexual and physical abuse and development of a functional GI disorder. Drossman et al. (26) found a 46% prevalence of such abuse in women seen for functional GI complaints. Similar studies have confirmed this finding (27,28). To investigate the possible relationship between abuse history and prevalence of functional dyspepsia, Talley subsequently surveyed 919 people in a community sample. Twenty-seven percent of respondents reported sexual, physical, verbal, or emotional abuse. When the data were adjusted to exclude irritable bowel syndrome by logistic regression analysis, Talley demonstrated an association between abuse, including verbal, emotional, physical, and sexual abuse, occurring during childhood or adulthood and development of functional dyspepsia (53).

To determine the prevalence of psychiatric comorbidity in dyspepsia, Magni and colleagues (29) compared 30 patients with dyspepsia of unknown origin to 20 patients with structural lesions as determined by upper endoscopy. In patients with dyspepsia of unknown origin, an 87% prevalence of axis I psychiatric disorders was found. Generalized anxiety disorder was most common, followed by simple phobia, atypical anxiety disorder, hypochondriasis, and adjustment disorder with anxious mood. Only one dyspeptic patient was diagnosed with an axis II diagnosis, histrionic personality disorder. The differences between the dyspepsia and organic groups were statistically significant for all psychiatric diagnoses.

Talley and colleagues (30) also investigated the relationship between psychosocial variables and NUD. Seventy-six patients with "essential dyspepsia" were compared to a sociodemographically matched dyspepsia-free community sample of controls. Dyspeptic patients were more prone to anxiety as measured by the Costello-Comrey Personality Questionnaire, and transient feelings of anxiety related to an acute situation (*state anxiety*) and chronic anxiety experienced in a more constitutional way (*trait anxiety*) as measured by the Spielberger State-Trait Anxiety Scale. Depression, evaluated by the Beck Depression Inventory, was elevated in the dyspeptic group compared with controls. In patients with peptic ulcer disease, the level of anxiety was the same in NUD patients and those with documented peptic ulcer disease. Depression levels were elevated in a similar way in both groups. These elevations were statistically significant for both the anxiety and the depression diagnoses. Lower socioeconomic status in both dyspeptic and control groups was associated with excess levels of depression and anxiety. No statistically significant differences were seen in depression and anxiety ratings when the subjects were retested about 4 months later. Talley concluded that patients with essential dyspepsia and duodenal ulcer showed similar levels of anxiety and depression, and that they had significantly more anxiety, neuroticism, and depression than did controls. The psychological scores did not vary over time and were not affected by change in the patients' symptom status.

To better evaluate the effect of major life events as possible sources of stress-induced dyspepsia, Talley and Piper (31) compared 290 consecutive outpatients with dyspepsia to sociodemographically matched controls from the general community. Subjects were administered the Holmes and Rahe Scale, which measures intensity of life changes, and the Paykel Life Change Scale, which measures the number of life events, level of distress, or overall life change. Only patients with evidence of gastritis or duodenitis visible on endoscopy differed significantly from controls in the total life change scores as measured by the Paykel Life Change Scale. This study did not support the hypothesis that there was a relationship between major life events or life changes and the development of functional dyspepsia.

The reasons for an excess prevalence of anxiety, neuroticism, and depression in patients with NUD remain poorly understood. It is not clear how emotional distress can generate dyspeptic symptoms. To investigate this relationship, Camilleri and coworkers (32) performed an experimental study of 16 patients with functional dyspepsia, defined as the presence of two or more symptoms, including epigastric pain, early satiety, postprandial bloating, nausea, vomiting, and regurgitation. The purpose of this experimental design was to assess the integrity of the systemic autonomic response as measured by heart rate, blood pressure, and skin conductance; the release of presumed hormonal mediators of stress (β-endorphins and catecholamines); and the sensitivity of the gastric antrum to experimental stress induced by transcutaneous electrical stimulation (TENS). No statistically significant difference was found between dyspeptics and healthy volunteers in the pattern of antral motility, although both groups experienced antral hypomotility in response to the stress. Finally, there were no differences in baseline blood pressure, heart rate, skin conductance, or plasma levels of β-endorphins and catecholamines. This study suggested that the neural pathways from the brain to the stomach in patients with functional dyspepsia were not abnormal, and they responded to acute artificial stress in a manner similar to that of normal controls.

Haug and coworkers (33) explored the relationship between vagal activity and its possible role as a mediating mechanism between psychological factors, antral dysmotility, and dyspeptic symptoms in patients with functional dyspepsia. They performed an experimental study of 21 patients with functional dyspepsia whose symptoms had been present for at least 3 months prior to entry into the study. Fifty-two percent of dyspeptic symptoms could be explained by an "inclusive analytic model which described state measurements of responsiveness rather than individual personality trait scores." After an experimental stressor was applied, this same inclusive model was able to correlate personality factors, as well as state measurements associated with changes in antral motility. Antral hypomotility was correlated with high neuroticism scores on the Eysenck Personality Questionnaire. Individuals with higher scores of neuroticism and other psychopathological traits were more likely to experience changes in vagal tone, which had an impact on antral motility. This effect became more pronounced during times of stress and, in turn, affected the patient's complaint of dyspepsia. Thus, a patient's psychological makeup appeared to play a role in the etiology of dyspeptic symptoms, and superimposed stress could further exacerbate that tendency. While these studies show that there is an intriguing association among neuroticism, complaints of NUD-like symptoms, and changes in motility, the exact nature of this relationship remains ill-defined.

C. Treatment of NUD

A wide variety of pharmacological agents have been evaluated in the treatment of NUD. These include motility agents that affect acid secretion and agents that interact with dopamine, erotonin, and other receptors. There are a number of difficulties associated with conducting drug treatment trials in NUD. First is the lack of a common terminology for diagnosing NUD. The poor correlation of symptoms and pathophysiology and the presence of multiple GI conditions that could give rise to NUD-like symptoms, such as gastric dysrhythmias or GERD, also complicate case inclusion for a treatment trial. Finally, the high correlation of psychiatric disorders and the tendency of NUD symptoms to spontaneously improve over time (34) make findings on outcomes subject to suspicion.

Kellow and colleagues (35) studied 61 dyspeptic patients in a double-blind trial of cisapride, which acts by stimulating the release of acetylcholine from the myenteric cholinergic nerves. It also interacts with serotonin receptors. Kellow recorded global evaluations of symptoms by both investigators and patients in a blinded manner both before and after treatment. There was no statistical difference between the treatment and placebo groups in symptom scores. However, the results suggested that there was a beneficial effect of cisapride over placebo in patients with "reflux-like dyspepsia." Motility agents such as cisapride, as well as the dopamine antagonists domperidone and metoclopramide, have all shown some value in NUD, particularly in patients with dysmotility-like dyspepsia (36–39).

Arienti et al. (40) studied 30 patients treated with the antiemetic agent levosulpiride compared to placebo in a randomized double-blind study. Levosulpiride affects both the central and peripheral nervous systems. Its effect is exerted at the pre- and postsynaptic DA_2 dopaminergic receptors, in both the submucosal and myenteric plexus. Arienti found that levosulpiride reduced dyspeptic symptoms significantly in the dyspeptic group over controls. No correlation was found between gastric emptying of either liquids or solids and dyspeptic symptoms assessed by symptom score. Arienti concluded that levosulpiride offered some benefit to patients with functional dyspepsia. However, the exact mechanism for this benefit remains unclear.

Loxiglumide, a cholecystokinin (CCK) antagonist, has been studied in patients with NUD and delayed gastric emptying. Li Bassi and colleagues (41) demonstrated the ability of loxiglumide to improve solid–liquid gastric emptying in patients with NUD. However, the prokinetic effect of loxiglumide has not been confirmed by other investigators (42).

The selective muscarinic antagonist pirenzepine, which selectively bonds to the M_1 muscarinic receptor, has been evaluated in NUD. In one study (43), pirenzepine produced improvement in symptoms in approximately one-quarter of dyspeptic patients, but its usefulness is limited by its significant side-effect profile. The synthetic prostaglandin misoprostol's usefulness in NUD is also severely limited by its side-effect profile, which actually tends to worsen symptoms in NUD patients (44).

Given the high prevalence of psychiatric comorbidity associated with NUD, one might expect a role for anxiolytic and antidepressant medications. However, the ability of benzodiazepines and tricyclic antidepressants to decrease lower-esophageal-sphincter pressure makes them unsuitable for patients with reflux-like dyspepsia. Likewise, the tendency of benzodiazepines and tricyclic antidepressants to retard gastric emptying makes them less than desirable in patients with NUD-related slow gastric emptying. The selective serotonin reuptake inhibitors (SSRIs) have a strong tendency to induce nausea and vomiting. This effect makes them less than ideal for NUD patients. Despite the potential advantages of prescribing psychiatric medications, no randomized controlled trials have been conducted to study the effects of psychotropic medications on NUD.

Studies of other agents have, by and large, been disappointing. Studies with prostaglandin analogs; somatostatin analogs; cholecystokinin antagonists; and macrolides such as erythromycin, anticholinergics, sucralfate, and ondansetron, a serotonin type 3 receptor antagonist, have shown no benefit (45). In one trial, gonadotropin-releasing hormone analogs such as leuprolide significantly improved symptom scores over a 3-month period (46). Fedotozine, a kappa opioid receptor agonist, was found in a large trial to be superior to placebo in reducing dyspeptic symptoms (47,48). The literature on antisecretory agents, i.e., H_2 blockers, and proton pump inhibitors has failed to show any consistent benefit (49). Lastly, antacids have been shown to be no better than placebo in randomized control trials (50).

Clearly, the medical management of nonulcer dyspepsia is still evolving. Significant difficulties with the design of trials, particularly with inclusion criteria, symptom scoring, and outcome measures, hamper this research. Likewise, the approach to patients who have significant psychosocial problems in combination with their dyspeptic symptoms needs better definition. Psychotherapy, particularly cognitive-based therapy, has been shown to be useful in the treatment of irritable bowel syndrome (51,52). The literature on the use of behavioral interventions in NUD is scant. although one recent study (54) demonstrated improvement in both psychological and GI symptoms in patients receiving 4 months of cognitive psychotherapy, compared to a control group that received only telephone follow-up. The promising literature demonstrating the efficacy of psychotherapy in IBS does suggest the possible applicability of this model to the treatment of NUD. Clearly, NUD is a common disorder that continues to be a diagnostic and therapeutic challenge and provides a fruitful arena for research.

REFERENCES

1. Meyer JH. Motility of the stomach and gastroduodenal junction. In: Johnson LR, ed. Physiology of the Gastrointestinal Tract. 2nd ed. New York: Raven Press, 1987.
2. Hall KE, El-Sharkey T, Diamant NE. Vagal control of postprandial upper gastrointestinal motility. Am J Physiol 1986; 250:G501–G510.
3. Koch KL, Stern RM, Vasey MW, et al. Gastric dysrhythmias and nausea of pregnancy. Dig Dis Sci 1990; 35:961–968.
4. You CH, Lee KY, Chey WY, et al. Electrogastrographic study of patients with unexplained nausea, bloating and vomiting. Gastroenterology 1980; 79:311–314.
5. You CH, Chey WY, Lee KY, et al. Gastric and small intestinal myoelectrical dysrhythmia associated with chronic intractable nausea and vomiting. Ann Intern Med 1981; 95:449–451.
6. Cucchiara S, Riezzo G, Minella R, et al. Electrogastrography in non-ulcer dyspepsia. Arch Dis Childhood 1992; 67:613–617.
7. Mitchell CM, Drossman DA. Survey of the AGA membership relating to patients with functional gastrointestinal disorders. Gastroenterology 1987; 92:1282–1284.
8. Krag E. Non-ulcer dyspepsia introduction: epidemiological data. Scand J Gastroenterol 1982; 79:608.
9. Tibblin G. Introduction to the epidemiology of dyspepsia. Scand J Gastroenterol 1985; 20(suppl 109):29–33.
10. Agreus L, Svardsudd K, Tibblin G, et al. The epidemiology of dyspepsia: symptom clusters and demographic characteristics (abstr). Gastroenterology 1991; A1.
11. Health and Public Policy Committee, American College of Physicians. Endoscopy in the evaluation of dyspepsia. Ann Intern Med 1985; 102:266–269.
12. Talley NJ, Weaver AL, Tesmer DL, et al. Lack of discriminant value of dyspepsia subgroups in patients referred for upper endoscopy. Gastroenterology 1993; 105:1378–1386.
13. Talley NJ, Colin-Jones DG, Koch KL, et al. Functional dyspepsia: a classification with guidelines for diagnosis and management. Gastroenterol Int 1991; 4:145–160.
14. Crean GP, Holden RJ, Knill-Jones RP. A database on dyspepsia. Gut 1994; 35:191–202.
15. Talley NJ, Phillips SF. Non-ulcer dyspepsia: potential causes and pathophysiology. Ann Intern Med 1988; 108:865–879.

16. Vatn MH, Fausa O, Gjone E. Diagnostic value of gastrointestinal endoscopy in patients with uncharacteristic abdominal disorders. Scand J Gastroenterol 1985; 20:636–640.
17. Desai HG, Amarapurkar Dn. New look at chronic gastritis. J Clin Gastroenterol 1992; 14:278–280.
18. Dooley CP, Cohen H, Fitzgibbons PL, et al. Prevalence of *Helicobacter pylori* infection and histologic gastritis in asymptomatic persons. N Engl J Med 1989; 321:1562.
19. Tucci A, Corinaldesi R, Stanghellini CT, et al. *Helicobacter pylori* infection and gastric function in patients with chronic idiopathic dyspepsia. Gastroenterology 1992; 103:768–774.
20. Frazzoni M, Lonardo A, Grisenndi A, Della Casa G, Pulvirenti M, Ferrari AM, et al. Are routine duodenal and antral biopsies useful in the management of functional dyspepsia? A diagnostic and therapeutic study. J Clin Gastroenterol 1993; 17:101–108.
21. Pieramico O, Ditschuneit H, Malfertheiner P. Gastrointestinal motility in patients with non-ulcer dyspepsia: a role for *Helicobacter pylori* infection? Am J Gastroenterol 1993; 88:364–368.
22. McQuaid KR. Endoscopy-negative dyspepsia: hold those forceps! J Clin Gastroenterol 1993; 17:97–100.
23. Veldhuyzen van Zanten SJ, Sherman PM. *Helicobacter pylori* and duodenal ulcer, gastric cancer, and nonulcer dyspepsia: a review. Can Med Assoc J 1994; 150:189–198.
24. Talley NJ. A critique of therapeutic trials in *Helicobacter pylori*–positive functional dyspepsia. Gastroenterology 1994; 106:1174–1183.
25. Talley NJ, Jones M. Psychosocial and childhood factors in essential dyspepsia. Scand J Gastroenterol 1988; 23:341–346.
26. Drossman DA, Leserman J, N achman G, et al. Sexual and physical abuse in women with functional or organic gastrointestinal disorders. Ann Intern Med 1990; 113:828–833.
27. Arnold R, Rogers D, Cook D. Medical problems of adults who were sexually abused in childhood. Br Med J 1990; 300:705–708.
28. Walker EA, Katon Wj, Harrop-Griffiths J, et al. Relationship of chronic pelvic pain to psychiatric diagnoses and childhood sexual abuse. Am J Psychiatry 1988; 145:75–80.
29. Magni G, DiMario F, Bernasconi G, et al. DSM-III diagnoses associated with dyspepsia of unknown cause. Am J Psychiatry 1987; 144:1222–1223.
30. Talley NJ, Fung LH, Gilligan I, et al. Association of anxiety, neuroticism and depression with dyspepsia of unknown cause: a case-control study. Gastroenterology 1986; 90:886–892.
31. Talley NJ, Piper DW. Major life event stress and dyspepsia of unknown cause: a case control study. Gut 1986; 27:127–134.
32. Camilleri M, Malagelada JR, Kao PC, et al. Gastric and autonomic responses to stress in functional dyspepsia. Dig Dis Sci 1986; 31:1169–1177.
33. Haug TT, Svebak S, Hausken T, et al. Low vagal activity as mediating mechanism

for the relationship between personality factors and gastric symptoms in functional dyspepsia. Psychosom Med 1994; 56:181–186.
34. Talley NJ, McNeil D, Hayden A, et al. Prognosis of chronic unexplained dyspepsia. Gastroenterology 1987; 92:1060–1066.
35. Kellow JE, Cowan H, Shuter B, et al. Effiacy of cisapride therapy in functional dyspepsia. Aliment Pharmacol Ther 1995; 9:153–160.
36. Bradette M, Pare P, Douville P, et al. Visceral perception in health and functional dyspepsia: crossover study of gastric distensions with placebo and domperidone. Dig Dis Sci 1991; 36:52–58.
37. Talley NJ, Drug treatment of functional dyspepsia. Scand J Gastroenterol 1991; 26:47–60.
38. Van Outryve M, De Nutte N, Van Eeghem P, et al. Efficacy of cisapride in functional dyspepsia resistant to domperidone or metoclopramide: a double-blind, placebo-controlled study. Scand J Gastroenterol 1993; suppl 195:47–52.
39. Jian R, Ducrot F, Ruskone A, et al. Symptomatic radionuclide and therapeutic assessment of chronic idiopathic dyspepsia: a double-blind placebo-controlled evaluation of cisapride. Dig Dis Sci 1989; 34:657–664.
40. Arienti V, Corazza GR, Sorge M, et al. The effects of levosulpiride on gastric and gall-bladder emptying in functional dyspepsia. Aliment Pharmacol Ther 1994; 8:631–638.
41. Li Bassi S, Rovati LC, Giacovelli G, et al. Effects of loxiglumide, a cholecystokinin antagonist, in non-ulcer dyspepsia (abstr). Gastroenterology 1990; 98:77A.
42. Corazziari E, Ricci R, Biliotti D, et al. Oral administration of loxiglumide (CCK antagonist) inhibits postprandial gallbladder contraction without affecting gastric emptying. Dig Dis Sci 1990; 35:50–54.
43. Dobrilla G, Comberlato M, Steele a, et al. Drug treatment of functional dyspepsia: a met-analysis of randomized controlled clinical trials. J Clin Gastroenterol 1989; 11:169–177.
44. Hausken T, Stene-Larsen G, Lange O, et al. Misoprostol treatment exacerbates abdominal discomfort in patients with non-ulcer dyspepsia and erosive prepyloric changes: a double-blind placebo-controlled multicentre study. Scand J Gastroenterol 1990; 25:1028–1033.
45. Gudjonsson H, Oddsson E, Bjornsson S, et al. Efficacy of sucralfate in treatment of non-ulcer dyspepsia: a double-blind placebo-controlled study. Scand J Gastroenterol 1993; 28:969–972.
46. Mathias JR, Clench MH, Reeves-Darby VG, et al. Effect of leuprolide acetate in patients with moderate to severe functional bowel disease. Dig Dis Sci 1994; 39:1155–1162.
47. Fraitag B, Homerin M, Hecketseiler P. Double-blind dose-response multicenter comparison of fedotozine and placebo in treatment of nonulcer dyspepsia. Dig Dis Sci 1994; 39:1072–1077.
48. Galmiche JP, de Meynard C, Abitbol JL, et al. Effects of fedotozine in chronic idiopathic dyspepsia: a double blind, placebo controlled multicentre study (abstr). Gastroenterology 1994; 106:A502.
49. Stanghellini V, Malagelada JR, Zinsmeister AR, et al. Stress-induced gastroduode-

nal motor disturbances in humans: possible humoral mechanisms. Gastroenterology 1983; 85:83–91.
50. Talley NJ. Drug treatment of functional dyspepsia. Scand J Gastroenterol 1991; 26:47–60.
51. Guthrie E, Creed FH, Dawson D, et al. A controlled trial of psychological treatment for the irritable bowel syndrome. Gastroenterology 1991; 100:450–457.
52. Guthrie E, Creed FH, Dawson D, et al. A randomised controlled trial of psychotherapy in patients with refractory irritable bowel syndrome. Br J Psychiatry 1993; 163:315–321.
53. Talley NJ, Fett SL, Zinmeister AR, et al. Gastrointestinal tract symptoms and self-reported abuse: a population based study. Gastroenterology 1994; 107:1040–1049.
54. Haug TT, Wilhelmsen I, Svebak S, et al. Psychotherapy in functional dyspepsia. J Psychosom Res 1994; 38(7):735–744.

9

Irritable Bowel Syndrome

Douglas A. Drossman
University of North Carolina at Chapel Hill
Chapel Hill, North Carolina

I. DEFINITION

The irritable bowel syndrome (IBS) is the most common GI disorder seen by primary-care physicians and specialists in gastroenterology and psychiatry. It is classified as a functional bowel disorder (see Chapter 30), since the symptoms relate to disturbances in intestinal motility or sensation. It is also considered the prototype of the functional GI disorders; most of the scientific literature on these disorders involves study of IBS.

IBS is characterized by symptoms of pain and disturbed defecation (diarrhea or constipation) and/or symptoms of bloatedness and distension (1,2). In addition, there should be no biochemical or pathological evidence of other disease to explain these symptoms. Management of patients with IBS is challenging, since objective diagnostic criteria and specific treatment do not exist. This chapter summarizes the epidemiological, physiological, and psychological features of the disorder, presents the ("Rome") criteria for diagnosis, and reviews current treatment approaches (3).

II. EPIDEMIOLOGY

In Western countries, 10–20% of persons suffer from IBS, and most (>60%) do not seek medical attention (4–7). Of those who do visit physicians, 75–80% are female. However, this may be influenced by cultural factors; in India, where men see physicians more often in general, the ratio is reversed (8). The disorder has been reported to comprise 12% of family practice and 28% of gastroenterology practice (9).

III. PATHOPHYSIOLOGICAL BASIS OF SYMPTOMS

Research to date suggests that physical or psychological stimuli produce motility changes and altered bowel patterns in healthy subjects and IBS patients. In other words, there is no specific stimulus or response pattern characteristic for IBS. However, IBS patients differ from normal subjects by having an increased motility response in the large and small intestine and increased symptoms to various stimuli (e.g., food, pentagastrin, CCK, rectal distension, physical/psychological stress) (3,10). In other words, patients appear to overrespond to factors that normally affect intestinal function. A variety of biological factors (altered myoelectric activity, neurotransmitters, gut opiate receptors, etc.) may predispose this increased motor reactivity to stimuli.

In addition, IBS patients have a lower sensation threshold and pain tolerance (11–13). They perceive stimuli sooner and, qualitatively, report different symptoms (14). This increased sensitivity (visceral sensitivity hypothesis) helps explain why patients report pain symptoms even when intestinal motility is not abnormally increased.

It is now believed that IBS and other functional GI disorders are caused by dysregulation of central-enteric nervous system pathways (the “brain–gut axis”) (15), enhancement of nociceptive activity in the myenteric plexus (16), or both (17). The richly innervated nerve plexes and neuroendocrine associations in the enteric nervous system, and certain brain centers (18, 19) such as the locus coeruleus (20), are the “hard wiring” that associate psychological distress with intestinal dysfunction. Furthermore, the peptide neurotransmitters (e.g, substance P, calcitonin gene–related polypeptide, and the enkephalins), found in the gut and brain, are the modulators that affect pain perception, intestinal function, and behavior (21).

IV. PSYCHOSOCIAL EFFECTS ON SYMPTOM-REPORTING AND HEALTH OUTCOME

Acute stress can lead to an increased frequency of reporting of bowel symptoms, and this has been reported by college students (5) and survivors of the Holocaust (22). Furthermore, patients with IBS who are seen in referral practices exhibit more psychosocial disturbances [life stress (23), psychiatric diagnoses (24), abuse histories (25) illness behaviors (26,27), and abnormal personality patterns (28)] than healthy or medical comparison groups. However, these disturbances do not relate to the disorder per se. Recent evidence indicates that most individuals with IBS are not psychologically different from normals (28, 29). However, psychosocial factors strongly influence the experience of the illness and subsequent behaviors (illness behavior), which affects symptom-reporting and health-care-seeking.

To test this contention, we evaluated the prevalence and effects of a major psychosocial stressor, sexual- or physical-abuse history, among women seen in the gastroenterology clinic at the University of North Carolina. Of 228 eligible women, 206 completed the confidential questionnaire (90% response rate), and 89 (44%) reported some type of sexual or physical abuse, including unwanted intercourse (22%) and frequent physical beatings (7%). The frequency of abuse was higher among those diagnosed with functional (mostly IBS) compared to structural (organic) diagnoses (sexual abuse 53% vs. 37%; frequent physical abuse 13% vs. 2%). In support of the contention that abuse affects health outcome, we found that patients with abuse history had: 1) more frequent and severe symptoms, including pelvic pain (16% vs. 6% nonabused) and nongastrointestinal symptoms (7.1 vs. 5.8 symptoms), 2) more frequent physician visits (4.2 vs. 3.3 visits/6 months), and 3) more lifetime surgeries (2.8 vs. 2.0 surgeries).

These data support the notion that psychological disturbance leads to more refractory illness in IBS (as well as other disorders). This can explain the selective referral of patients with abuse history or other psychosocial disturbances to specialty practices (30–32). One study in a Health Maintenance Organization, using our questionnaire, supports this observation. The frequency of rape/incest, ranged from 5% in HMO members without IBS to 10% in those with mild IBS to 22% with severe IBS (33), and this compares to 31% in our UNC referral GI patient population (25).

From these data, it is proposed that sociocultural factors, family beliefs, personality, major life stress, and previous experiences with illness affect how an individual will react to a disorder such as IBS. These factors can affect the severity of the symptoms reported, the degree of psychological destress and quality of life, the frequency of health-care visits, and even the risk of iatrogenic complications (25, 28, 29, 34–39). These effects may also be modified or "buffered" through certain (e.g., problem-based) coping strategies (37, 40, 41), by adequate social-support networks (42, 43), and by the physician–patient interaction (21, 44). So, while psychosocial factors are not etiological for the disorder, clinical attention to their contributing effects are likely to yield a better outcome than would occur with treatment of the symptoms alone.

V. DIAGNOSIS

The diagnosis of IBS is based on the positive identification of symptoms consistent with the disorder, and by excluding other etiologies that produce similar symptoms. If another etiology is found to explain the patient's symptoms (e.g., lactase deficiency, collagenous colitis, pelvic dyssynergia), the patient may not have IBS, and more specific treatment is undertaken. However, given the high prevalence of IBS symptoms in the population, it is also likely that IBS may co-exist with other disorders. In these situations, treatment depends on assessing the role of all contributing factors.

The use of symptom-based criteria aids the diagnosis greatly. Table 1 lists the multinational consensus ("Rome") criteria for IBS (1,2,45). These criteria were established after careful review of existing epidemiological and clinical studies. While designed primarily for clinical research, they serve as quidelines for the physician in clinical practice.

The diagnostic studies selected must be individualized, and a complete discussion is beyond the scope of this chapter. It should be recognized that a complete history and physical examination are most important, and diagnostic tests serve only to exclude other disorders. The differential diagnoses for patients with chronic ore recurrent bowel dysfunction are listed in Table 2. Their selection is determined by symptom type (e.g., diarrhea and constipation will have different evaluations), chronicity and symptom trajectory (e.g., longstanding stable symptoms may require less evaluation than recent, severe, or progressing symptoms), age of the patient (older patients are at greater risk for other types of bowel disorders), and associated clinical features (e.g., fever, weight loss, abnormal blood tests, blood in stool, etc., require a more complete assessment). Table

TABLE 1 Diagnostic Criteria for IBS (1,2,45)

Continuous or recurrent symptoms for at least 3 months of:

1. Abdominal pain or discomfort, relieved with defecation, associated with a change in the frequency of consistency of stool

   and

2. An irregular (varying) pattern of defecation at least 25% of the time (two or more) of:
   a. Altered stool frequency
   b. Altered stool form (hard or loose/watery stool)
   c. Altered stool passage (straining or urgency, feeling of incomplete evacuation)
   d. Passage of mucus
   e. Bloating or feeling of abdominal distension

Source: Ref 3.

TABLE 2 Differential Diagnosis of Chronic/Recurrent Bowel Dysfunction

1. Irritable bowel syndrome
2. Lactase deficiency
3. Drugs
   a. Laxative/cathartics
   b. Magnesium-containing antacids
4. Bacterial infection
   a. Salmonella species
   b. *Campylobacter jejuni*
   c. *Yersinia enterocolitica*
   d. *Clostridium difficile*
5. Parasitic infection
   a. *Giardia lamblia*
   b. *Entamoeba histolytica*
6. Inflammatory bowel disease
   a. Crohn's disease
   b. Ulcerative colitis
7. Malabsorption
   a. Chronic pancreatitis
   b. Celiac sprue
   c. Postgastrectomy syndromes[a]
8. Metabolic disorders
   a. Diabetes mellitus
   b. Thyrotoxicosis
9. Endocrine-producing tumors
   a. Gastrinoma
   b. Carcinoid
   c. VIPoma
10. Psychiatric disorders
    a. Depression
    b. Somatization disorders
11. Intestinal pseudo-obstruction
    a. Primary visceral myopathy/neuropathy
    b. Secondary myopathy/neuropathy (e.g., scleroderma, diabetes)
12. Other colonic diseases
    a. Microscopic/collagenous colitis; mast-cell disease
    b. Villous adenoma
13. Opportunistic infections in immunocompromised host

[a]Related to vagotomy, incomplete mixing of bile salts and pancreatic enzymes with food, or development of celiac sprue.

3 lists some of the studies that can be obtained depending on the symptom type, but they serve only as quidelines. Care should be taken to avoid unnecessary studies out of uncertainty or patient demands ("furor medicus") (46).

In most cases, symptom-based criteria and a few screening tests lead to a confident diagnosis. Studies indicate a missed diagnosis rate of 3% or less for patients diagnosed in this manner who are followed up to 6 years (47,48).

TABLE 3 Diagnostic Evaluation of Chronic/Recurrent Bowel Dysfunction

A. Initial screening evaluation
   1. History and physical examination[a]
   2. Pelvic examination
   3. Sigmoidoscopy[a]
   4. Stool testing[a] (blood, ova/parasites, fecal PMNs, culture[b])
   5. Complete blood count[a]
   6. Sedimentation rate[a]
   7. Electrolytes (if vomiting or diarrhea present)
   8. Urinalysis

B. Optional studies (only as clinically indicated)
   1. Further Bowel Assessment
      a. Colonoscopy or barium enema
      b. UGI series/small-bowel study or enteroclysis
   2. Predominant pain
      a. Serum amylase
      b. Liver chemistries
      c. Flat plate and upright of abdomen
      d. Abdominal ultrasound/CT
   3. Predominant pain
      a. Inspection of stool (fat, laxatives)
      b. Quantitation of stool (weight <250 g/24 hr, 72-hr fast)
      c. Serum elctrolytes
      d. Calcium, phosphorus, magnesium, alkaline phosphates
      e. Thyroid-function tests
      f. Serum peptides (gastrin, VIP, 5HIAA, etc.)
      g. Serum carotene
      h. Serology for *E. histolytica*
      i. Duodenal aspiration (Giardia)
      j. Small-bowel biopsy
      k. Abdominal CT
      l. Rectal biopsy (microscopic/collagenous colitis, mast cells)
      m. Enteroclysis

[a]Recommended by consensus criteria (1,45,81).
[b]Bacterial culture should be ordered if fever or fecal PMNs present.

VI. TREATMENT

Once the diagnosis has been made, ttreatment is directed toward ameliorating symptoms, modifying factors that exacerbate them, and helping the patient adapt to what is a chronic disorder. No drug or specific treatment plan is of proven value (49). The following recommendations are derived from experience and review of treatment trials in IBS (3).

A. General Approach

The patient should have a primary-care physician for continuity and to minimize unneeded diagnostic procedures, offer symptomatic treatment, and educate, counsel and provide psychological support. The establishment of a good physician–patient relationship is at least as important as any specific treatment in producing clinical improvement.

It is also important to determine the immediate reasons for the patient's visit, which may not always be volunteered. Careful open-ended questioning (e.g., "What led you to see me at this time?") can elicit important information. Possible causes include: 1) new exacerbating factors (dietary change, concurrent medical disorder, side effects of new medication), 2) personal concern about a serious disease (recent family death from GI disease), 3) environmental stressors, 4) psychiatric comorbidity (depression, anxiety), 5) impairment in daily function (recent inability to work or socialize), or 6) a "hidden agenda," such as narcotic or laxative abuse, pending disability, unconscious secondary gain, or somatic representation of psychosocial conflict.

It should also be recognized that the illness in IBS exists on a continuum (Table 4) (3, 27) that depends not only on the severity of the pain but on its constancy, its association with physiological events [e.g., worsened with eating or

TABLE 4 Continuum of Illness Severity in IBS

	Mild	Moderate	Severe
Estimated prevalence (%)	70	25	5
Clinical setting	Primary	Secondary	Tertiary
Physiologic correlation	+++	++	+
Symptom constancy	0	+	+++
Activity disruption	0	+	+++
Health-care use	+	++	+++
Illness behavior	0	+	+++
Psychiatric diagnoses	0	+	+++

0 = generally absent; + = mild; ++ = moderate; ;+++ = severe.
Source: Ref. 3.

during menses (50, 51), relieved by defecation or not], the degree of disruption in daily activity, the patient's illness behavior, and associated psychological disturbance. Consideration of all these factors, as illustrated below, will help in planning treatment.

B. Treatment of Mild Symptoms

Patients with mild or infrequent symptoms are usually seen in primary-care practices and have no significant functional impairment or psychological disturbance. These patients may have concerns about the implications of their symptoms, but they do not make frequent physician visits and usually maintain normal activity levels. Treatment is directed toward education, reassurance, and achievement of a healthier lifestyle.

Education

It is usually helpful to explain that IBS is a very real disorder in which the intestine is overly sensitive to a variety of stimuli such as food, hormonal changes (such as during menses), and stress. Pain resulting from spasm or stretching of the gut, from a sensitive gut, or both, can be experienced anywhere in the abdomen (52) and is associated with changes in bowel function (53,54). Both physiological and psychological factors interact to produce symptoms. Patients are relieved to learn that, while chronic, the condition does not presage serious illness, require surgery, or shorten life expectancy.

Reassurance

The physician should elicit patient concerns such as fear of a serious disease and possible surgery or feelings of helplessness and lack of control imposed by disease. Reassurance after an appropriate evaluation can be an effective therapeutic intervention, and in some cases is all that is required. However, reassurance will not be helpful if it is communicated in a perfunctory manner and before necessary tests have been completed.

Diet

If certain foods such as lactose, caffeine, fatty foods, alcohol, sorbitol gum, and beans exacerbate symptoms, they should be eliminated to see if symptoms abate. All patients should ingest ample amounts of fiber (20–25 g/day), either through diet or with commercial bulking supplements, and controlled trials do show some improvement in constipation and, perhaps, abdominal pain (55). However, bloating and gaseousness may occur due to colonic metabolism of nondigestible fiber; this usually improves over time. Benefit is based on improvement in stool consistency and frequency, and an insufficient dose is a frequent cause of failure. Synthetic fibers such as polycarbophil or methylcellulose theoretically produce less bloating, but their efficacy has not been adequately evaluated.

C. Treatment of Moderate Symptoms

A smaller proportion of patients reporting moderate symptoms have intermittent disruptions in activity (e.g., missing social functions, work, or school), and they often identify a close relationship between syptoms and inciting events such as dietary indiscretion, travel, or distressing experiences. They are usually more psychologically distressed than patients with mild symptoms. For this group, additional treatment options are recommended.

Symptom Monitoring and Modification

The patient can keep a symptom diary for 1 to 2 weeks in which the time, severity, and presence of associated factors are recorded (56). This method may identify exacerbating factors, such as lactose intolerance, excess caffeine or dietary fat, or specific stressors not previously considered. Dietary and behavioral modifications are then discussed, negotiated, and implemented in a manner that permits the patient's participation and, as symptoms improve, increases his or her sense of control over the illness.

Pharmacotherapy Directed at Specific Symptoms

In general, prescription medication is not routinely recommended since IBS is a chronic disorder and most drugs have side effects and variable efficacy. However, if a symptom is distressing enough or impairs daily function, a drug targeted at that symptom can be prescribed for a limited time.

Predominant Pain The anticholinergic ("antispasmodic") drugs are most frequently used to treat the pain symptoms of IBS. While they reduce the cholinergically mediated colonic motor response to a meal (57), a clear relationship between pain symptoms and gut motility has not been confirmed. They are most effective for patients with postprandial episodes of pain (e.g., dicyclomine 10–20 mg). Other agents, such as peppermint-oil capsules, trimebutine, and mebeverine, have been used in Europe but are of uncertain benefit.

Predominant Diarrhea Loperamide (2 to 4 mg q.i.d.), an opioid, increases intestinal transit time, facilitates water and ion absorption, and strengthens rectal-sphincter tone, thereby ameliorating the diarrhea, urgency, and fecal soiling of patients with IBS (58). It is preferred over narcotics since it does not cross the blood–brain barrier. Cholestyramine may be considered in patients who may have bile acid induced diarrhea, particularly if they have had a cholecystectomy (59, 60).

Predominant Constipation Dietary fiber is the standard long-term treatment method for constipation-predominant IBS. Bowel retraining (61) can also be helpful in reconditioning "habit" constipation. Cisapride, a recently approved prokinetic drug, could be considered for more severe episodes of constipation. The drug facilitates acetylcholine release from the myenteric plexus, and some studies report efficacy for constipation (62) and constipation-predominant IBS (63). Chronic use of stimulant laxatives should be discouraged.

Behavioral Treatments

Behavioral interventions may also help motivated patients with moderate to severe symptoms, particularly if they can associate symptoms with stressors, and if they experience a stress-induced health-promoting behaviors, offer a sense of control in the treatment, and improve pain tolerance (61). The choice of treatment depends on cost, availability, and patient motivation.

Relaxation Techniques Relaxation response, meditation, autogenic training, and generalized biofeedback may reduce sympathetic nervous system activity and produce skeletal-muscle relaxation. The relaxation response technique is simple: In a quiet and comfortable environment, the patient focuses on an image, word, or phrase, removes distractions, and uses slow breathing to achieve a state of deep relaxation. Biofeedback, which uses skeletal-muscle EMG monitoring, is relatively expensive, but it appeals to some patients. Clinical trials in IBS suggest promising benefit from relaxation techniques (64).

Hypnosis Hypnosis is more commonly used in England. It has been reported to be effective in treating patients with IBS (65,66), and it may reduce pain perception in the gut (67). It is more effective for patients without associated psychopathology (65).

Psychotherapy

Psychotherapy should be considered for patients having moderate symptom distress and/or functional impairment. However, some medical patients view a recommendation of psychotherapy with a negative attribution (i.e., "in my head") or as a rejection by the medical physician. Therefore, the medical physician must present this approach in a manner that is relevant to the patient (for example, to help him or her achieve better control over the symptoms), and as part of an overall treatment plan with continued medical care.

Insight-Oriented Therapy Short- or long-term insight therapy work best when patients are interested in understanding and modifying psychosocial stressors, or their physical or psychic consequences. In a controlled study of 101 IBS outpatients (68), the study group receiving 12 weeks of psychotherapy with medical treatment showed greater reduction is psychological distress and bowel symptoms than those treated only medically. Improvement continued 1 year after the psychotherapy treatment. The therapy was presumed to help the patient cope with psychological stressors exacerbating the symptoms.

Cognitive-Behavioral Therapy Cognitive-behavioral treatment helps the patient to identify stressors and cognitions that increase distress, and develop new ways of coping with the stress by modifying actions or restructuring the thoughts. In one study (64), cognitive-behavioral therapy, IBS education, and relaxation training led to over 50% improvement in symptoms in almost two-thirds of those treated.

Other Psychotherapies In one uncontrolled trial (69), group therapy led to improved emotional symptoms, but physical symptoms remained. Family counseling may help when family dysfunction contributes to symptom exacerbation but has not been adequately studied. Recent data indicate that a multicomponent treatment plan is optimal (64,70). In one study (70), a combined program of relaxation, psychotherapy, and medical treatment led to improvement in diarrhea and abdominal pain. Good prognostic factors included: 1) a short duration of bowel complaints, 2) few sites of abdominal pain, 3) the absence of constant pain, and 4) overt symptoms of anxiety or depression.

D. Treatment of Severe Symptoms

A very small subset of IBS patients with severe symptoms behave more like patients with chronic pain, since they have continuous refractory abdominal pain that does not correlate with gut physiology (e.g., is made worse by meals or relieved by defecation). Psychiatric comorbidity (anxiety, depression, somatization), disability, and chronic illness behaviors (27) are common. These patients are unable to acknowledge psychological contributions to the illness, and they believe that a serious disease is being overlooked. They often hold unrealistic expectations to be "cured" and insist on unneeded diagnostic studies and treatments. These patients frequently see gastroenterology consultants, and are usually unresponsive to traditional psychotherapy (70) or to pharmacotherapy directed at the gut. Treatment employs behavioral techniques and the use of psychoactive drugs.

Recommendations for the Medical Physician

The patient with severe or intractable symptoms needs an ongoing relationship with the medical physician for psychosocial support and to prevent "doctor-shopping" and overinvestigation. The physician may feel pressured to comply with unreasonable patient demands or to assume full responsibility for care. Some recommendations can be made (61): 1) perform diagnostic and therapeutic measures based on objective findings and/or observations over time rather than in response to patient demands, 2) set realistic goals to improve function and quality of life rather than to cure, 3) provide therapeutic options to shift responsibility for treatment to the patient, and 4) demonstrate a commitment to the patient's well-being rather than to treat the disease. This approach reduces patient tendencies to focus on symptoms ("organ recital") in order to keep physicians interested. Brief, regular appointments with the primary-care physician, and less frequently with the consultant, are palliative since they reinforce the patient's perception of the physician's interest.

Psychopharmacological Agents

Antidepressants control chronic abdominal pain via central analgesia (71), anticholinergic action on the gut, or relief of depression. While data on IBS are limited (72,73), well-designed trials of patients having other chronic pain syndromes show clinical benefit (74–76). Antidepressants should be considered for unremitting pain and impaired daily functioning, or for coexistent symptoms of panic or major or atypical depression. Even without depressive symptoms, these agents may help when the pain is dominant and consuming. The tertiary amine tricyclic agents or the serotonin reuptake inhibitors (SRIs) have a theoretical advantage because of their enhancing effect on brain serotonin, which blocks pain perception (77,78). The more sedating drugs (e.g., amitriptyline, doxepin) can be given when there is sleep disturbance, and the SRIs can be used when sedating or anticholinergic side effects are not well tolerated. A poor clinical response may be due to insufficient dose or failure to adjust the dosage based on therapeutic response or side effects (79). Benzodiazepine-type anxiolytics occasionally help ameliorate brief episodes of stress-related symptom flares. However, they are not recommended for continuous treatment because of the risk of drug interactions, habituation, or withdrawal rebound.

Referral to Pain-Treatment Centers

Pain-treatment centers should be considered when patients are unresponsive to usual treatments and when they are seriously disabled. One controlled study (80) showed that an interdisciplinary pain-management program decreased pain scores for patients with chronic pelvic pain, decreased anxiety and depression, and improved psychosocial functioning 6 months after treatment.

REFERENCES

1. Drossman DA, Thompson WG, Talley NJ, Funch-Jensen P, Janssens J, Whitehead WE. Identification of subgroups of functional bowel disorders. Gastroenterol Int 1990; 3:159–172.
2. Thompson WG, Creed F, Drossman DA, Heaton KW, Mazzacca G. Functional bowel disorders and chronic functional abdominal pain. Gastroenterol Int 1992; 5:75–91.
3. Drossman DA, Thomson WG. The irritable bowel syndrome: Review and a

graduated, multicomponent treatment approach. Ann Intern Med 1992; 116: 1009–1016.
4. Thompson WG, Heaton KW. Functional bowel disorders in apparently healthy people. Gastroenterology 1980; 79:283–288.
5. Drossman DA, Sandler RS, McKee DC, Lovitz AJ. Bowel patterns among subjects not seeking health care: Use of a questionnaire to identify a population with bowel dysfunction. Gastroenterology 1982; 83:529–534.
6. Bommelaer G, Rouch M, Dapoigny M, Pais D, Loisy P, Gualino M, Tournut R. Epidemiology of functional bowel disorders in apparently healthy people. Gastroenterol Clin Biol 1986; 10:7–12.
7. Drossman DA, Li Z, Andruzzi E, Temple R, Talley NJ, Thompson WG, Whitehead WE, Janssens J, Funch-Jensen P, Corazziari E, Richter JE, Koch GG. U.S. Householder Survey of Functional GI Disorders: Prevalence, Sociodemography and Health Impact. Dig Dis Sci 1993; 38:1569–1580.
8. Pimparkar BD. Irritable colon syndrome. J Indian Med Assoc 1970; 54:95–102.
9. Mitchell CM, Drossman DA. Survey of the AGA membership relating to patients with functional gastrointestinal disorders. Gastroenterology 1987; 92:1282–1284.
10. Thompson WG. The irritable bowel. Gut 1984; 25:305–320.
11. Whithead WE, Holtkotter B, Enck P, Hoelzl R, Holmes KD, Anthony J, Shabsin HS, Schuster MM. Tolerance for rectosigmoid distension in irritable bowel syndrome. Gastroenterology 1990; 98:1187–1192.
12. Sun WM, Read NW, Prior A, Daly JA, Cheah SK, Grundy D. Sensory and motor responses to rectal distension vary according to rate and pattern of balloon inflation. Gastroenterology 1990; 99:1008-1015.
13. Kellow JE, Phillips SF, miller LJ, Zinsmeister AR. Dysmotility of the small intestine in irritable bowel syndrome. Gut 1988; 29:1236–1243.
14. Heaton KW, Gosh S. Relation between stool form on a seven point scale and symptoms of urgency, straining, and incomplete evacuation: a new way of looking at irritable bowel syndrome (abstr). Gut 1989; 30:A1465.
15. Mayer EA, Raybould HE. Role of visceral afferent mechanisms in functional bowel disorders. Gastroenterology 1990; 99:1688–1704.
16. Cervero F, Jaenig W. Visceral nociceptors: a new world order? Trends Neurosci 1992; 15:374–378.
17. Drossman DA. The functional gastrointestinal disorders and their diagnosis: A coming of age. In: Drossman DA, Richter JE, Talley NJ, Thompson WG, Corazziari E, Whitehead WE, eds. The Functional Gastrointestinal Disorders: Diagnosis, Pathophysiology and treatment. Boston: Little, Brown, 1994:1–23.
18. Baber NS, Dourish CT, Hill DR. The role of CCK, caerulein, and CCK antaganists in nociception. Pain 1989; 39:307–328.
19. Bueno L. Fioramonti J. Action of opiates on gastrointestinal function. Baillieres Clin Gastroenterol 1988; 2:123–139.
20. Svensson TH. Peripheral, autonomic regulation of locus coeruleus nordrenergic neurons in brain: Putative implications for psychiatry and psychopharmacology. Psychopharmacology 1987; 92:1–7.
21. Drossman DA. Psychosocial considerations in gastroenterology. In: Sleisenger

MH, Fordtran JS, Scharschmidt BF, Feldman M, eds. Gastrointestinal Disease: Pathophysiology, Diagnosis, Management. Philadelphia: WB Saunders, 1993: 3–17.
22. Stermer E, Bar H, Levy N. Chronic functional gastrointestinal symptoms in Holocaust survivors. Am J. Gastroenterol 1991; 86:417-422.
23. Creed FH, Craig T. Farmer RG. Functional abdominal pain, psychiatric illness and life events. Gut 1988; 29:235–242.
24. Walker EA, Roy-Byrne PP, Katon WJ. Irritable bowel syndrome and psychiatric illness. Am J Psychiatry 1990; 147(5):565–572.
25. Drossman DA, Leserman J, Nachman G, Li Z, Gluck H, Toomey TC, Mitchell CM. Sexual and physical abuse in women with functional or organic gastrointestinal disorders. Ann Intern Med 1990; 113:828-833.
26. Whithead WE, Winget C. Fedoravicius AS, Wooley S, Blackwell B. Learned illness behavior in patients with irritable bowel syndrome and peptic ulcer. Dig Dis Sci 1982; 27:202–208.
27. Drossman DA. Illness behaviour in the irritable bowel syndrome. Gastroenterol Int 1991; 4:77–81.
28. Drossman DA, McKee DC, Sandler RS, Mitchell CM, Cramer EM, Lowman BC, Burger AL. Psychosocial factors in the irritable bowel syndrome: A multivariate study of patients and nonpatients with irritable bowel syndrome. Gastroenterology 1988; 95:701–708.
29. Whitehead WE, Bosmajian L, Zonderman AB, Costa PTJ, Schuster MM. Symptoms of psychologic distress associated with irritable bowel syndrome: Comparison of community and medical clinic samples. Gastroenterology 1988; 95:709–714.
30. Walker EA, Katon Wj, Roy-Byrne PP, Jemelka RP, Russo J. Histories of Sexual victimization in patients with irritable bowel syndrome or inflammatory bowel disease. Am J Psychiatry 1993; 150:1502–1506.
31. Talley NJ, Kramlinger KG, Burton MC, Colwell Lj, Zinsmeister AR. Psychiatric disorders and childhood abuse in the irritable bowel syndrome. Eur J Gastroenterol Hepatol 1993; 5:647–654.
32. Scarinci IC, Haile JM, Bradley LA, Richter JE. Altered pain perception and psychosocial features among women with gastrointestinal disorders and history of abuse: A preliminary model. Am J Med 1994; 97:108–118.
33. Longstreth GF, Wolde-Tsadik G. Irritable bowel-type symptoms in HMO examinees: prevalence, demographics, and clinical correlates. Dig Dis Sci 1993; 38:1581–1589.
34. Burns DG. The risk of abdominal surgery in irritable bowel syndrome. South Afr Med J 1986; 70:91.
35. Smith RC, Greenbaum DS, Vancouver JB, Henry RC, Reinhart MA, Greenbaum RB, Dean HA, Mayle JE. Psychosocial factors are associated with health care seeking rather than diagnosis in irritable bowel syndrome. Gastroenterology 1990; 98:293–301.
36. Drossman DA, Patrick DL, Mitchell CM, Zagami EA, Appelbaum MI. Health related quality of life in inflammatory bowel disease: Functional status and patient worries and concerns. Dig Dis Sci 1989; 34:1379–1386.
37. Drossman DA, Leserman J, Mitchell CM, Li Z, Zagami EA, Patrick DL. Health

status and health care use in persons with inflammatory bowel disease: A national sample. Dig Dis Sci 1991; 36:1746–1755.
38. Arnold RP, Rogers D, Cook DAG. Medical problems of adults who were sexually abused in childhood. Br Med J 1990; 300: 705–708.
39. Katon W, Von Korff M, Lin E, Lipscomb P, Russo J, Wagner E, Polk E. Distressed high utilizers of medical care: DSM-III-R diagnoses and treatment needs. Gen Hosp Psychiatry 1990; 12:355–362.
40. Lazarus RS, Folkman S. Stress, Appraisal, and Coping. New York: Springer, 1984.
41. Bradley LA, Richter JE, Scarinci IC, Haile JM, Schan CA. Psychosocial and psychophysical assessments of patients with unexplained chest pain. Am J Med 1992; 92:65S–73S.
42. Jamison RN, Virts KL. The influence of family support on chronic pain. Behav Res Ther 1990; 28:283–287.
43. Berkman LF, Leo-Summers L, Horwitz RI. Emotional support and survival after myocardial infarction: A prospective, population-based study of the elderly. Ann Intern Med 1992; 117:1003–1009.
44. Simpson M, Buckman R, Stewart M, Maguire P, Lipkin M, Novack D, Till J. Doctor-patient communication: the Toronto consensus statement. Br Med J 1991; 303:1385–1387.
45. Drossman DA, Richter JE, Talley NJ, Thompson WG, Corazziari E, Whitehead WE, eds. The Functional Gastrointestinal Disorders: Diagnosis, Pathophysiology and Treatment. Boston: Little, Brown, 1994.
46. Devaul RA, Faillace LA. Peristent pain and illness insistence—A medical profile of proneness to surgery. Am J Surg 1978; 135:828–833.
47. Svendsen JH, Munck LK, Andersen JR. Irritable bowel syndrome: Prognosis and diagnostic safety. A 5-year follow up study. Scand J Gastroenterol 1985; 20:415–418.
48. Harvey RF, Mauad Ec, Brown AM. Prognosis in the irritable bowel syndrome: a five-year prospective study. Lancet 1987; i:963–965.
49. Klein KB. Controlled treatment trials in the irritable bowel syndrome: a critique. Gastroenterology 1988; 95:232–241.
50. Heitkemper MM, Jarrett M. Pattern of gastrointestinal and somatic symptoms across the menstrual cycle. Gastroenterology 1992; 102:505–513.
51. Crowell MD, Dubin NH, Robinson JC, Cheskin LJ, Schuster MM, Heller BR, Whitehead WE. Functional bowel disorders in women with dysmenorrhea. Am J Gastroenterol 1994; 89:1973–1977.
52. Swarbrick ET, Hegarty JE, Bat L, Williams CB, Dawson AM. Site of pain from the irritable bowel syndrome. Lancet 1980; ii:443–446.
53. Manning AP, Thompson WG, Heaton KW, Morris AF. Towards positive diagnosis of the irritable bowel. Br Med J 1978; 2:653–654.
54. Kruis W. Thieme CH, Weinzierl M, Schussler P, Hall J, Paulus W. A diagnostic score for the irritable bowel syndrome: Its value in the exclusion of organic disease. Gastroenterology 1984; 87:1–7.
55. Heaton KW. Role of dietary fibre in irritable bowel syndrome. In: Read NW, ed. Irritable Bowel Syndrome. London: Grune & Stratton, 1985:203–222.

56. Shimberg EF. Relief from IBS. New York: M Evans, 1988.
57. Sullivan MA, Cohen S. Snape WJ. Colonic myoelectrical activity in irritable-bowel syndrome. N Engl J. Med 1978; 298:878–883.
58. Cann PA, Read NW, Holdsworth CD, Barends D. Role of loperamide and placebo in management of irritable bowel syndrome. Dig Dis Sci 1984; 29:239–247.
59. Thaysen EH, Pedersen L. Idiopathic bile salt catharsis. Gut 1976; 17:965–970.
60. Sciarretta G. Fagioli G, Furno A, Vicini G, Cecchetti L, Grigolo B, Verri A, Malaguti P. 75Se HCAT test in the detection of bile acid malabsorption in functional diarrhoea and its correlation with small bowel transit. Gut 1987; 28:970–975.
61. Drossman DA. Psychosocial factors in the care of patients with gastrointestinal disorders. In: Yamada T, ed. Textbook of Gastroenterology. Philadelphia: JB Lippincott, 1995.
62. Mueller-Lissner SA. Treatment of chronic constipation with cisapride and placebo. Gut 1987; 28:1033–1038.
63. Van Outryve M, Milo R, Toussaint J, Van Eeghem PV. "Prokinetic" treatment of constipation-predominant irritable bowel syndrome: A placebo-controlled study of cisapride. J Clin Gastroenterol 1991; 13:49–57.
64. Schwarz SP, Taylor AE, Scharff L, Blanchard EB. Behaviorally treated irritable bowel syndrome patients: A four-year follow-up. Behav Res Ther 1990; 28:331–335.
65. Whorwell PJ, Prior A, Colgan SM. Hypnotherapy in severe irritable bowel syndrome: further experience. Gut 1987; 28:423–425.
66. Harvey FR, Hinton RA, Gunary RM, Barry RE. Individual and group hypnotherapy in treatment of refractory irritable bowel syndrome. Lancet 1989; i:424–425.
67. Prior A, Colgan SM, Whorwell PJ. Changes in rectal sensitivity after hypnotherapy in patients with irritable bowel syndrome. Gut 1990; 31:896–898.
68. Svedlund J, Sjodin I, Ottosson JO, Dotevall G. Controlled study of psychotherapy in irritable bowel syndrome. Lancet 1983; ii:589–591.
69. Wise TN, Cooper JN, Ahmed S. The efficacy of group therapy for patients with irritable bowel syndrome. Psychosomatics 1982; 23:465–469.
70. Guthrie E, Creed F, Dawson D, Tomenson B. A controlled trial of psychological treatment for the irritable bowel syndrome. Gastroenterology 1991; 100:450–457.
71. Aronoff GM, Wagner JM, Spangler ASJ. Chemical interventions for pain. J Consult Clin Psychol 1986; 54:769–775.
72. Heefner JD, Wilder RM, Wilson JD. Irritable colon and depression. Psychosomatics 1978; 19:540-547.
73. Greenbaum DS, Mayle JE, Vanegeren LE, Jerome JA, Major JW, Greenbaum RB, Matson RW, STein GE, Dean HA, Halvorsen NA, Rosen LW. The effects of desipramine on IBS compared with atropine and placebo. Dig Dis Sci 1987; 32: 257–266.
74. Ward NG, Bloom VL, FRiedel RO. The effectiveness of tricyclic antidepressants in the treatment of coesisting pain and depression. Pain 1979; 7:331–341.
75. Hameroff SR, Weiss JL, Lerman JC, Cork RC, WATTS KS, Crago BR, Newman CP, Womble JR, Davis TP. Doxepin's effects on chronic pain and depression: A controlled study. J Clin Psychiatry 1984; 45:47–52.

76. Pilowsky I, Barrow CG. A controlled study of psychotherapy and amitriptyline used individually and in combination in the treatment of chronic intractable, "psychogenic" pain. Pain 1990; 40:3–19.
77. Eberhard G. Von Knorring L, Nilsson HL, Sundquist U, Bjorling G. Linder H, Svard KO, Tysk L. A double-blind randomized study of clomipramine versus maprolitine in patients with idiopathic pain syndromes. Neuropsychobiology 1988; 19:25–34.
78. Tura B, Tura SM. The analgesic effect of tricyclic antidepressants. Brain Res 1990; 518:19–22.
79. Cakkues AL, Popkin MK. Antidepressant treatment of medical-surgical inpatients by nonpsychiatric physicians. Arch Gen Psychiatry 1987; 44:157–160.
80. Kames LD, Rapkin AJ, Naliboff BD, Afifi S, Ferrer-Brechner T. Effectiveness of an interdisciplinary pain management program for the treatment of chronic pelvic pain. Pain 1990: 41(1):41–46.
81. Dotevall G. Peptic ulcer, noxious stress, and *Campylobacter pylori.* Gastroenterology 1990; 98:252–253.

10

Chronic Idiopathic Constipation

Arnold Wald
University of Pittsburgh School of Medicine
and University of Pittsburgh Medical Center
Pittsburgh, Pennsylvania

I. DEFINITIONS

Constipation is a symptom for which treatment is often provided on the basis of a patient's subjective interpretation that there is a disturbance in bowel function. Not unexpectedly, the definition of constipation has different meanings for different persons. For some, it means that stools are too hard or too small; for others, stools are too difficult to expel or occur too infrequently. The first three complaints are difficult to quantify in clinical practice; the last can be measured and compared to bowel frequency in the general population in a given country or region.

Many physicians define constipation as a stool frequency consistently less than three per week. This is based on epidemiological studies that indicate that 98% of adults in the United States or the United Kingdom have stool frequencies of three per week or greater (1,2). Yet this definition is insufficient, as up to 60% of subjects in a community survey who reported themselves to be constipated had daily bowel movements (3)! These individuals most frequently complained of defecatory straining or a sense of incomplete evacuation, complaints that occur far more frequently that do those of infrequent defecation. An international working committee (4) has recommended the following operational definitions of constipation (known informally as the "Rome criteria"):

A. Either two or more of the following complaints present for at least 12 months:
   1. Straining with at least 25% of bowel movements when not taking laxatives
   2. A feeling of incomplete evacuation after at least 25% of bowel movements when not taking laxatives
   3. Hard or pellet stools on at least 25% of bowel movements when not taking laxatives
   4. Stools less frequent than three per week without laxatives

or

B. Fewer than two bowel movements per week on average, present for at least 12 months

II. EPIDEMIOLOGY

Self-reported constipation in the United States is more prevalent in women, nonwhites, and those over age 60. After adjusting for these factors, constipation is more prevalent in those with little daily activity or exercise, low income, and poor education (5,6). Surveys of physician visits for constipation in the United States, England, and Wales have also found more visits by women than men, nonwhites than whites, those with lower compared to higher incomes, and persons with less that 12 years of education (7). In both countries, prevalence rates rise with age, most dramatically in persons 65 years of age or older (6,7). However, despite the belief of many physicians, self-reported constipation has not been significantly correlated with either fluid or fiber intake (5,8).

III. SECONDARY CAUSES OF CONSTIPATION

Because colonic and anorectal motor functions are coordinated by both enteric nerves and the extrinsic innervation by sympathetic and parasympathetic nerves, it is not surprising that diseases of the central and peripheral nervous systems are often associated with constipation (9; Table 1). The distal colon receives parasympathetic innervation from the sacral nerves that pass through the pelvis and enter the bowel wall in the rectum. Transection of these nerves or lesions in the cauda equina may produce constipation associated with hypomotility, colonic dilatation, decreased rectal tone and sensation, stasis of the distal colon, and impaired defecation. Similar findings may occur with injury to the lumbosacral spine, with meningomyelocele, and following low spinal anesthesia.

Table 1 Some Secondary Causes of Chronic Constipation

Neurogenic Disorders	Non-neurogenic disorders
Peripheral	Diabetes mellitus
Hirschsprung's disease	Hypothyroidism
Chagas' disease	Hypercalcemia, hypocalcemia
Autonomic neuropathy	Pregnancy
Intestinal pseudo-obstruction (myopathy, neuropathy)	Porphyria
	Panhypopituitarism
Central	Systemic sclerosis
Multiple sclerosis	Myotonic dystrophy
Spinal-cord injury	
Parkinson's disease	

Constipation may also occur following high spinal-cord damage, but, in contrast to lower cord damage, colonic reflexes are intact and defecation can often be triggered by digital stimulation of the anal canal.

The prevalence of constipation in multiple sclerosis is high (10) and may be worsened by physical inactivity or use of medications with constipating side effects. Severely constipated patients with advanced multiple sclerosis appear to have absent colonic motor responses after eating a meal and other characteristic changes that may result from interruption of normal cortical inhibition of colonic motor activity.

Hirschsprung's disease is a congenital disorder characterized by obstipation from birth and colonic dilatation proximal to a spastic nonpropulsive segment of distal bowel. Functional obstruction of the distal bowel is due to absent intramural ganglion cells of the submucosal and myenteric plexuses, a result of arrest of caudal migration of neural crest cells during embryonic development.

Finally, constipation can be caused or exacerbated by various drugs (9; Table 2).

IV. MEDICAL EVALUATION

A. History

The workup of a patient with constipation depends on the chronicity and severity of the complaint. In general, a relatively short history of a recent change in bowel habits in an adult makes exclusion of a neoplasm or another structural abnormality a high priority. On the other hand, a long history of unremitting severe constipation, especially if it is resistant to dietary measures or mild laxatives, should prompt more comprehensive testing to provide both structural and functional information about colorectal activity (see below).

The pattern of symptoms may suggest various categories of bowel dys-

TABLE 2 Drugs Associated with Constipation

Analgesics
Anticholinergics
Antispasmodics
Antidepressants
Antipsychotics
Cation-containing agents
Iron supplements
Aluminum (antacids, sucralfate)
Calcium (antacids, supplements)
Metallic intoxication (arsenic, lead, mercury)
Neurally active agents
Opiates
Antihypertensives
Ganglionic blockers
Vinca alkaloids
Anticonvulsants
Calcium channel blockers

function and also identify complaints based on patient misconceptions or misperceptions. These include whether there is infrequent defecation or defecatory difficulties such as excessive straining, discomfort, or a sense of incomplete evacuation. Inquiry concerning laxative use and its duration is important, as are questions concerning gastrointestinal complaints in other family members and parental views on laxatives and bowel habits. One critical question concerns the onset of the complaint. For example, constipation that is present from birth or the neonatal period suggests a congenital disorder, whereas onset in later life indicates an acquired abnormality. A careful assessment for possible affective disorders, emotional distress, and use of mood-altering drugs may identify factors that potentially contribute to subjective complaints in the patient.

If the patient is a child, inquiry should be made concerning nightmares, enuresis, school performance, and intrafamilial tensions. In addition, a history of bowel disturbances in the family should be elicited, as there is a greater incidence of constipation in one or both parents of children with fecal soiling associated with constipation (encopresis).

B. Physical Examination

The examiner should search for perineal disease or deformity, anterior location of the anal orifice, atrophy of the gluteal muscles, and rectal prolapse. Digital examination of the rectum may elicit pain from an anal fissure, detect anal stenosis, assess tone and strength of the anal canal, or palpate a rectal mass or fecal impaction. Asking the patient to strain may assist in identifying a rectocele bulging anteriorly into the vagina or a rectal prolapse. Perineal sensation should be assessed as well as reflex contraction of the anal canal following pinprick of the perianal area ("anal wink").

C. Studies of Colorectal Structure and Function

Endoscopy

Flexible sigmoidoscopy and colonoscopy are superior techniques for assessing bowel mucosa and intraluminal characteristics. They may detect lesions that narrow or occlude the bowel and identify melanosis coli, a brown-black discoloration of the bowel mucosa that is characteristic of chronic use of anthraquinone laxatives. A solitary ulcer may be present on the anterior rectal wall in patients with excessive defecatory straining.

Structural causes of constipation are more likely to be found in someone with a short history of complaints or when there has been a recent change in bowel habits rather than in a patient with longstanding constipation. Certainly, endoscopic studies should not be performed repeatedly in patients with chronic stable complaints, because they are expensive and time-consuming and occasionally cause complications.

Radiographic Studies

Barium radiographs are an important complement to sigmoidoscopy in detecting organic lesions. They can identify the characteristic narrowed denervated bowel segment in classic Hirschsprung's disease (9). A simple plain film of the abdomen can detect stool retention in the colon, indicate megacolon, and monitor bowel-cleansing regimens in patients with fecal retention. Barium radiographs may also identify colonic hypersegmentation, which is suggestive of spasticity of the large intestine.

Defecography is a technique in which barium thickened to a consistency approximating stool is introduced into the rectum (11). Evacuation of the barium can be monitored by fluoroscopy or videotape while the patient sits on a specially constructed commode. Assessment of the anorectal structures, including the anorectal angle, are obtained at rest and during expulsion of the barium mixture. Anatomical abnormalities such as rectoceles and intussusceptions may also be apparent during straining. However, as there is great variability among radiologists with respect to interpreting these studies, more experience with this technique is needed before dicisions can be made with confidence on the basis of radiographic findings.

Marker Studies

Colonic transit studies are most useful when evaluating patients whose major complaint is infrequent defecation (12). The subject ingests a high-fiber diet (20 to 30 g per day) while abstaining from laxatives, enemas, and medications that may affect bowel function. Radiopaque markers are swallowed, and their passage through the colon is monitored by abdominal radiographs. Markers are counted in the right, left, and rectosigmoid colons, which are defined by certain anatomical landmarks, and are followed as they move distally until expelled.

Patients with slow colonic transit can be categorized according to patterns of marker movement. In *colonic inertia*, transit in the right colon is delayed. This pattern can occur because of decreased propulsion (*hypomotility*) or because of increased nonpropulsive contraction waves in the left colon and retropulsion of markers from the left to the right colon (*spastic constipation*). A second pattern of slow transit is *outlet delay*, in which markers progress normally through the proximal colon but stagnate in the rectum. This pattern is observed in many children with idiopathic constipation, in elderly patients with fecal impaction and or megarectum, and in some adults with dyschezia. Finally, a third pattern, *hindgut delay*, has been described, in which markers move normally through the right colon but are delayed through the left and rectosigmoid colons. The pathophysiology and clinical importance of this pattern are uncertain.

Many patients with chronic constipation, even those who complain of intractable symptoms, have normal colonic transit. These patients may consciously or unconsciously misrepresent their bowel habits and, *as a group*, exhibit psychological profiles different from those of patients with slow-transit constipation (13). Using the Hopkins Symptom Checklist, a self-rating inventory in which the subject indicates how distressed he or she is for each of 90 symptoms, constipated patients with normal colonic transit scored significantly higher in eight of the nine clinical subscales and in the global symptoms index than did patients with slow colonic transit and control patients (nonconstipated patients who were about to undergo endoscopy or colonoscopy). All but one of the constipated patients with normal transit scored in the abnormal range in the global symptoms index and the somatization, anxiety, and depression subscales, in contrast to only a minority of patients in the two other groups. These findings have potentially important ramifications with respect to treatment approaches (see below).

Motility

Anorectal manometry may provide useful information in some patients with severe constipation. The most useful parameters are rectal sensation and compliance, reflexive relaxation of the internal anal sphincter, and manometric patterns produced upon attempted expulsion of the apparatus (pseudodefecation). Satisfactory measurements of anal-sphincter pressures can be obtained with open-tipped perfused catheters, direct on-line pressure transducers, and air- or water-filled balloons of various sizes and configurations.

The manometric demonstration that the internal anal sphincter relaxes following rectal distension excludes Hirshsprung's disease from diagnostic consideration (14). Manometry can also identify abnormal sphincteric responses during attempted expulsion (15,16). Pressures recorded by the rectal balloon inflated with air provide some indication of intraabdominal pressures generated during expulsion efforts, while pressure recordings of the anal-sphincter transducers indicate relaxation or inappropriate contraction of the external anal sphincter. Manometry may be supplemented for diagnostic purposes by electromyographic (EMG) studies of the external sphincter and puborectalis muscles using concentric-needle or surface-electrode recordings.

If rectal sensation is impaired, as often occurs in patients with severe constipation, it is helpful to know whether there is increased rectal compliance or megarectum. Rectal compliance can be measured by sequentially inflating a balloon placed in the rectum and measuring pressures at each level of distension. One should indicate the volume at which the first urge to expel the balloon occurs and also any symptoms elicited with increasing inflation of the balloon. Patients with "spastic constipation" often have low compliance and tolerate distension poorly, in contrast to patients with megarectum.

V. CLINICAL PRESENTATIONS AND TREATMENT

When evaluating a patient with idiopathic chronic constipation, the physician should attempt to place that patient into a pathophysiological category. Diagnostic studies and treatment depend, in part, on the clinical presentation. For clinical purposes, it is often useful to group patients according to age at presentation, recognizing that underlying pathogenetic mechanisms will vary from patient to patient and within age categories.

A. Constipation in Children

Idiopathic constipation in children is frequently associated with fecal impaction and dilatation of the rectum and sigmoid colon (4). Many have slow colonic transit, usually in the distal colon and rectum (17), which is consistent with either voluntary withholding behavior or an anorectal disorder. Abdominal pain is not prominent, stools are large and infrequent, and defecation is often uncomfortable. In children with severe retention, fecal soiling may develop. Several reports indicate that many constipated children with fecal soiling exhibit pelvic-floor dyssynergia (16,18). This may be a learned behavior which is acquired at an earlier age, perhaps when attempts to evacuate a large fecal bolus were associated with anal discomfort or a fissure (see below).

Encopresis

The most common type of fecal incontinence in childhood occurs in association with chronic constipation. It is present in approximately 1.5% of second-graders, with a strong male predominance Most children exhibit "overflow incontinence" caused by the movement of liquid stool around fecal impactions and through a distended internal anal sphincter. Although early studies considered encopresis a psychogenic disorder, more recent theories have implicated both psychological and physiological factors. The importance of each to the pathogenesis and maintenance of encopresis remains controversial. Conventional medical treatment is based on the assumption that a physiological predisposition to constipation places many of these children at risk for developing encopresis. Yet psychosocial factors may determine which "at-risk" children develop symptoms and also may affect therapeutic responses (19).

Psychological Issues Familial and environmental risk factors were analyzed by Bellman (20) in her study of over 9000 children with encopresis in Stockholm. She found that 1.3% of biological mothers, 15% of fathers, and 8.7% of the brothers of encopretic children had a history of encopresis, in contrast to its infrequency in family members of the matched control group. Although these and similar observations by other investigators (21) suggest a possible familial predisposition to bowel disturbances, other explanations include the possible influence of parental behavior in the development of encopresis or factors such as a lifestyle that may limit the availability of toileting times to children and thereby promote fecal retention.

Inappropriate toilet-training has been implicated as an important factor in the development of encopresis. Several investigators (20,22,23) have noted that the mothers of these children were inconsistent in their toilet-training approaches, alternating between excessive rigidity and permissiveness. It is not possible to determine whether such parental behaviors were causal or were in response to difficulties experienced during toilet training.

Stressful events appeared to be precipitating factors in 70% of children who develop encopresis after successful toilet-training (20). These included starting school, the birth of a sibling, or parental separation or divorce. Hoag et al. (23) noted that three of five boys developed encopresis following the birth of siblings to mothers who were ill at the time. They found that soiling was exacerbated during periods of family turmoil, an observation also made by others (22).

Some investigators believe that encopresis is a learned behavior that is maintained by the presence of secondary gain. Youngsters may use soiling to either avoid unpleasant events (e.g., school) or obtain parental attention (parents must take time to assist the child to clean both the soiled clothing and his or her body). Behavioral factors may also affect treatment success (24).

Nevertheless, the importance of behavioral factors in the etiology of encopresis is uncertain. Much controversy centers on differences in the reported frequency and severity of behavioral disorders in encopretic children and whether they precede soiling or occur because of the underlying bowel dysfunction. Differences in the incidence and severity of psychological/behavioral disorders among various studies may be due to differences in study populations. For example, children with encopresis who were evaluated in psychiatric settings have exhibited significant psychological dysfunction whereas those referred to medical settings were less likely to do so. Gabel et al. (25) found only mild behavioral dysfunction in 55 encopretic children referred to a pediatric medical clinic. Similar observations in encopretic children treated in medical settings have been made by others (21,26). In contrast, Bellman (20) reported more anxiety, less tolerance for demands, submission in the face of peer aggression, less control of aggressive impulses, and more academic difficulties among encopretic children than matched controls.

Landman et al. (27), using a measure of locus of control (the extent to which one perceives that an event is contingent on one's own behavior), found that children with encopresis tended to feel less in control of life events and had lower self-esteem than did children with other chronic illnesses such as recurrent abdominal pain, enuresis, or chronic headache. Although others have made similar observations, they concluded that these personality characteristics developed because of negative experiences associated with soiling (22,23). Consistent with this interpretation, Levine and Bakow (28) found that successfully treated children became better adjusted and exhibited no evidence of symptom substitution as long as 3 years after therapy. Whereas this might imply that behavioral factors do not necessarily predispose a child toward encopresis, one consequence of fecal soiling is the development of poor coping skills, low self-esteem, and passivity, which are potentially reversible with successful therapy.

Physiological Aspects In addition to possible behavioral abnormalities, many children with overflow incontinence exhibit abnormalities of anorectal function. As a result of chronic stool retention, the rectum may become dilated, sensory feedback from the bowel may become impaired, and the rectal wall may be stretched and unable to sufficiently contract for complete evacuation (16). Increased water absorption from retained fecal material produces harder and larger feces. The associated painful defecation may result in avoidance of toilet use or the unconscious inhibition of defecation. This concept is supported by the demonstration of an abnormal defecation pattern in 40–60% of encopretic children (16,18). This pattern is characterized by contraction of the external anal sphincter and/or puborectalis muscle during attempted expulsion of the anorectal manometry apparatus (simulated defecation) and may represent a learned behavior since it can be normalized using biofeedback techniques. Consequently, after bowel-cleansing, children may need to relearn to recognize and appropriately respond to rectal distension by initiating appropriate defecation responses.

Treatment

Acknowledging the role of both psychological and physiological components in encopresis, treatment has encompassed both medical and behavioral strategies. Medical approaches begin with enemas or suppositories to relieve constipation. Laxatives or high-fiber diets are then used to promote regular evacuation and to maintain continence. Behavioral interventions have included habit training with positive reinforcement for appropriate toileting, cleanliness training that requires that children clean their clothing and body following soiling episodes, and toilet desensitization. Parker and Whitehead (29) noted that most published experiences either are single-case reports or involve small treatment groups (fewer than 10 children), and none contained adequate control groups.

Despite a paucity of studies that compare different medical and behavioral treatment interventions, combined medical and behavioral treatments in larger subject samples have been reported. Levine and Bakow (28) reported a success rate of 78% utilizing parent counseling, initial bowel-cleansing with enemas and/or suppositories, extended use of mineral oil and oral laxatives to promote regular defecation, and habit training by having the child attempt to defecate on the toilet after breakfast or dinner each day. Lowery et al (21) reported a long-term success rate of 61% using a similar protocol that also included contingent use of enemas if the child failed to defecate for 2 consecutive days, more structured praise and tangible reinforcers following bowel movements and for accident-free periods, and handling accidents in a nonpunitive manner. Similarly, Christophersen and Rainey (30) successfully utilized cleanliness and habit training together with daily enemas or suppositories to maintain rectal sensitivity and promote defecation. Unfortunately, there have been no component analyses to ascertain the most important aspects of these treatment regimens.

Another promising behavioral approach to encopresis has incorporated the use of biofeedback techniques. Wald et al. (31) used biofeedback to teach relaxation of the external anal sphincter during defecation and compared outcomes to those in children receiving conventional mineral oil. Children with abnormal defecation patterns tended to do better with biofeedback, whereas children with normal defecation patterns responded better to conventional therapy. Although biofeedback may have no advantages when used as initial treatment, it may prove useful when encopresis is resistant to conventional medical and/or behavioral interventions (see Chapter 16).

B. Constipation in Young to Middle-Aged Adults

In contrast to childhood constipation, which occurs equally in boys and girls, chronic constipation in young to middle-aged adults occurs more often in women. Patients may complain of infrequent defecation, excessive straining when defecating, or both. Patients can be grouped according to clinical characteristics, studies of bowel function, and psychological profiles.

Physiological Types

Spastic constipation, also known as constipation-predominant irritable bowel syndrome (32), is a common cause of idiopathic constipation in this age group. It is characterized by the presence of abdominal pain, especially in the lower abdomen, and passage of small, hard stools, often with excessive straining and a sense of incomplete evacuation (see Chapter 9). These patients frequently complain of abdominal bloating and upper-gastrointestinal symptoms such as heartburn, dysphagia, and nausea. Others have clinical features suggestive of *hypotonic constipation*. They complain of infrequent defecation but do not experience abdominal pain or symptoms characteristic of spastic constipation. Often, these patients date onset of symptoms from their mid- to late teens or early 20s, and constipation is frequently unremitting.

Finally, some individuals complain predominantly of *dyschezia*, characterized by difficulty in passing stools (2). They tend to be somewhat older women who have problems evacuating solid stool; some have difficulty expelling liquids as well. These patients are heterogeneous with respect to colorectal function and psychological profiles.

Psychological Issues

The influence of behavioral and psychological factors on colonic function in patients with chronic functional constipation has not been extensively studied; moreover, the literature on the subject is somewhat contradictory. Several small but well-controlled studies suggest that stool output in nonconstipated male volunteers is influenced by personality factors (33) and that voluntary suppression of defecation can influence both stool frequency and colonic transit (34). In one small study of male volunteers aged 18 to 50 years (33), total dietary fiber was predictive of stool weight but not frequency of defecation; however, larger stools were produced by subjects who were more socially outgoing, less anxious, and more optimistic as measured by the Minnesota Multiphasic Personality Inventory (MMPI). The authors suggested that personality factors may predispose an individual to disorders for which fiber might be effective or protective. Since dietary fiber appeared to influence stool production independently of effects thought to be due to personality, those persons with low stool output might be particularly benefited by dietary fiber. In another study of male volunteers (34), voluntary suppression of the urge to defecate resulted in fewer and smaller stools as well as substantial slowing of colonic transit, especially in the distal colon. These findings support the commonly held concept that habitual suppression of the urge to defecate may lead to chronic constipation (35).

A number of surveys have shown that self-reported constipation and stool frequency are correlated with abnormal scores of self-administered psychometric tests (4). For example, after analyzing a survey of over 14,000 adults in the United States, Everhart and associates (2) concluded that symptoms of depression constituted an independent risk factor for self-reported constipation. Similarly, unspecified psychological distress correlated with self-reports of constipation in a survey of over 200 elderly persons living at home (36). These surveys did not evaluate patients seeking medical attention for constipation, which itself may be associated with increased psychological distress in individuals with functional gastrointestinal symptoms.

There have been relatively few studies that evaluate psychological parameters of patients who seek medical attention for severe chronic constipation. An early study (37) reported that constipated patients with normal transit often exhibited evidence of psychosocial disturbances, including the use of antidepressant medications and ongoing psychiatric counseling; in contrast, patients with slow colonic transit uncommonly manifested evidence of psychological dysfunction. Using a prospectively obtained, self-administered behavioral instrument, the SCL-90-R (38), Wald and colleagues (13) demonstrated that constipated patients with normal colonic transit had significantly higher scores for psychological distress than did those with slow transit, and that the latter had psychological profiles similar to those of a control group. Subsequently, similar findings were obtained in a somewhat larger group of constipated patients (39); moreover, the SCL-90-R instrument was noted to have certain advantages over the MMPI for clinical purposes. It provides information similar to the MMPI with which to measure behavioral profiles of patients in an office setting, but it can be completed and scored more rapidly and easily. These studies suggest that patients who complain of severe idiopathic constipation may be broadly separated into two groups based on colonic transit and psychological profiles, and that different therapeutic approaches may be required: one behaviorally and psychologically based (for those with normal transit) and the other focused on modification of disordered colonic transit.

These findings were somewhat at variance with those of Devroede and colleagues (40), who measured the personality characteristics of 38 women with slow-transit constipation. They found no correlation between stool frequency and personality but did find that high levels of anxiety significantly correlated with slow transit of markers through the right colon. They also noted that women with a pattern of colonic inertia did not exhibit this association, which was restricted to those with slowing of the distal colon (hindgut delay). The reasons for the inconsistent findings between this study and those previously cited are unknown.

The importance of psychological screening of severely constipated patients was also emphasized in a recent report of 21 patients who underwent subtotal colectomy for intractable symptoms (41). Preoperative scores for anxiety and depression were significantly higher in the eight patients who had an unsatisfactory outcome than in the 13 who showed clinical benefit from the procedure. As the results of the colonic transit studies were not provided, it is possible that some or all of the patients who had a poor outcome had normal colonic transit.

It is undoubtedly too simplistic to divide chronically constipated patients into precisely defined subgroups on the basis of psychological and physiological patterns. However, the literature does suggest that measuring psychological distress as well as colonic function is both prudent and necessary when evaluating adult patients with chronic servere functional constipation.

Treatment

Dietary Approaches Dietary adjustments are the first line of intervention for most adults with idiopathic constipation. Although constipation appears to result from dietary-fiber inadequacy in some individuals, there is no evidence that most constipated patients consume less fiber than do nonconstipated individuals (2,4). However, many constipated individuals do respond when fiber intake is increased to between 20 and 30 g per day, although whether this represents a purely physiological effect is not entirely clear.

Fiber components are not equivalent in their ability to modify stool characteristics and bowel habit. For example, wheat bran is most effective in increasing stool weight, followed by fruits and vegetables, oats, mucilages, corn, cellulose, soya, and pectin. The "bulking" effect of fiber is not related entirely to water-retention capabilities or mechanical factors but also to colonic microbial ecology and interaction with intraluminal contents. Fiber supplements may help those with low fiber intake and patients with "spastic constipation," in whom fiber intake should be increased gradually to avoid undue cramping and bloating. If there is a fecal impaction, it should be removed before starting fiber supplementation. Patients with obstructive lesions anywhere in the gastrointestinal tract should not be given fiber supplements. Fiber is not indicated in patients with megacolon or megarectum, who are better managed by reducing colonic contents and periodic timed evacuation.

Behavioral Approaches One behavioral approach is the use of *biofeedback* to correct inappropriate contraction of the pelvic-floor muscles and external anal sphincter during defecation (see Chapter 16). Studies have employed EMG recordings using anal plugs or anorectal manometers to monitor external anal-sphincter pressures during attempted expulsion of the apparatus (31,42). The patient watches the recordings of EMG or pressure responses and is told to modify inappropriate responses through trial-and-error efforts. Improvement has been reported in constipated adults receiving biofeedback for rectosphincteric dyssynergia, but these studies are small and uncontrolled. Biofeedback warrants further evaluation in such patients and may prove helpful to some. It may be important to assess behavioral parameters in candidate patients, as some reports suggest that biofeedback has a higher failure rate in patients with psychosocial distress.

Laxatives Laxatives are classified into five groups on the basis of their presumed mode of action. Except for bulk laxatives and hyperosmolar agents, chronic laxative use should be discouraged in young to middle-aged adults.

The *bulk-forming laxatives* consist of natural (psyllium) or synthetic polysaccharides or cellulose derivatives that act in a manner similar to dietary fiber. Because fluid intake should be increased with these preparations, caution should be exercised in patients who require severe fluid restriction.

Docusate salts are anionic surfactants that lower the surface tension of stool to allow mixing of aqueous and fatty substances. This softens stool to permit easier defecation. Recent studies failed to demonstrate changes in stool water content, stool weight, frequency of defecation, or colonic transit times when docusates were given in currently recommended doses (43).

Hyperosmolar agents include nonabsorbable sugars such as lactulose and sorbitol. Sorbitol and lactulose are degraded by colonic bacteria to low-molecular-weight acids that increase stool acidity and osmolarity. Doses should be adjusted to reduce side effects and modulate defecation.

Saline laxatives include magnesium salts and mixed electrolyte solutions containing polyethylene glycol that exert an osmotic effect to increase intraluminal water content. Magnesium salts may stimulate the release of cholecystokinin to increase intestinal motor activity but should be avoided in patients with renal insufficiency because of the danger of magnesium toxicity (44).

Stimulant laxatives include castor oil, anthraquinones (cascara sagrada, senna, and casanthranol), and diphenylmethanes (phenolphthalein and bisacodyl). Castor oil is hydrolyzed by intestinal lipases to ricinoleic acid, which stimulates intestinal secretion and intestinal motility. Anthraquinone laxatives increase fluid and electrolyte accumulation in the distal ileum and colon and are pharmacologically activated when they come in contact with intestinal microorganisms. Pathological changes in the colon produced by chronic anthraquinone use include melanosis coli, a benign and reversible condition, and possible damage to the myenteric plexus (45). Bisacodyl and phenolphthalein act directly to stimulate colonic motor activity and inhibit glucose and sodium absorption to increase intraluminal fluid content.

In general, the chronic use of phenolphthalein, anthracene glycosides, and other stimulant laxatives should be avoided, although concerns about the risk of damage to the myenteric plexus may be exaggerated. Certainly, the chronic use of these agents may result in abdominal cramps, fluid and electrolyte disturbances, malabsorption, and psychological dependency. As these agents are readily available as over-the-counter medications, efforts must be made to educate patients and convince them to minimize their use of these agents.

Prokinetic Agents The use of drugs to enhance colonic transit by increasing propulsive motor activity has been hampered somewhat by our limited knowledge concerning the control of colonic motility and the pathophysiology of severe idiopathic constipation. *Cholinergic agents* such as bethanechol and neostigmine have been used with little success and moderate side effects in patients with the pattern of colonic inertia (9).

A new class of drugs that stimulate gastrointestinal motor activity to enhance transit of intraluminal contents are the *prokinetic agents*. Metoclopramide exerts little effect on colonic motility and is not effective in constipated patients. Cisapride is a newer prokinetic agent that appears to enhance transit through the proximal colon in humans and has been shown to stimulate distal colonic motility and improve rectal sensation in chronically constipated patients (46). Although some studies have reported clinical improvement with the drug (47), others report disappointing results in patients with severe idiopathic constipation.

Several patients with severe constipation have been treated successfully with *opioid-receptor antagonists*. Naloxone has been found to accelerate transit in various parts of the colon in normal volunteers (48) and may increase stool volumes in elderly constipated individuals when compared to placebo (49). Further studies are required to assess this class of agents.

Surgical Treatment In carefully selected patients with colonic inertia, subtotal colectomy with ileorectal anastomosis can be dramatically beneficial in ameliorating incapacitating symptoms that are unresponsive to medical management (50). Before surgery is undertaken, it is important to document that the disorder is confined to the large intestine by performing radiological and/or manometric studies to establish normal esophageal, gastric, and small-intestinal motor function.

Constipation in Patients with Eating Disorders (see Chapter 11)

Anorexia nervosa and bulimia nervosa are related eating disorders that affect 2–7% of women and a smaller portion of men (51). Abdominal bloating, cramps, and constipation are frequent in this population (52), as is the high frequency of abuse of laxatives and diuretics. In a study of 10 anorectic and 18 bulimic patients, colonic transit was found to be significantly prolonged in both groups compared to healthy controls, although there was much variability and transit times in both groups overlapped those of the control population (51). Transit times were not related to caloric intake at the time of testing, or to laxative abuse or use of anticholinergic medications. The authors speculated that delayed gut transit may predispose to eating disorders in one of two ways. First, rectal distension reflexively inhibits gastric emptying (53), which might interfere with normal satiety mechanisms. Second, subjective sensations of bloating might aggravate a patient's fear of fatness. At present, there is no support for either of these hypotheses in patients with eating disorders.

C. Constipation in the Elderly

Constipation is a frequently expressed concern for elderly persons, and the number of physician visits for constipation rises steeply among people over age 65 years (5,6). Moreover, many healthy elderly persons use laxatives regularly and often inappropriately. Most elderly individuals with chronic constipation had similar complaints when they were younger (54). Others develop constipation due to colonic or systemic disorders or as a side effect of medications. There are little data to suggest that aging alone significantly affects colonic motor function.

Institutionalized Elderly

Fecal impaction is a significant problem in elderly individuals who are institutionalized (55). Mental confustion, immobility, or inadequate toilet arrangements may contribute to failure to act on the urge to defecate, and dyschezia may occur when the fecal bolus becomes too large or uncomfortable to pass. The development of megarectum blunts rectal sensation; this often persists after disimpaction (56) and predisposes such patients to reaccumulate feces unless scrupulous toileting programs are instituted. Fecal impaction is the most common cause of spurious diarrhea and of fecal incontinence in the institutionalized elderly (57).

Ambulatory Elderly

Surprisingly little is known about constipation in the ambulatory elderly population. However, population surveys of constipation that address only frequency of defecation overlook the fact that many constipated elderly patients complain of excessive straining when defecating (36,58). These complaints may be exaggerated by depression and social isolation (59), use of constipating medications, or illnesses associated with chronic constipation.

Psychological Issues

Among the predisposing causes of constipation in the elderly are psychological distress, depression, and dementia, which are associated with increased self-reporting of constipation (2,36). One hypothesis to explain these findings is that psychological factors such as anxiety and depression may result in symptom distortion or exaggeration, or excessive preoccupation with bodily functions. Another explanation is that depression and dementia predispose to constipation, in part because such patients ignore the urge to defecate, a hypothesis supported by the previously mentioned study concerning the effects of voluntary suppression of defecation on colonic function (34).

Laxative Use and Abuse

Another aspect of this problem is the documentation that laxative use by elderly people often bears little relationship to either bowel frequency or the presence of defecatory straining. Indeed, one-fifth to one-third of regular laxative users do not consider themselves to be constipated (1,59), but rather have a misguided belief that regular purgation is beneficial to their health (60). Habitual rather than surreptitious laxative abuse is more often found in the elderly (61); this perpetuates a cycle in which laxatives empty the colon of stool that normally would pass into the rectum and signal an urge to defecate. Because the colon has been emptied, the patient often has no urge to defecate for several days; this in turn makes the anxious patient use more laxatives and perpetuates the cycle. Unfortunately, such practices may extend to institutionalized patients; several studies have documented that approximately three-fourths of all hospitalized elderly persons or nursing-home residents are prescribed at least one type of laxative (62).

Treatment of Constipation in the Elderly

Many elderly individuals use laxatives regularly and often excessively and inappropriately. Education as to what are normal bowel habits and that daily defecation or purgation is not necessary for good health should be addressed to any patient who complains of constipation (61). A careful psychological assessment to exclude depression, dementia, or excessive preoccupation with bodily functions is also important during the initial assessment and in formulating a therapeutic strategy. Finally, a careful review of all medications that potentially have constipating side effects should be carried out so that attempts to eliminate, reduce, or substitute them with nonconstipating alternatives can be made.

Behavioral Approaches Further assessment and advice about toileting habits are often helpful. In institutional settings, attention should be given to comfort and privacy, with adequate time allotted to attempt defecation after breakfast or other meals to take advantage of the gastrocolonic response that occurs with eating. Elevating the legs when seated on the toilet may assist patients with weakened abdominal and pelvic-floor muscles. If stools are hard and defecatory straining is to be minimized, docusates may help to soften stools, although they have no demonstrable laxative activity (43).

Fiber Although there is little if any evidence that constipated patients eat less fiber than do nonconstipated individuals, most physicians believe that a common cause of chronic constipation in the elderly is improper diet. The addition of bran to the diet of normal individuals increases stool weight, shortens colonic transit time, and increases frequency of defecation (63). Wheat bran appears to be most effective in shortening transit times; numerous reports have documented that constipation is reduced in the institutionalized elderly following the addition of dietary fiber and fluids in a controlled fashion (64,65). In these studies, bran supplements from 6 to 20 g daily were well tolerated by patients. During the initial stages of bran supplementation, patients may complain of abdominal discomfort or excessive flatulence, but these symptoms usually improve with time. In general, bran administered in the form of cereals, breads, and biscuits appears to be somewhat better tolerated than psyllium and other bulk-forming preparations, whose taste and consistency tend to reduce patient compliance.

Osmotic Agents Of the many laxatives available, lactulose or sorbitol is recommended for chronic use if fiber supplements are ineffective or poorly tolerated (66). The effective daily dose ranges from 7.5 to 30 ml. Polyethylene glycol electrolyte solution (8 to 16 oz per day) may be effective as well, although published studies are methodologically flawed (67). Mineral oil should be avoided because it may lead to aspiration with lipid pneumonia and perhaps to deficiencies of fat-soluble vitamins.

Stimulant Laxatives The chronic use of stimulant laxatives has been discouraged. Avoidance of these drugs may be more important in younger individuals, because of the potential for long-term side effects, than in the elderly. Certainly, the stimulant laxatives are the most commonly abused cathartics, and their chronic use may lead to abdominal cramps, fluid and electrolyte disturbances, malasorption, and cathartic colon (68). Unfortunately, these agents are readily available as over-the-counter medications, and the elderly are often unwilling to change patterns of use they have enagaged in for many years. With such individuals, it seems reasonable to achieve a compromise by limiting use of these cathartics to once or twice weekly. Such an approach should help to minimize adverse effects.

Treatment of Fecal Impactions Prevention and treatment of fecal impactions are important in managing institutionalized elderly people. In cases of fecal impaction, enemas should be administered daily until there is no evidence of impaction; this is followed by sorbitol, perhaps combined with senna, until there is no radiographic evidence of stool retention (61). Prophylactic measures such as daily sorbitol may be used to prevent recurrent impaction. If this is impractical or unsuccessful, enemas once or twice weekly may be required to prevent recurrent impaction.

D. Constipation in Patients with Profound Psychiatric Illness

Severe constipation, often with fecal retention and megacolon, have been described in patients with serious psychiatric illness, particularly schizophrenia and depression. Often, they are institutionalized and may develop constipation because their illness somewhat reduces the urge to defecate or because they simply ignore it. Psychopharmacological agents may contribute to this condition as well.

Management consists of disimpaction, colonic cleansing with enemas and laxatives, and attempts to reestablish a normal toilet routine, similar to the approach used in children with constipation or encopresis. In some patients with megacolon, polyethylene glycol solution (8 to 16 oz per day) is more helpful than lactulose or cathartics.

ACKNOWLEDGMENT

I wish to thank Ms. Helen Gibson for her expert preparation of the manuscript.

REFERENCES

1. Connell, AM, Hilton C, Irvin G, Lennard-Jones JE, Misiewicz JJ. Variations in bowel habit in two population samples. Br Med J 1965; 2:1095–1099.
2. Everhart JE, Go VLW, Johannes RS, et al. A longitudinal survey of self-reported bowel habits in the United States. Dig Dis Sci 1989; 34:1153–1162.
3. Sandler RS, Drossman DA. Bowel habits in young adults not seeking health care. Dig Dis Sci 1987; 32:841–845.
4. Whitehead WE, Chaussade S, Corazziari E, Kumar D. Report of an international workshop on management of constipation. Gastroenterol Int 1991; 4(3):99–113.
5. Sandler RS, Jordan MC, Shelton BJ. Demographic and dietary determinants of constipation in the US population. J Public Health 1990; 80:185–189.
6. Johanson JF, Sonnenberg A, Koch TR. Clinical epidemiology of chronic constipation. J Clin Gastroenterol 1989; 11(5):525–536.
7. Sonnenberg A, Koch TR. Physician visits in the United States for constipation: 1958 to 1986. Dig Dis Sci 1989; 34:606–611.
8. Sonnenberg A, Koch TR. Epidemiology of constipation in the United States. Dis Colon Rectum 1989; 32:1–8.
9. Wald A. Constipation. In: Winawer SJ, ed. Management of Gastrointestinal Diseases. New York: Gower Medical Publishing, 1992:33.1–33.24.
10. Hinds JP, Wald A. Colonic and anorectal dysfunction associated with multiple sclerosis. Am J Gastroenterol 1989; 84:587–595.
11. Mahieu P, Pringot J, Bodart P. Defecography. II. Contributions to the diagnosis of defecation disorders. Gastrointest Radiol 1984; 9:253–261.
12. Metcalf AM, Phillips SF, Zinsmeister AR, et al. Simplified assessment of segmental colonic transit. Gastroenterology 1987; 92:40–47.
13. Wald A, Hinds JP, Caruana BJ. Psychological and physiological characteristics of patients with severe idiopathic constipation. Gastroenterology 1989; 97:932–937.
14. Tobon F, Reid NCRW, Talbert JL, Schuster MM. Nonsurgical test for the diagnosis of Hirschsprung's disease. N Engl J Med 1968; 278:188–194.
15. Preston DM, Lennard-Jones JE. Anismus in chronic constipation. Dig Dis Sci 1985; 30:413–418.

16. Wald A, Chandra R, Chiponis D, Gabel S. Anorectal function and continence mechanisms in childhood encopresis. J Pediatr Gastroenterol Nutr 1986; 5:346–351.
17. Corazziari E, Cucchiara S, Staiano A, et al. Gastrointestinal transit time, frequency of defecation and anorectal manometry in healthy and constipated children. J Pediatrics 1985; 106:379–382.
18. Loening-Baucke VA, Cruikshank BM. Abnormal defecation dynamics in chronically constipated children with encopresis. J Pediatrics 1986; 108:562–566.
19. Wald A, Handen BL. Behavioral aspects of disorders of defecation and fecal continence. Ann Behav Med 1987; 9(3):19–23.
20. Bellman MM. Studies on encopresis. Acta Paediatrica Scandinavia 1966; 56(suppl 170):1–151.
21. Lowery SP, Srour JW, Whitehead WE, et al. Habit training as treatment of encopresis secondary to chronic constipation. J Pediatr Gastroenterol Nutr 1985; 4:397–401.
22. Bemporad JR, Kresch RA, Asnes R, Wilson A. Chronic neurotic encopresis as a paradigm of a multifactorial psychiatric disorder. J Nerv Ment Disord 1987; 166:472–479.
23. Hoag JM, Norriss NG, Himeno ET, Jacobs J. The encopretic child and his family. J Am Acad Child Psychiatry 1971; 10:242–256.
24. Levine MD. Encopresis: Its potentiation, evaluation, and alleviation. Pediatr Clin North Am 1982; 29(2):315–331.
25. Gabel S, Hegedus AM. Wald A, Chandra R, Chiponis D. Prevalence of behavior problems and mental health utilization among encopretic children: Implications for behavioral pediatrics. Development Behav Pediatrics 1986; 7:293–297.
26. Wolters WHG, Wauters EAK. A study of somatopsychic vulnerability in encopretic children. Psychother Psychosom 1975; 26:27–34.
27. Landman GB, Rappaport L, Fenton T, Levine M. Locus of control and self-esteem in children with encopresis. Development Behav Pediatrics 1986; 7:111–113.
28. Levine MD, Bakow H. Children with encopresis: A study of treatment outcome. Pediatrics 1976; 58:845–852.
29. Parker L, Whitehead WE. Treatment of urinary and fecal incontinence in children. In: Russo DR, Varni JW, eds. Behavioral Pediatrics: Research and Practice. New York: Plenum Press, 1982:143–174.
30. Christopherson ER, Rainey SK. Management of encopresis through a pediatric outpatient clinic. J Ped Psychol 1976; 4:38–41.
31. Wald A, Chandra R, Gabel S, Chiponis D. Evaluation of biofeedback in childhood encopresis. J Pediatr Gastroenterol Nutr 1987; 6:554–558.
32. Whitehead WE, Engel BT, Schuster MM. Irritable bowel syndrome: Physiological and psychological differences between diarrhea-predominant and constipation-predominant patients. Dig Dis Sci 1980; 25:404–413.
33. Tucker DM, Sandstead HH, Logan GM, et al. Dietary fiber and personality factors as determinants of stool output. Gastroenterology 1981; 81:879–883.
34. Klauser AG, Voderhoizer WA, Heinrich CA, et al. Behavioral modification of colonic function: Can constipation be learned? Dig Dis Sci 1990; 35(10):1271–1275.
35. Phillips S. Disorders of gastrointestinal motility. In: Wyngaarden JB, Lloyd HS, eds. Cecil Textbook of Medicine. 18th ed. Philadelphia: WB Saunders; 1988:714–725.

36. Whitehead WE, Drinkwater D, Cheskin LJ, Heller BR, Schuster MM. Constipation in the elderly living at home: Definition, prevalence and relationship to life style and health status. J Am Geriatr Soc 1989; 37:423–429.
37. Wald A. Colonic transit and anorectal manometry in chronic idiopathic constipation. Arch Intern Med 1986; 146:1713–1716.
38. Derogatis LR, Rickels K, Rock K, Rock AF. The SCL-90 and the MMPI: A step in the validation of a new self-report scale. Br J Psychiatry 1976; 128:280–289.
39. Wald A, Burgio K, Holeva K, Locher J. Psychological evaluation of patients with severe idiopathic constipation: Which instrument to use? Am J Gastroenterol 1992; 87:977–980.
40. Devroede G, Girand G, Bouchoucha M, et al. Idiopathic constipation by colonic dysfunction: Relationship with personality and anxiety. Dig Dis Sci 1989; 34:1428–1433.
41. Fisher SE, Breckan K, Andrews HA, Keighley MRB. Psychiatric screening for patients with faecal incontinence or chronic constipation referred for surgical treatment. Br J Surg 1989; 76:352–355.
42. Bleijenberg G, Kuijpers HC. Treatment of the spastic pelvic floor syndrome with biofeedback. Dis Colon Rectum 1987; 30:108–111.
43. Chapman RU, Sillery J, Fontana DD, Matthys C, Saunders DR. Effect of oral dioctyl sodium sulfosuccinate on intake-output studies of human small and large intestine. Gastrenterology 1985; 89:489–493.
44. Sekas G. The use and abuse of laxatives: Recognizing the abusive patient. Practical Gastroenterol 1987; 11:33–39.
45. Smith B. Pathologic changes in the colon produced by anthroquinone purgatives. Dis Colon Rectum 1973; 16:455–458.
46. Krevsky B, Mauer A, Malmud LS, Fisher RS. Cisapride accelerates colonic transit in constipated patients with colonic inertia. Am J Gastroenterol 1989; 84:882–887.
47. Muller-Lissner SA and The Bavarian Constipation Study Group. Treatment of chronic constipation with cisapride and placebo. Gut 1987; 28:1033–1038.
48. Kaufman PN, Krevsky B, Malmud LS, et al. Role of opiate receptors in the regulation of colonic transit. Gastroenterology 1988; 94:1351–1356.
49. Kreek MJ, Paris P, Bartol MA, Mueller D. Effects of short-term oral administration of the specific opioid antagonist naloxone on fecal evacuation in geriatric patients. Gastroenterology 1984; 86:1144.
50. Pemberton JH, Rath DM, Ilstrup DM. Evaluation and surgical treatment of severe chronic constipation. Ann Surg 1991; 214:403–413.
51. Kamal N, Chami T, Andersen A, et al. Delayed gastrointestinal transit times in anorexia nervosa and bulimia nervosa. Gastroenterology 1991; 101:1320–1324.
52. Waldholz BD, Andersen AE. Gastrointestinal symptoms in anorexia nervosa: A prospective study. Gastroenterology 1990; 98:1415–1419.
53. Youle MS, Read NW. Effect of painless rectal distension on gastrointestinal transit of solid meal. Dig Dis Sci 1984; 29:902–906.
54. Wald A. Constipation and fecal incontinence in the elderly. Gastroenterol Clin North Am 1990; 19:405–418.
55. Wrenn K. Fecal impaction. N Engl J Med 1989; 321:658–662.

56. Read NW, Abouzekry L, Read MG, Howell P, Ottewell D, Donnelly TC. Anorectal function in elderly patients with fecal impaction. Gastroenterology 1985; 89:959–966.
57. Szurszewski JH, Holt PR, Schuster MM. Proceedings of a workshop entitled "Neuromuscular Function and Dysfunction of the Gastrointestinal Tract in Aging." Dig Dis Sci 1989; 34:1135–1146.
58. Talley NJ, O'Keefe EA, Zinsmeister AR, Melton LJ. Prevalence of gastrointestinal symptoms and functional bowel disorders in the elderly: A population-based study. Gastroenterology 1992; 102:895–901.
59. Donald IP, Smith RG, Cruikshank JG, Elton RA, Stoddary ME. A study of constipation in the elderly living at home. Gerontology 1985; 31:112–118.
60. Moore-Gillon V. Constipation: What does the patient mean? J Roy Soc Med 1984; 77:108–110.
61. Harari D, Gurwitz JH, Minaker KL. Constipation in the elderly. J Am Geriatr Soc 1993; 41:1130–1140.
62. Kinnunen O. Study of constipation in a geriatric hospital, day hospital, old people's home and at home. Aging 1991; 3:161–170.
63. Burkitt DP, Walker ARP, Painter NS. Effect of dietary fibre on stool and transit times and its role in the causation of disease. Lancet 1972; ii:1408–1411.
64. Hope AK, Down EC. Dietary fiber and fluid in the control of constipation in a nursing home population. Med J Australia 1986; 144:306–307.
65. Hull C, Greco RS, Brooks DC. Alleviation of constipation in the elderly by dietary fiber supplementation. J Am Geriatr Soc 1980; 28:410–414.
66. Lederle FA, Busch DL, Mattox KM, West MJ, Aske DM. Cost-effective treatment of constipation in the elderly: A randomized double-blind comparison of sorbitol and lactulose. Am J Med 1990; 89:597–601.
67. Andorsky RI, Goldner F. Colonic lavage solution (polyethylene glycol electrolyte lavage solution) as a treatment for chronic constipation: A double-blind, placebo-controlled study. Am J Gastroenterol 1990; 85:261–265.
68. Wald A. Constipation in elderly patients: Pathogenesis and management. Drugs Aging 1993; 3(3):220–231.

11

Gastrointestinal Aspects of Eating Disorders

Bruce D. Waldholtz
Eastern Virginia Medical School
Norfolk, Virginia

Arnold E. Andersen
University of Iowa College of Medicine
Iowa City, Iowa

I. INTRODUCTION

Anorexia nervosa and bulimia are psychiatric disorders that often result in gastrointestinal (GI) symptoms and complications (1,2). These gastrointestinal symptoms may cause significant distress and interfere with psychiatric treatment unless dealt with effectively (3,4). Comprehensive treatment of gastrointestinal symptoms, on the other hand, increases the therapeutic alliance and allows the treatment team to move to the central goals of behavior change and reevaluation of the commitment to weight loss as a central source of self-esteem, identity, and mood regulation.

In each patient it is important to consider whether GI symptoms are 1) expected findings associated with the natural history of the eating disorder, 2) due to treatment, such as refeeding, or 3) due to underlying coexistent or prior GI disease.

The goals of this chapter are to:

1. Review common GI symptoms of eating disorders described in the literature and based on our experience with several hundred inpatients
2. Examine esophageal and gastric symptomatology as a cause or consequence of anorexia nervosa
3. Examine constipation and laxative abuse, their significance and treatment, as a frequent "vicious circle" of medical symptomatology and behavioral dysfunction
4. Review clinical studies on the time course of GI symptoms from weight loss or binge–purge behavior and the resolution of these symptoms with treatment
5. Suggest how to formulate a treatment plan for patients with anorexia nervosa and bulimia nervosa, including guidelines for refeeding or interruption of binge–purge behaviors and suggestions for when further GI studies are needed

II. DIAGNOSIS, EPIDEMIOLOGY, AND ETIOLOGY

Table 1 summarizes diagnostic criteria for anorexia nervosa, bulimia nervosa, and eating disorders not otherwise specified, also known as atypical eating disorders, including a newer diagnostic subtype, binge eating disorder. Anorexia and bulimia nervosa are two sides of the same coin. Both disorders begin by attempts at weight loss in more than 95% of cases. In anorexia nervosa, the weight loss is sustained and then leads to the formal diagnosis of anorexia nervosa when weight becomes less than 85% of normal and is associated with an overvaluation of thinness and a phobic fear of fatness, plus abnormality of reproductive-hormone functioning (more than 3 months of amenorrhea in women or a decrease in sexual drive and functioning in men). These individuals are often very persevering in temperament, with anxious, perfectionistic, and obsessional features (5). Anorexia is divided into a pure food-restricting subtype (ANR) and a bulimic subtype (ANB), the latter being present when patients binge or purge during a significant part of their anorexic disorder.

In contrast, bulimia nervosa represents, in many ways, a failed attempt at anorexia nervosa. In these individuals, hunger breaks through the attempt at weight loss. Initially, hunger-based binges overtake the patient's attempt at slimming, producing great psychological stress because the binges represent exactly the opposite of what the dieter was trying to achieve. Soon, however, the binges undergo a transition, becoming driven by their ability to give relief from emotional distress. A formal diagnosis of bulimia nervosa is made when binge episodes occur approximately twice a week for 3 or more months, in association with the same psychopathology as anorexia nervosa, and when followed by compensatory attempts at avoiding weight gain such as self-induced vomiting,

TABLE 1 Diagnostic Criteria for Anorexia Nervosa, Bulimia Nervosa, and Eating Disorders Not Otherwise Specified (Atypical Eating Disorders), Including Binge Eating Disorder

A. Anorexia nervosa, food restricting subtype (ANR)
   1. Self-induced weight loss or failure to gain weight normally, with resulting weight more than 15% below normal, through food restriction without binge or purge behavior
   2. An inappropriate, excessive fear of fatness and pursuit of thinness
   3. Reproductive hormone abnormality: for females, 3 months of secondary amenorrhea, or primary amenhorrhea; for males, decreased sexual drive and function, associated with lowered testosterone
   4. Usually associated with distorted body image
B. Anorexia nervosa, bulimic subtype (ANB)—see 1–4 above, plus:
   5. Binge episodes and/or purging by vomiting, laxative, diuretic abuse, compensatory fasting, or excessive exercise after binge eating
C. Bulimia nervosa at normal weight (BN)
   1. Anorexia nervosa criteria for weight not fulfilled
   2. Presence of binge episodes—usually large amount of food, often high in fats and sweets, generally eaten quickly and privately while feeling out of control, to the point of physical and/or psychological discomfort, social interruption, or running out of food; followed by guilt and self-blame—two episodes per week for 3 months on average
   3. Preoccupation with desire to be thinner or different in shape and/or irrational fear of becoming fat
   4. Generally, distortion of body image, body rejection, excess dissatisfaction with body size and/or shape.
   5. Binges followed by efforts to compensate for excess food intake by at least one of the following:
      a. Self-induced vomiting
      b. Periods of food restriction
      c. Laxative, diuretic, emetine (Ipecac), or diet-pill abuse
D. Eating disorders not otherwise specified (EDNOS)—milder versions of anorexia or bulimia that do not currently meet full criteria; for example, only one binge episode a week or binges for less than 3 months; weight loss less than 15% for anorexia; weight loss more than 15% but no amenorrhea, etc.
   1. Major EDNOS subtype: binge eating disorder—binge episodes with typical psychopathology, at normal or overweight, with no postbinge compensating behaviors.

medication abuse, compulsive exercise, or rigorous fasting. Reproductive-hormone abnormality may be present, but is not required. These criteria represent the current standardized consensus for diagnosis, but will undoubtedly continue to evolve. The definition of a binge remains elusive, but in practice, these episodes typically consist of the ingestion of large amounts of food, eaten rapidly to the point of medical and/or psychological distress, and are followed by guilt, and by compensatory attempts to avoid weight gain.

The proposed new diagnostic category of *binge eating disorder* is considered a form of atypical eating disorder in the new psychiatric diagnostic manual (6), but has gained widespread acceptance by many clinicians and researchers as a separate subtype. This variant is characterized by episodes of binge eating along with preoccupying fear of weight gain, but without any compensatory purging or fasting afterward. It tends to occur in older individuals (in their 30s and 40s) who are more passive in personality, nurturing of others but not of themselves, and low in self-esteem. They are typically mildly (20–40%) to moderately (40–60%) overweight, less often severely (60–100%) or morbidly obese (>100% excess).

The true onset of eating disorders begins in childhood even though symptoms generally manifest themselves in adolescence or later. Children and adolescents in this country, and most of the Western democracies, are subjected to a relentless gender-divergent process of socialization regarding body size and shape. By the sixth grade, approximately half of girls feel fat. Nylander (7) has shown that more than 70% of Swedish young women between 14 and 21 years of age feel fat enough to diet. Even when women are 10% or more under average weight, 50% still feel fat and would like to reduce. There appears to be at least a 15% threshold difference in the percent of ideal body weight between men and women regarding the point at which they feel fat and begin to diet. While most people accept that height and intelligence are distributed in a bell-shaped curve, there is not the same acceptance that weight has a broad normal distribution around an average. To be healthy but incidentally 20% above average weight is almost always unacceptable in an upper-middle-class family. There is increasing divergence between norms and ideals versus actual weight of the population, with the population weight slowly increasing and idealized norms decreasing for women.

The prevalence of eating disorders in the population may be different in number and type from cases referred to treatment centers. Prevalence rates also depend on current diagnostic criteria. A reasonable current estimate is that between 0.5 and 1% of college-bound white females meet full criteria for full anorexia nervosa and up to 5% may experience a transient or milder form. Two to four percent meet full criteria for bulimia nervosa (8), while up to 15% experience some form of bulimic symptomatology short of full criteria. A substantial, not well defined number of individuals meet criteria for atypical forms of eating disorders or for newly emerging diagnoses such as binge eating disorder, which is found in approximately 25% of persons with medical obesity.

Theander (9) has documented up to 19% excess mortality in a 30-year follow-up of eating-disordered patients compared to a matched population. These rates of death attributable to eating disorders appear to have decreased recently, especially acute fatality, but still remain substantial and may occur years to decades after the onset of illness. Three groups that are often overlooked in diagnosis are males (10), minorities (11), and matrons (in study average age was 59 years) (12). Age of onset may be as young as 7 years or older than 70 years, even though most cases do begin between 13 and 21 years of age.

The history of eating disorders is replete with disproven or unproven theories of single causation. The current consensus is that eating disorders are a probabilistic outcome of the number and severity of specific risk factors present. In addition to a sociocultural environment that promotes slimness and/or shape change as a means of dealing with developmental issues, eating disorders have been quantitatively related to other specific variables. There is a 10-fold greater incidence in females compared to males. A rigorous ballet school was shown to have a sevenfold higher than average occurrence rate of anorexia nervosa and 50% occurrence of amenhorrea (13). Individuals with a family history of depressive illness have four to five times as much probability of developing an eating disorder as those without a similar history.

A history of familial obesity leads to an increased probability of bulimia nervosa, as do certain personality features or participation in interest groups associated with weight loss, such as modeling or wrestling. The following equation summarizes, in very general form, the risk-factor probability of a specific individual's developing an eating disorder:

$$P_i = k \times p_g \times f(x_1, x_2, x_3 \ldots x_n)$$

where:

P_i = individual risk
p_g = risk by gender
$x_1, x_2, x_3 \ldots x_n$ = specific quantitative factors documented to increase risk

The exact way in which statistically proven psychosocial factors contribute to the onset and maintenance of eating disorders is not known, but clinical experience suggests that some factors lead to increased sensitivity to criticisms of self (low self-esteem), while others (depressive symptoms) pave the way by creating a negative body image that may be improved by self-starving or binge eating (see Table 2).

Even for those individuals who do not develop formal eating disorders, most women and a substantial minority of men in our society carry a psychological and social burden throughout life of continually feeling fat beyond objective measurements, and base an excessive proportion of their self-esteem, personal adequacy, and mood state on artificially low norms for body weight or, for men especially, impossible-to-achieve ideals of shape or height.

TABLE 2 Risk Factors That Increase Probability of Developing an Eating Disorder

A. Epidemiology
    1. Lives in a society that values slimness
    2. Female gender
    3. Membership in an interest group that encourages thinness—ballet, modeling, cheerleading, gymnastics, wrestling
    4. Adolescence or young adulthood
B. Dieting behavior
C. Comorbidity
    1. Vulnerable personality
        a. Anorexia: perfectionistic, self-critical, "external locus of control"
        b. Bulimia: impulsive, dramatic, borderline
    2. Personal history of mood disorder (OCD)
D. Developmental
    1. Childhood obesity with teasing, criticism
    2. Possibly history of sexual or physical abuse
    3. Early puberty, with weight greater than that of peers
E. Family
    1. Family pattern of enmeshed functioning
    2. Family history of:
        a. Mood disorder
        b. Obesity

A. Effects of Starvation

A number of papers have described common physiological changes in anorexia nervosa, including the bulimic subtype, during starvation (3,4,14–22). A generalized metabolic slowdown occurs in the starved anorexia nervosa patient, reflected in resulting bradycardia, hypotension, and hypothermia. This adaptive hypometabolic state may resemble the euthyroid-sick syndrome, in which peripheral conversion of thyroxin to triiodothyronine is decreased (20), or result in a frankly hypothyroid patient with bradycardia. The mechanism of hypothermia present in starvation from anorexia is not well understood but most likely represents hypothalamic dysfunction.

Amenorrhea occurs with sufficient weight loss, patients having decreased gonadotropin-releasing hormone (21). Interestingly, menses may stop early in the dieting process or after varying amounts of weight loss, stimulating unresolved controversy as to whether primary preexisting hypothalamic abnormality exists.

Hypercholesterolemia in anorexia nervosa was described by Klienfelter in 1965 (22), when he reviewed 98 patients with anorexia nervosa referred to Johns Hopkins Hospital over a 30-year period. He found significantly elevated cholesterol in some patients, with a mean value of 260 mg/dl despite their starved state, but no correlation was noted between cholesterol levels and duration of symptoms. The mechanism for this phenomenon remains unknown, occurring in the absence of thyroid dysfunction.

The eating behavior of these patients accounts for much of their medical symptomatology, either directly or indirectly. Self-induced vomiting or medication abuse after binge eating represents the other main factor contributing to medical symptomatology beside self-starvation. Table 3 summarizes in schematic form the differences in abnormal eating behavior among the various diagnostic categories. Some of these are based on firm research studies while others rest on clinical experience.

B. A Survey of the GI-Tract Findings in Eating Disorders

Oropharyngeal Effects

One subtle feature of anorexia nervosa or bulimia is damage to the enamel and dentin of teeth, especially the lingual surface, due to self-induced vomiting. This may be detected incidentally in normal-weight bulimic patients who present with potentially life-threatening hypokalemia from vomiting but no other physical

TABLE 3 Relative Frequency of Abnormal Eating Behavior in Typical Eating-Disordered Patients (by Subtype)

	ANR	ANB	BN	BED
Self-starvation	+++	++	+[a]	0
Secret eating	+[b]	+++	+++	++
"Grazing"	0	0	0	+++
Binge eating	0	+++	+++	++
Secret disposal of food	+++	++	+[c]	0
Hoarding food	+	++	+++	0
Stealing food	+	++	+++	0
Self-induced vomiting	+[d]	+++	+++	0
Laxative abuse	+	++	+++	0
Diuretic abuse	0	+	+	0
Compulsive exercise	+++	++	+	0
Ipecac abuse	0	+	++	0
Diet-pill abuse	0	+	++	0

[a]After binge episodes.
[b]Often before sleep.
[c]During restricting phase after binges.
[d]Without binges.

findings. Dentists are increasingly identifying this pattern and referring patients for treatment of the causative eating disorder. Some patients may damage the skin over the knuckles due to self-induced vomiting (Russell's sign) and this should be noted when present. Telangiectasisas of the facies may occur in patients with forceful vomiting. Patients may present with parotid hypertrophy ("chipmunk facies"), with symptomatic distress or no complaints.

The amylase elevation recorded in many patients with anorexia nervosa may actually be salivary in origin, not necessarily related to upper-abdominal discomfort (23,24). In addition, parotid gland enlargement may occur and may persist despite weight restoration, contributing to the elevated amylase level. Parotid enlargement occurs in association with both ANB and bulimia at normal weight even in the absence of alcohol use. However, pancreatitis may occur in these patients in association with underlying alcohol abuse, particularly if patients drink while depressed or to be less fearful of eating or if gallstones are present, for which patients may be at an increased risk secondary to significant weight loss (24,25).

Esophagus

Esophageal complications occur due to 1) reflux secondary to self-induced vomiting, 2) possible underlying esophageal motility dysfunction, and 3) eating-disorder-induced esophageal dysmotility with reversible peristaltic-type changes (20). Patients with bulimic features may rarely develop acute Mallory-Weiss tears, but more commonly develop the routine complications of significant reflux, that is, esophagitis, esophageal ulceration, and strictures or dysphasia (19). Studies are not in agreement about the frequency of significant esophageal complications (3,26).

Stacher et al. (27), for example, reported a high incidence of esophageal motility disorders in anorexia nervosa. Clouse (28) noted esophageal motility disturbances in many patients with depression and somatization disorders. Depressed anorectics may have reversible esophageal motility disorders that may improve with treatment of associated depression and/or weight restoration. In addition to Mallory-Weiss tears, rarely Boerhaave's syndrome can occur in any patient with persistent retching and self-induced vomiting.

Stomach

Delayed gastric emptying is one of the most important GI features in anorexia nervosa. Analysis of studies supports the conclusion that it is primarily a complication of weight loss rather than a cause of the disease itself, as has been postulated (3,29–34). Reports by Keys and others from experimental starvation studies around World War II demonstrated delayed gastric emptying on upper-GI x-rays and even reports of gastric rupture with rapid refeeding (35). There have been reports of gastric rupture with anorexia nervosa (36). A number of studies have demonstrated delayed gastric emptying on nuclear scans (30–34). However, in contrast to frequent complaints of gastric symptoms in nonanorectic patients with gastroparesis, such as bloating, fullness, vomiting, and postprandial pain, studies in patients with anorexia have not shown a good correlation between the results of emptying scans and subjective symptoms (30–34). We have shown improvement in bloating and other symptoms of gastroparesis from anorexia nervosa during nutritional rehabilitation despite consuming the 3500 to 4500 calories required daily to achieve adequate weight gain in these patients 93). Rigaud et al. also demonstrated improved gastric emptying with weight gain (29).

Improvement in gastric emptying has also been shown with medications, including bethanechol, metoclopramide, and cisapride, the latter released in 1993 (32–34,37). Metoclopramide, used at a dose of 5–10 mg 1/2 hour before meals and at bedtime, is a dopamine antagonist that not only promotes gastric emptying but also suppresses nausea and vomiting by a separate mechanism. However, its central-nervous-system side effects can include fatigue, anxiety, extrapyramidal complications, or depression, which may limit its use.

Bethanechol at a dose of 10–25 mg q.i.d. has also been shown to increase gastric emptying in anorexia nervosa (37). Neither domperidone nor cisapride, a recently released prokinetic drug, crosses the blood–brain barrier, causing fewer central-nervous-system side effects than metoclopramide. Domperidone acts via an antidopaminergic mechanism. Cisapride works by increasing the release of acetylcholine from postganglionic neurons, and is taken 15 minutes before meals and at bedtime. This medication was approved for the symptomatic relief of nocturnal heartburn due to gastroesophageal reflux and not specifically for anorexic gastroparesis.

In addition, erythromycin has been shown to improve gastric emptying in diabetic gastroparesis, but has not been studied in gastroparesis associated with anorexia nervosa. It improves gastric emptying for solids and liquids by acting as a motilin-receptor agonist, a hormone responsible for phase III contractions during the intradigestive motor complex (38). While studies demonstrate that these agents can improve gastric emptying in patients with gastroparesis from diabetes or possibly in anorexia nervosa, the routine use of these agents cannot be recommended in anorexia nervosa until studies demonstrate them to be effective. On a case-by-case basis, cisapride may be usefully employed.

The underlying pathophysiological gastric process in patients with anorexia nervosa is not a preexisting defect in gastric emptying that, if improved, will cure the disease, but rather (18,20) a primary psychiatric disorder with associated starvation and reversible gastroparesis (3,29). No patient in our series required prokinetic agents despite all of their severe intestinal symptoms; each substantially improved with weight gain alone (3). We provided continued medical education and reassurance to patients that their symptoms of gastroparesis would improve along with periodic medical follow-up, explaining the common occurrence and expected improvement of their symptoms. While our patients often expressed concern about bloating and fullness, their understanding of this process and the experiencing of gradual improvement, as predicted by us with time, allowed expectant management only, without the use of prokinetic agents.

Small Intestine

The small bowel has not been well studied in anorexia nervosa. Delayed motility has been documented throughout the entire GI tract, as determined by breath-hydrogen tests (4) although whether this is due to a delay in the small bowel, the colon, or a combined defect is not known. Primary malabsorption does not appear to occur, as diarrhea is not frequently seen without laxative abuse.

Large Intestine and Laxative Abuse

Large-intestine symptomatology is common in starving anorectics and generally improves with weight retoration. Dysfunction may be due not only to decreased intake but also to globally diminished autonomic body function and, where applicable, to side effects of prolonged laxative abuse, causing a cathartic colon. Many eating-disordered patients abuse laxatives due to the incorrect assumption that the laxatives will cause weight loss. Bo-Linn et al. (39) showed that even with 6 liters daily of diarrhea fluid from GoLytely purge, patients could not cause significant decrease in nutrient absorption. We inform our patients of this study during the process of refeeding and normalization of eating so that they can understand that they are not likely to lose weight by this method. Associated diuretic use may also, via electrolyte changes and dehydration, contribute to constipation.

Persistent diarrhea may require evaluation for laxative abuse, not only in eating disorders but in any patient with unexplained diarrhea. Stools can be tested for phenolphthalein by alkalization using one drop of 1N sodium hydroxide (NaOH) with 3 ml of stool supernate, which results in a positive pink to red color if present. The presence of melanosis coli on sigmoidoscopy suggests prolonged use of laxatives. Of note, melanosis coli can occur in the sigmoid from anthracin (senna, cascara, and aloe), but not with phenolphthalein or bisacodyl, which are diphenolic laxatives (40).

Constipation is a common complaint of these patients, and we should remember that diarrhea secondary to laxative abuse and diarrhea around constipation should certainly be considered in the differential diagnosis of any current diarrhea (3,40,41).

III. PRACTICE GUIDELINES: MEDICAL ASPECTS

A. General Medical Principles and Approach to the Patient

While anorexia nervosa and bulimia are probably psychiatric in origin, they may have a prolonged phase that is substantially medical, marked by frequent GI symptoms that can interfere with therapy. A careful general medical—and specifically GI—evaluation, beginning with a history and physical, is the most useful initial procedure preceding selective specialized studies for these patients.

The internist or gastroenterologist plays a vital supportive and collaborative role in treatment of eating disorders. Weight loss and/or binge–purge behavior are generally self-induced and unlikely to be due to an underlying or coincidental second medical disease. However, both the frequent secondary GI symptoms and less frequent primary GI disorders must be evaluated and treated in the context of knowledge of which symptoms are part of the natural history of eating disorders and expected to be self-improving—often distressing, but not medically serious and requiring no specific GI intervention—as opposed to unexpected atypical conditions requiring investigation and treatment. Just as a patient trusts her psychiatrist's reassurance that she will not be allowed to become fat, the medical consultant confirms which expected symptoms, such as severe bloating and constipation, have a high likelihood of spontaneous, gradual improvement, thereby establishing the patient's trust during refeeding and allowing her to accept transient medical symptoms and freeing the focus for psychological and behavioral treatment.

When the central psychopathological fear of fatness and self-induced starvation are present, medical tests may be useful to document the severity of the medical complications. However, only in rare cases are they needed to evaluate for the existence of comorbid disorders—or, even more uncommon, preceding GI conditions, such as peptic ulcer disease—to explain weight loss in a patient with an eating disorder. These medical tests are not needed for diagnosis to rule out GI disorders in typical cases. Critical time can be wasted in such endeavors, with resulting additional iatrogenic weight loss and excessive patient focus on somatic symptoms, unless there is a strong clinnical suspicion of preceding underlying GI disease. For example, it would be unlikely that a patient with weight loss and extreme fear of fatness and constipation would have coexisting Crohn's disease causing small-intetine malabsorption.

Assurance from both the psychiatrist and the gastroenterologist is needed to persuade the patient that many symptoms, including cramping, bloating, and constipation, improve with weight restoration and will gradually resolve. Firm assurance is made by both the psychiatrist and the gastroenterologist that the patient "will not be allowed to become overweight."

B. Medical History

Initial medical history serves to identify the presence and severity of physical, especially GI, symptoms. It is important to determine if GI symptoms were present prior to an eating disorder, including ulcers, reflux, irritable bowel syndrome, diarrhea or constipation, or preexisting altered bowel pattern. It should also be determined whether there was prior surgery or a history of prior alcohol or other drug abuse, or even physical or sexual abuse. Drossman et al. (42) documented a higher incidence of irritable-bowel-type problems in individuals subjected to previous sexual abuse, often years before. These findings were supported by the work of Walker et al. (43). Although the issue has not been settled, Pope and Hudson (44) did not find evidence to support the widespread concern that childhood sexual abuse is a risk factor in bulimia nervosa.

C. Physical Examination

The physical examination is of great importance in detecting the frequently occurring physical consequences of starvation, vomiting, medication abuse, or overexercise and in searching for coexisting independent disease. In the presence of anxiety, depression, and other comorbid psychiatric problems, it is important to make clear to the patient the contribution to care of a general physical examination and to have a same-gender attendant present to reassure the patient and to protect the physician. Generally vaginal examination will be deferred in non-sexually-active women. Rectal exam is performed as needed, with awareness of psychological reactions to examination.

Common physical abnormalities include parotid enlargement, erosion of dental enamel, excoriations on the backs of the hands from self-induced vomiting, hypotension, bradycardia, loss of scalp hair, growth of lanugo (fine, downy) hair, loss of muscle mass, muscle weakness, abdominal distension, fecal impaction or ileus, and possibly pitting edema along with decreased reflexes. When they are present, starvation-caused or -accentuated findings are generally reversible. Patients may be reassured that they will continue to feel better with weight restoration and can reasonably expect improvement of these physical findings.

D. Laboratory Studies

Multiple abnormalities in hematological and blood-chemistry studies may occur and contribute to both GI and general medical symptoms. Leukopenia, anemia, or thrombocytopenia may occur due to decreased bone-marrow production. Specific folate- or B_{12}-deficiency anemias are less common (16). A pretreatment pseudonormal hematocrit may appear to decrease as secondary dehydration is corrected during the early phase of treatment.

Hypercholesterolemia and elevated beta-carotene are also seen, but the significance and etiology are not known (22). In addition, as noted before, hyperamylasemia may be present and is generally due to parotid enlargement rather than pancreatitis. Hypophosphatemia has been reported independent of purging (45) and can result in profound weakness. Multiple electrolyte abnormalities, including hypokalemia and alkalosis secondary to vomiting or other purging, also occurs frequently.

The hematological abnormalities in food-restricting anorexia nervosa are generally due to starvation itself and improve with time. Anemia is not from iron deficiency due to menstruation since amenorrhea is present. If iron deficiency is present, especially in the amenorrheic patients, it calls for evaluation of GI blood loss.

Constipation and generalized decreased GI motility may occur from hypokalemia. Metabolic correction may lead to symptomatic improvement. Starvation alone can cause transient, generally reversible, changes in hepatic enzymes. However, it is important to evaluate for less easily reversible underlying chronic liver disease, such as hepatitis or cirrhosis. All patients should be evaluated, in addition to a CBC, with an SMA-18 that includes SGOT, SGPT, alkaline phosphatase, and total bilirubin. A direct bilirubin may be needed if the total bilirubin is elevated. If any liver studies are abnormal, a PT and PTT should be done. The possibility of coexisting hepatitis in a new patient with abnormal transaminases must be evaluated by requesting studies for hepatitis A-IgM, hepatitis B surface antigen, hepatitis B surface antibody, hepatitis B core antibody, and hepatitis C antibody. An underlying hepatitis may cause fatigue and anorexia independent of the eating disorder. In addition, if these are negative, iron, TIBC, and a ferritin level should be checked to evaluate for hemochromatosis. A copper and ceruloplasmin level will determine the unlikely possibility of a chronic active hepatitis from Wilson's disease.

Elevations in total bilirubin may occur in patients having a form of Gilbert's syndrome with indirect hyperbilirubinemia due to fasting, which can result in clinical jaundice. If the fasting total bilirubin is elevated, a postprandial total, indirect, and direct fraction should be obtained. If the total bilirubin falls with eating and is mainly indirect, no further hepatic evaluation is needed.

Gallstones likewise may be a complication of weight loss from dieting although the incidence in anorexia is not known and, if present, may be coincidental (45). Actigall (Ursodiol) may prevent gallstones with rapid weight loss, but the routine use of this agent could not be recommended (25).

In addition to elevations of hepatic enzymes that occur with starvation during anorexia nervosa, these patients may also be at risk of "nonalcoholic steatohepatitis," as previously reported in diabetes, obesity, or hypercholesterolemia (25). The possible occurrence of "alcoholic hepatitis" in a patient with bulimia may present in the absence of the diagnosis of alcoholism. Cueller and VanThiel (15) described a bulimic patient who was not alcoholic but drank two cans of beer fewer than five times per week. A biopsy showed micro- and macronodular cirrhosis and alcoholic hepatitis. It is not known whether this vulnerability results from the weight loss itself or a possibly greater risk of liver disease in bulimics.

E. Radiological Studies

Gastric emptying studies are useful clinically with recurrent vomiting that is not self-induced or with persistent bloating not responding to nutritional rehabilitation but that is limiting intake, especially if the patient does not tolerate prokinetic agents. Gastric emptying studies using radiolabeled meals of solids, liquids, or combined components can measure emptying over time. For example, a patient may ingest a technetium-labeled meal and scanning may be done with a gamma camera at 10–15-minute intervals until a curve is constructed and the $t_{1/2}$ (time for one-half of the meal to empty) determined for that particular meal. In some of the studies mentioned above, the patient can then repeat the emptying studies using a pharmacological agent to see if there is improvement (32–34).

If noninduced vomiting occurs, patients may have retained food from gastroparesis. Patients with poor emptying on nuclear-medicine scan who do not respond to a brief trial of smaller meals or prokinetic agents may require an upper-endoscopy or upper-GI series to rule out pyloric obstruction from peptic disease. Upper-GI and small-bowel series should be strongly considered in any patient who has heme-positive stools and iron deficiency, atypical for anorexia nervosa alone, to rule out Crohn's disease. It is particularly important since many patients with Crohn's disease are between the ages of 15 and 35. This series may also be needed if we are concerned about the possibility of a patient vomiting from a specific GI process causing the vomiting or pain. An abdominal x-ray may occasionally be ordered to evaluate for gastric retention or ileus. Total transit time for the entire GI tract may be estimated by radiological methods employing observble radiopaque markers. A Sitzmark study, using a gelatin capsule around radiopaque markers, is commercially available (Konsyl Pharmaceutical Inc.). GI transit time can be estimated by obtaining a flat plate 5 days later to note presence and number of markers (46). Most markers will be passed by 5 days.

F. Specialized Tests: Endoscopy, Motility Studies, and pH Probes

Endoscopic evaluation may be needed for a patient 1) with preexisting disease (such as peptic ulcer disease) causing epigastric pain and bloating, to rule out a recurrence of peptic ulcer, 2) if routine supportive nutritional and psychotherapeutic measures do not result in symptomatic GI improvement or adequate weight gain, or 3) if gastropesophageal reflux symptoms persist, including heartburn, vomiting, or dysphagia, despite vigorous supportive care. All may need to be evaluated with endoscopy, as these symptoms may interfere with the ability to restore weight or to reestablish normal eating in the patient.

Esophageal motility studies may be useful in patients with persistent dysphagia if they have a negative upper-endoscopy as is seen in some patients with a psychological causation of a motility disorder (18,28). Patients who complain persistently of heartburn and have had aspiration but do not have significant esophagitis on endoscopy may, in fact, have intermittent reflux causing severe symptoms. In these cases, a 24-hour pH probe is useful to document exposure of the esophagus to the acid pH.

IV. EVALUATION AND TREATMENT: TYPICAL CASES

A. Bloating

A 25-year-old woman was referred for gastroenterological evaluation after a 20-pound weight loss over the previous 6 months. She complained of multiple episodes of daily vomiting with epigastric pain, distension, and discomfort along with associated heartburn. She had no odynophagia or melena and took antacids without relief. She underwent an upper-endoscopy that was normal. When questioned, she admitted that she experienced episodes of binging followed by self-induced vomiting associated with a fear of fatness. She was referred for evaluation and was subsequently hospitalized, where she was initially prescribed 1200 calories per day. She complained of severe bloating by midmeal but had no distension on physical examination. She was changed to five smaller meals per day for the next 2 weeks and had resolution of her bloating. Gradually she was able to tolerate 1700 calories per day over the next 3 weeks, followed by further increases to above 3000 kilocalories per day until adequate weight was restored.

B. Epigastric Distress

A 15-year-old white female outpatient was undergoing outpatient psychotherapy treatment for anorexia nervosa with associated depressive symptoms. She lost 15 pounds and complained of epigastric fullness and pain which interfered with further eating so that she had not restored any weight. She was switched to five smaller meals per day and experienced improvement in her symptoms. She received reassurance from both the psychiatrist and the gastroenterologist, and was told that her symptoms were common and should improve with time. Over the next 2–3 weeks, she gradually improved and was able to have her calories increased with progressive weight restoration to a healthy goal range while hospitalized.

C. "Heartburn"

A 37-year-old black woman with a 17-year history of anorexia nervosa and alcohol abuse (four beers per day) experienced a recent weight loss of 10 pounds as well as mild depressive symptoms. She complained of heartburn and mild dysphagia, with food "sticking" in the lower chest. Her physical examination was unremarkable. She was placed on cimetidine 400 mg p.o. b.i.d., with only slight improvement after 2 weeks. Endoscopy revealed moderate distal esophagitis but no stricture, and she was changed to Prilosec (omeprazole) 20 mg per day. The patient did not drink alcohol at this time or complain of additional emesis. She did not improve and continued to lose weight. Cisapride 10 mg before meals and at bedtime was added. She lost several pounds over the next 2 weeks. On repeat questioning, she admitted that she was losing weight not just because she felt depressed and lost appetite, but because she restricted food intake—mildly obese, she believed that her life would improve if she looked slimmer. She was referred for psychiatric evaluation, and then improved with a combination of psychotherapy and antidepressants over the next few months, but admitted that some of her vomiting had been self-induced. She was later able to have her GI medications tapered, with no further recurrence of GI symptoms. Because this patient had an associated depression, cisapride, which does not cause CNS symptoms, was used instead of metoclopramide.

D. Constipation

A 17-year-old food-restricting anorectic was admitted to the hospital with a 30-pound weight loss—from 120 pounds to 90 pounds. She complained of severe constipation and had been taking multiple oral laxatives at home. She took these believing that she would lose weight and that they would make her bowels move better.

Physical examination was remarkable only for an emaciated female. Her Hemoccult was negative. Her abdominal examination was normal. She was instructed that the laxatives would probably not contribute significantly to weight loss and that her constipation was likely due to decreased food and fluid intake. After she had been placed on eight to 10 glasses of fluid per day along with an initial 1200 calories, her bowel pattern gradually improved. The 1200-calorie diet was low in fat and salt. To avoid refeeding enema, it was gradually increased by 500 calories every 6 days in gradual steps until the maintenance phase of 3500 calories was reached (3,47).

E. Parotid Enlargement

A 23-year-old white woman with normal-weight bulimia nervosa was hospitalized for the fifth time with moderate weight loss and recurrent self-induced vomiting. She complained of heartburn at night and after most meals, but no dysphagia. Physical examination revealed parotid-gland enlargement and excoriation of the back of her fingers. She was given cimetidine 400 mg p.o. b.i.d. during the initial week of hospitalization. GI symptoms resolved after her previous self-induced emesis was interrupted, without further recurrence. She was thereby freed to focus on her cognitive behavioral psychotherapy program for bulimia nervosa.

V. OVERALL GUIDELINES

A. Internal Medicine

1. Both internal-medicine and gastroenterology consultants play vital roles in the treatment of eating-disorder patients, to evaluate for illness-induced GI disease, to help with the management of refeeding symptoms or symptoms

secondary to interruption of a binge–purge behavior cycle, and to manage preexisting medical disorders. This joint approach is very useful not only from the psychiatrist's perspective but also from the patient's viewpoint, to understand the major changes in GI function that her body has undergone and other body-system changes due to the weight loss and/or binge–purge behaviors. Patients are reassured and informed about these changes and receive encouragement from the entire medical team that they will improve and symptoms will be managed medically to minimize discomfort and distraction from psychological care.

2. For inpatients with weight loss meeting criteria for anorexia nervosa, complete bowel examination is not necessary. Earlier suggestions for extensive GI workup came from an older study expressing concern that patients thought to have anorexia nervosa might actually have Crohn's disease (48). These patients were probably misdiagnosed regarding their primary disorder and most likely had Crohn's disease all along; older reports did not specifically require the psychopathology of a morbid fear of fatness and the relentless pursuit of thinness to make a diagnosis of anorexia nervosa.

In our experience, patients with Crohn's disease do not have a fear of fatness or a fear of gaining weight but in fact are distressed by their weight loss. They try to eat frequently despite their pain. They do not distort body size. When self-induced weight loss and morbid fear of fatness are present, a primary medical causation for symptomatology is rarely found.

Extended medical evaluation of all anorectic patients' disease is therefore not necessary unless they fail to gain weight or have other factors such as Hemoccult-positive stool, elevated sed. rate, or objective abdominal distension (3).

3. Patients with prior known and treated GI disease such as reflux or peptic ulcer disease will likely need to continue such treatment, sometimes modified or intensified due to exacerbation of their symptoms with weight loss. This may occur, for example, in a patient with preexisting reflux who in addition develops gastroparesis from anorexia. She may then experience exacerbation of the reflux because of acid sitting in the stomach. If there are prior peptic ulcers resulting from pyloric narrowing, reflux may be manifested by increased symptomatology due to decreased gastric emptying.

4. Conditions requiring further evaluation with endoscopy, pH monitoring, and barium studies include the following:

a. For Hemoccult-positive stools, diagnoses of straining from hemorrhoids, peptic ulcer disease, or Crohn's disease need to be considered.
b. Persistent vomiting, reflux, or aspiration, if not relieved with H2 blockers and motility-promoting agents, requires evaluation for peptic ulcer disease and/or mechanical gastric outlet of obstruction.

5. Bloating and constipation. Bloating often responds to reassurance and dietary changes to include:

a. Five smaller meals per day.
b. Encouraging sufficient liquid to allow for softer, larger bowel movements, along with adequate fiber, gradually increasing to 25–30 mg per day of fiber.
c. If needed, briefly change to a liquid supplement such as Ensure instead of solid food, with subsequent return to "normal food eaten normally."
d. Finally, use metoclopramide 10 mg 1/2 hr a.c. plus q.h.s. or, if depressive or anxiety symptoms are present, the newer agent cisapride may be used, 10 mg 15 min a.c. plus q.h.s., or bethanechol 25 mg q.i.d.
e. Constipation may improve with oral refeeding and electrolyte normalization. If not, the addition of Peri-Colace 100 mg p.o. b.i.d. (Mead Johnson Pharmaceuticals, Evansville, Indiana) may be needed along with the addition of at least eight glasses of liquid per day.
f. Both anorectics and bulimics generally will experience improvement from GI symptoms as a result of treatment of the eating disorder, but upon discharge from hospitalization will still have more GI symptoms than controls (3). While generally improved at discharge, they are not normal yet and may require 3 to 6 months for complete improvement. Further studies need to be performed on these patients to determine if symptoms persist and interfere with long-term follow-up and treatment. One future area of investigation may involve hormonal therapy. Cholecystokinin (CCK) may play a role in decreased food intake. Both central receptor mechanisms and peripheral mechanisms via gastric/pyloric CCK may be involved (49–51).

B. Psychiatry

1. The etiology of anorexia nervosa and bulimia nervosa remains unknown. They appear to be "biopsychosocial" disorders that involve interactive symptomatology in medical and psychiatric functioning, all in the context of relentless sociocultural norms promoting slimness and shape change. Although increasing information is available concerning specific quantitative risk factors, premature closure on concepts of etiology will lead to lopsided treatment.

2. Anorexia nervosa and bulimia nervosa are really two sides of the same coin. Both disorders begin, in more than 95% of cases, when an individual decides to diet to achieve weight loss and/or shape change, usually for psychological and social rather than medical reasons. The anorectic patient classically decreases in weight until a medically serious state of starvation is reached and is self-sustaining. Bulimia nervosa, in many ways, represents a failed attempt at anorexia nervosa, with appetite breaking through in the form of a binge despite the attempt at restriction. Current research suggests that those patients who go on

to bulimic, rather than strictly anorectic, symptomatology have different physiological and psychological vulnerabilities, being less tolerant of hunger, less persevering in temperament, and more impulsive in behavior.

3. The specific factors that *predispose* to eating disorders, *precipitate* the onset of the disorder, *sustain* the disorder, and *ameliorate* the disorder may, in fact, be quite different within the same individual over the course of time, and certainly vary between individuals. Overall, there appears to be a transition from a primarily psychosocial onset to later sustaining biomedical factors that is not yet well understood, but probably includes adaptive GI changes. The relatively successful progressive adaptation of the body to either severe weight loss or binge–purge behavior sometimes makes treatment more difficult because transient but sometimes significant medical symptomatology may be produced when normalization of weight and eating behavior is attempted. On the whole, however, prudent normalization of weight is necessary and highly beneficial, and patients' fears that overweight will be attained are not warranted.

4. Eating disorders generally progress through three stages. The first stage is the attempt at weight loss which occurs in 70% or more of young females. The second stage occurs when the individual meets criteria for the illnesses of anorexia nervosa or bulimia nervosa. This second stage represents a consolidation of widespread attempts at dieting and weight loss into an established syndrome in 2–5% of the population which then has a well-described and somewhat predictable course. The third stage represents a progression of the eating disorder into (a) a chronic, identity-giving disorder in which the individual becomes so closely identified with the symptomatology he or she finds it hard to imagine life without it; and (b), the body resists improvement in the disorder with the medical symptoms becoming relatively self-sustaining.

5. The principles of psychiatric treatment are as follows:

a. Treatment at its basics involves several logical steps. These include: 1) diagnostic confirmation of the eating disorder subtype, 2) identification of associated comorbid psychiatric conditions, 3) weight restoration, 4) where appropriate, interruption of binge–purge and other abnormal behaviors, 5) correction of cognitive distortions regarding the value of slimness and shape change, 6) encouraging normal social eating behavior, and 7) equipping the patient for gradual reintroduction into a society besotted with thinness, in conjunction with several years of experienced outpatient follow-up care. In addition to the shared features of biological and psychological dysfunction secondary to starvation and/or binge–purge behavior, each individual has a unique life story that enters into the predisposition onset and maintenance of this disorder through a central dynamic formulation.

b. Where anorexia nervosa is present, the overall condition of the individual whose weight has been severely lowered is primarily a medical disorder, consequent to the psychiatric initiation, with significant secondary nonspecific psychological and social changes due to starvation, in addition to the unique central psychopathology of the eating disorder. Until the individual is approximately 90% of ideal body weight, he or she has diminished, but not absent, capacity for meaningful technical psychotherapy of either the cognitive behavioral form or the dynamic types. Support, education, and preliminary attempts to persuade patients to rethink their commitment to thinness are potentially beneficial even at lower weights, but are less effective than when the patient is restored to normal weight and free of binge–purge behavior. There is good evidence that the brain size is diminished in anorexia nervosa and neuropsychological functioning is often profoundly changed despite seemingly normal participation in work or school, the last activities to suffer from starvation.

c. Most anorexia nervosa requires a stay in hospital as part of comprehensive treatment, while most bulimia nervosa may be treated out of hospital, but exceptions occur frequently in both conditions. Hospitalization, when necessary, is always part of a long-term treatment, with transition to partial hospitalization and/or outpatient care when feasible.

d. There are generally three crucial stages during which patients may wish to discontinue their treatment or relapse. The first challenge is gaining the person's commitment and cooperation to enter treatment and dealing with their fears and fantasies prior to beginning treatment. Often, entering treatment is a shock when the seriousness of the illness becomes apparent. The next crisis stage is when treatment is underway and patients recognize that weight is actually being restored and will probably rise to a truly healthy body weight, about which they are almost always conflicted and ambivalent. This midcourse crisis requires continued support and encouragement. Patients may benefit from speaking with others who have successfully accomplished full treatment and are leading normal lives. Lastly, discharge from inpatient care to infrequent or nonexpert follow-up often leads to relapse. This is also more probable if the treatment period is too short and consists only of reversal of medical symptoms.

e. For established cases of eating disorders, especially anorexia nervosa, team treatment is essential. Actually, two teams are involved: the treatment team in the hospital and the patient-and-family team in a partnership to decrease illness behavior and thinking and to encourage healthy attitudes and daily living free of excessive emphasis on slimness.

f. Men with eating disorders suffer from a lack of prompt recognition of their condition, sometimes with some stigma from professionals and from other eating-disordered patients. They required individualized psychosocial, and sometimes endocrine, preparation to return to the gender specific norms and roles in society that they experience from birth onward in a way different from that of the more typical female patient.

6. The following are guidelines for follow-up care.

a. Follow-up is crucial for virtually all eating disorders requiring inpatient care. The individual often has to return socially and psychologically to an earlier state of life where the eating disorder began and then develop the deferred social and psychological stages of maturation. Treatment includes follow-up for resolution of comorbid psychological disorders such as depressive illness, obsessive-compulsive states, and chronic medical states secondary to the eating disorder, such as osteopenia and menstrual irregularity.
b. Eating disorders have been, at times, casually linked to addictive disorders. While there are some superficial similarities, there are more important differences. First, abstention from the object of "addiction," namely food, cannot be part of the treatment of eating disorders. Second, individuals with eating disorders can truly be cured, not just improved. There is accumulating evidence that, in contrast to addictive disorders, eating-disordered individuals can gradually become free of virtually all their symptoms and move successfully into the common, almost normal, mildly distressed attitude of most women in our society who wish to lose a few pounds but do not undertake strenuously behavioral efforts to accomplish this goal. Studies suggest that 90% of individuals who do not die from their eating disorder will eventually be either improved or cured (9).

VI. CONCLUSIONS

Severe and persisting GI symptomatology is common in eating disorders. Early historical cases document the multiple GI complaints of emaciated patients. Historical reports have often used the term "hysterical" to indicate the psychological components of some of the medical symptomatology (52), but more recent evidence documents an important medical component. The syndrome of bulimia nervosa was not clearly described until 1979. Since then, the symptomatology from the characteristic binge episodes and compensatory self-induced purging due to vomiting or medication abuse (which occurs in 80% of bulimia nervosa patients) has been extensively studied. The preponderance of evidence available suggests that widespread GI symptomatology is common in eating disorders but best understood as an adaptive part of the natural history of the eating disorders or resulting from treatment. There is no evidence that preceding abnormal GI functioning is common or predisposes to eating disorders in the average patient.

The ability to form a therapeutic relationship with the patient often depends on getting beyond the medical symptomatology through expert handling of GI complaints. It is highly desirable for a clinician who has no medical training or no specific GI training to work with the same experienced gastroenterologist, one who has acquired a thorough working knowledge of eating-disordered patients and a deep appreciation of which symptoms are typical but not serious and usually self-improving, in contrast to those that are typical but potentially dangerous and require intervention or, finally, atypical and definitely require evaluation and treatment. Likewise, it is important for a gastroenterologist to have a high index of suspicion for eating disorders in patients who present with vague GI symptoms for medical evaluation with no mention of complaints associated with eating disorders.

In many ways, it is surprising not how poorly eating-disordered patients do medically, but how well they do, considering the extraordinary abuse the body is subjected to through self-induced starvation and/or binge–purge behavior as well as compulsive exercise. Eating disorders represent the diversion of the normal pattern of eating, regulated by the limbic system around a fairly narrow "set point," into a psychosocially driven pseudosolution for developmental issues or mood regulation. In contrast to addictive disorders, eating disorders cannot be treated by abstention from the substance involved, namely food. The patient needs to come to terms with the abnormal eating behavior and the underlying overvaluation of slimness that grows out of relentless sociocultural pressures toward weight loss, which, for a small percentage of the population, are not merely culturally normative sources of everyday distress but develop into fixed, self-sustaining psychiatric and medical disorders. Even though they are often misclassified as solely psychiatric disorders, the etiology of eating disorders remains unknown. Eating disorders represent a true intermix of psychiatric and medical symptomatology. The mechanisms sustaining established chronic severe eating disorders may well involve a substantial contribution of biomedical factors in contrast to the more clearly psychosocial predisposing and initiating factors. The physician's ability to handle the medical aspects of eating disorders generally leads to a more confident relationship with the patient, and the ability to move beyond endless discussions of weight, calorie intake, and medical distress into the real heart of treatment: the psychological work to make sense of, and to put behind the patient, the abnormal eating and thinking. The goal is for the patient to accept the challenge of living an age-appropriate, satisfying life in a society preoccupied with slimness yet surrounded by attractively packaged dense calories.

A purely medical or psychiatric approach seldom works as effectively as comprehensive integrated treatment of eating disorders. The most successful and effective outcome generally occurs with a coordinated team of medical, psychiatric, nursing, social work, dietary, and other health experts working together. A coordinated, integrated team effort prevents the common occurrence of splitting by patients who are ambivalent about treatment, especially weight restoration, and who often reproduce unconsciously the dynamics of their home environment in the treatment setting.

REFERENCES

1. American Psychiatric Association. Practice Guideline for Eating Disorders. Washington, DC: American Psychiatric Association, 1993.
2. Andersen A. Practical Comprehensive Treatment of Anorexia Nervosa and Bulimia. Baltimore: Johns Hopkins University Press, 1985.
3. Waldholtz B, Andersen A. Gastrointestinal symptoms in anorexia nervosa: A prospective study. Gastroenterology 1990; 98:1415–1419.
4. Kamal N, Chami T, Andersen AE, Roswell FA, Schuster M, Whitehead WE. Gastrointestinal transit times in anorexia nervosa and bulimia nervosa. Gastroenterology 1991; 101:1320–1324.
5. Casper RC, Hedeker D, McClough JF. Personality dimensions in eating disorders and their relevance for subtyping. J Am Acad Child Adolesc Psychiatry 1992; 31(5):830–840.
6. American Psychiatric Association. Diagnostic and Statistical Manual of Mental Disorders IV. Washington, DC: American Psychiatric Association, 1994.
7. Nylander, I. The feeling of being fat and dieting in a school population. Acta Socio-Medica Scand 1971; 1:17–26.
8. Kendler KS, MacLean C, Neale M, Kessler R, Heath A, Eaves L. The genetic epidemiology of bulimia nervosa. Am J Psychiatry 1991; 148:1627–1637.
9. Theander S. Chronicity in anorexia nervosa: Results from the Swedish long-term study. In: Herzog, Vandereycke, eds. The Course of Eating Disorders. New York: Springer-Verlag, 1992.
10. Andersen AE. Males with eating disorders. In: Yager J, Gwirtsman HE, Edelstein CK, eds. Special Problems in Managing Eating Disorders. Washington, DC: American Psychiatric Press, 1992:87–118.
11. Andersen AE, Hay A. Racial and socioeconomic influences in anorexia nervosa and bulimia. Int J Eating Disorders 1985; 4(4):479–487.
12. Andersen AE, Casper R, Beck D. Truly late onset of eating disorders: a study of 12 cases averaging 59 years old. 6th International Conference on Eating Disorders. 1994.
13. Garner DM, Rockert W, Olmsted MP, Johnson C, Coscina DV. Psychoeducational principles in the treatment of bulimia and anorexia nervosa. In: Garner, Garfinkel, eds. Handbook of Psychotherapy for Anorexia Nervosa and Bulimia. New York: Guilford Press, 1985.
14. Balaa MA, Drossman DA. Anorexia nervosa and bulimia: the eating disorders. Dis Mon 1985; 31:5–52.
15. Cuellar RE, VanThiel DH. Gastrointestinal complications of the eating disorders: anorexia nervosa and bulimia. Am J Gastroenterol 1986; 81:113.

16. Halmi KA, Falk JR. Physiologic changes in anorexia nervosa. Int J Eating Disorders 1981; 1:16–27.
17. Comerci GD. Medical complications of anorexia nervosa in bulimia nervosa. Med Clin North Am 1990; 74:293–1310.
18. Clouse R. Ann Intern Med 1983; 99:800–807.
19. Herzog D, Copeland P. N Engl Med 1985; 313:295–303.
20. Moshang TJ, Utiger R. Low triiodothyronine euthyroidism in anorexia nervosa. New York: Raven Press, 1977.
21. Vigersky R. The effect of cyproheptadine in anorexia nervosa: a double-blind trial. New York: Raven Press, 1977.
22. Klienfelter H. Clin Endocrinol 1965; 25:1520–1521.
23. Cox K, Cannon R, Ament M, Phillips H, Schaffer C. Biochemical and ultrasonic abnormalities of the pancreas in anorexia nervosa. Clin Endocrinol 1983; 28:225–229.
24. Humphries L, Adams O, Levitt M, McClean C. Hyperamylasemia in patients with eating disorders. Ann Intern Med 1987; 106:50–52.
25. Liddle L, Goldstein R, Saxton J. Gallstone formation during weight reduction dieting. Arch Intern Med 1989; 149:1750–1754.
26. Crowell M, Cheskin L, Musial F. Prevalence of gastrointestinal symptoms in obese and normal weight binge eaters. Am J Gastroenterol 1994; 89:387–391.
27. Stacher G, Kiss a, Wiesnagrotski S, Bergmann H, Hobarth J, Schneider C. Oesophageal and gastric motility disorders in patients characterized as having primary anorexia nervosa. Gut 1986; 27:1120.
28. Clouse R. Psychiatric disorders in patients with esophageal disease. Med Clin North Am 1991; 75:1081.
29. Rigaud D, Bedig G, Merrouchae M. Gastric emptying and anorexia nervosa is improved by completion of a renutrition program. Dig Dis Sci 1988; 33:1919–1925.
30. Dubois A, Gross H, Ebert M. Gastric emptying and secretion and primary anorexia nervosa. Gastroenterology 1979; 77:319–323.
31. McCallum R, Grill B, Lange R. Definition of a gastric emptying abnormality in patients with anorexia nervosa. Dig Dis Science 1985; 30:713–722.
32. Stacher G, Bergmann H, Wiesnagrotski S, Kiss A. Intravenous cisapride accelerates delayed gastric emptying and increases antral contraction amplitude in patients with primary anorexia nervosa. Gastroenterology 1987; 92:1000–1006.
33. Saila W, Lebwohl P. Metoclopramide-induced gastric emptying in patients with anorexia nervosa. Am J Gastroenterol 1980; 74:127–132.
34. Russell D, Freedman M, Feiglan D. Delayed gastric emptying and improvement with domperidone in a patient with anorexia nervosa. Am J Gastroenterol 1983; 140:1235–1236.
35. Keys A, Brozek J, Henscheo A. The Biology of Human Starvation. Minneapolis, MN: University of Minnesota Press, 1950.
36. Brook G. Acute gastric dilatation in anorexia nervosa. Br Med J 1977; 32:499.
37. Dubois A, Gross H, Richter J. Effect of bethanechol on gastric functions in primary anorexia nervosa. Dig Dis Sci 1981; 6:598–600.
38. Janssen S, Petters T., VanTrappen G. Improvement of gastric emptying in diabetic gastroparesis by erythromycin-preliminary studies. N Engl J Med 1990; 22:1028–1031.

39. Bo-Linn G, Santanaa C, Morawski S, Fordtran J. Purging and caloric absorption in bulimic patients and normal women. Ann Intern Med 1983; 99:14.
40. Fine K, Krejs G, Fordtran J. Gastrointestinal Disease. Philadelphia: WB Saunders, 1993.
41. Morris A, Turnberg L. Surreptitious laxative abuse. Gastroenterology 1979; 77:780.
42. Drossman D, Leserman J, Nachman G. Sexual and physical abuse in women with functional or organic gastrointestinal disorders. Ann Intern Med 1990; 113:828–833.
43. Walker EA, Katon WH, Roy-Byrne PP, Jemelka RP, Russo J. Histories of sexual victimization in patients with irritable bowel syndrome or inflammatory bowel disease. Am J Psychiatry 1993; 150(10):1502–1506.
44. Pope HG, Hudson JI. Is childhood sexual abuse a risk factor for bulimia nervosa? Am J Psychiatry 1992; 149(4):455–463.
45. Waldholtz B, Andersen A. Hypophosphatemia during starvation in anorexia nervosa. Int J Eating Disord 1988; 7:551–555.
46. Bouchocha M, Duevroede, Arhan, et al. What is the meaning of colorectal transit time measurement? Dis Colon Rectum 1992; 35(8):273.
47. Andersen A, Morse C, Santmyer K. Inpatient treatment of anorexia nervosa. In: Garner D, Garfinkel P, eds. Handbook of Psychotherapy for Anorexia Nervosa and Bulimia. New York: Guilford Press, 1985:311–343.
48. Grayboski J, Katz J, Sangree M, Herskovic T. Eleven adolescent girls with severe anorexia. Clin Pediatr 1968; 7:684–689.
49. Kissileff H, Pi-Sunyer F, Thornton J, Smith G. C-terminal octapeptide of cholecystokinin decreases food intake in men. Am J Clin Nutr 1981; 34:154.
50. Raybould H, Tache Y. Cholecystokinin inhibits gastric motility and emptying via a capsaicin sensitive vagal pathway. Am J Physiol 1988; 255:G242.
51. Cooper S, Barber D. SCH23390-induced hypophagia is blocked by the selective CCK-A receptor antagonist devazepide, but not by the CCK-B/gastrin receptor antagonist L-365,260. Brain Res Bull 1990; 24:631.
52. Lasegue. On hysterical anorexia. In: Andersen AE, ed. Practical Comprehensive Treatment of Anorexia Nervosa and Bulimia. Baltimore, MD: The Johns Hopkins University Press, 1873:19–27.

12

Chronic Abdominal Pain

Edward A. Walker
University of Washington
Seattle, Washington

I. INTRODUCTION

Despite continuing advances in sophisticated diagnostic technology, the majority of common symptoms presented in primary-care clinics remain medically unexplained. Kroenke (1) has shown that eight common symptoms (chest pain, abdominal pain, fatigue, shortness of breath, back pain, headache, anxiety, and depression) take up approximately 25% of all primary-care visits, yet an organic etiology can be found in only 16% of these patients.

Of these symptoms, abdominal pain appears to be one of the most common both in the general population and in primary-care clinics. The 1984 National Institute of Mental Health survey of 18,571 subjects in the general population found that approximately 25% of respondents reported that they had experienced significant distress from medically unexplained abdominal pain sometime in their lives (2). Although abdominal pain is also a common complaint in primary-care clinics, it is one of the most difficult to evaluate. A recent study of common presenting medical symptoms showed that 11% of primary-care visits were for abdominal pain; however, only one in 10 of these patients was found to have an organic etiology over a 1-year period, at an average cost of $1816 per evaluation (1).

Despite the high prevalence of this symptom, these data suggest that for the vast majority of abdominal pain cases an organic cause may never be found. New-onset abdominal pain may follow one of several courses: 1) a time-limited, acute episode with complete resolution, 2) a recurrent, waxing and waning pain syndrome associated with repeated, temporary disruption of social and occupational function, or 3) chronic abdominal pain for more than 6 months with disabling interference in the patient's life. It is chronic abdominal pain, with its associated disability, that is the focus of this chapter. Patients with chronic abdominal pain represent a heterogeneous group, and relatively little is known about them. Methodological problems hamper researchers while the management of these patients frustrates clinicians. In this chapter we attempt to review what is known about the characteristics of patients with chronic abdominal pain, examine the issue of disability in this population, and suggest practical management strategies.

II. THE ELUSIVE DEFINITION OF CHRONIC ABDOMINAL PAIN

The definition of chronic abdominal pain says more about what it is *not* than what it is. The current consensus among researchers is that chronic abdominal pain is unexplained pain in patients with minimal or absent organic pathology that has persisted for at least 6 months. Patients receive this diagnosis when a clinician decides that a "sufficient evaluation" has excluded likely physiological causes for the pain. There is a certain degree of imprecision in this, as clinicians may disagree on what constitutes a "sufficient" workup, and may even inadvertently neglect sources of pathology outside the clinician's specialty—e.g., a gastroenterologist may fail to consider gynecological disease, or a gynecologist may not investigate gastrointestinal (GI) pathology.

Chronic abdominal pain is an umbrella term that encompasses several forms of mysterious abdominal distress. In the literature it has been used to refer to patients with pain-predominant irritable bowel syndrome (IBS), functional abdominal pain (patients who report pain referred to GI sources yet who do not meet criteria for IBS), chronic pelvic pain (CPP), and functional dyspepsia. This process of *diagnosis by exclusion* continues to be methodologically problematic since chronic abdominal pain patients are definitionally a heterogenous group, and conclusions drawn about them are unavoidably subject to a large degree of variability.

Research on patients with chronic abdominal pain has been stymied by seemingly insurmountable definitional problems and paradoxes. Merely establishing a working definition that minimizes false negatives and positives is difficult. Consider that:

1. At least some patients at first classified with chronic abdominal pain (absent or minimal abdominal pathology) will eventually be found to have occult or prodromal organic pathology that will manifest itself at a later date as the natural history of the underlying disease progresses (this number is probably small, however, because of the 6-month period during which most pathophysiological processes can be discovered).
2. Conversely, at least some patients who are found to have organic pathology will eventually develop comorbid chronic abdominal pain (i.e., there is no reason that a patient with inflammatory bowel disease or endometriosis could not also have pain mediated by the same mechanisms as chronic abdominal pain in addition to, or instead of, the nociceptive inputs of the organic pathology).
3. The recurrent and changing nature of some types of chronic abdominal pain makes longitudinal study of these patients difficult (some forms of chronic abdominal pain are reported as continuous while others have a waxing and waning course with variable severity, and it is not certain whether these represent differences in kind or degree.
4. Various distinct "quasi-physiological" subtypes of chronic abdominal pain are possible. (As we will see below, women with CPP report abdominal discomfort that they believe to be distinct from their gynecological distress and attribute to GI causes; likewise, women with IBS also report CPP that they recognize as distinct from their IBS, suggesting that multiple forms of chronic abdominal pain may coexist simultaneously or interchangeably.)

Still another problem in defining chronic abdominal pain is the assessment of severity. Not all patients who experience chronic abdominal pain feel it is severe enough to seek medical help (3). Moreover, some patients who do feel their discomfort is severe enough to warrant treatment become disabled by their pain whereas others do not. The development of disability, as we shall see later, appears to be an important factor in the establishment and maintenance of chronic abdominal pain, and predicts both high medical utilization and poor treatment outcome.

These definitional issues complicate our understanding of this disorder. From a research standpoint, these methodological problems make comparison of studies difficult. We therefore need to accept the imprecision of our present definitions and, for the purpose of this chapter, declare chronic abdominal pain to be 6 or more months of abdominal pain with minimal or absent organic pathology. In this definition, abdominal pain includes pain reported anywhere in the abdomen, including both GI (IBS, functional abdominal pain, and functional dyspepsia) and gynecological (CPP) disorders. Although musculoskeletal (trigger points), rheumatic (fibromyalgia), and urinary tract (functional bladder pain) disorders could also conceivably be linked to abdominal pain, we do not address these syndromes in this chapter.

III. RELIANCE ON PHYSIOLOGICAL DEFINITIONS

The dilemma of *diagnosis by exclusion* yields evaluations that are perceived by both clinicians and patients as expensive and frustrating. Attempts at prospective diagnosis using physiological symptom patterns (similar to the Manning criteria for IBS) (4) have had limited success in chronic abdominal pain, largely due to their unfortunate reliance on biomedical symptom patterns.

In contrast to the lack of consensus on the pathophysiology of chronic abdominal pain, there has been an explosion of interest in psychosocial factors that are likely involved in the initiation or maintenance of this disorder. Separate literatures have emerged from gynecology and internal medicine detailing the psychological symptoms and psychiatric histories of patients with chronic abdominal pain. The most robust data are associations with current and lifetime psychiatric disorders, somatization, and prior emotional, sexual, and physical trauma.

A. Current and Lifetime Psychiatric Disorders

Several studies have documented higher current and lifetime prevalence rates for selected psychiatric disorders in patients with chronic abdominal pain when compared to medical controls. The two most frequent forms of abdominal pain are CPP and IBS.

Chronic Pelvic Pain

CPP is a common disorder in gynecological practice. Although precise prevalence data are scarce, two studies have suggested that approximately one-third of women experience intermittent discomfort from pelvic pain, and possibly as many as 14% have experienced 6 or more months of pain (5).

We have done two studies using sequential samples of women scheduled for diagnostic laparoscopy comparing women diagnosed with CPP and those seeking tubal ligation or infertility evaluation (6,7). Structured psychiatric, family-history, and sexual-trauma interviews as well as psychological self-report measures were administered to the pain and nonpain groups, and laparoscopy reports were blindly rated by a gynecologist. When compared with women undergoing laparoscopy for tubal ligation and infertility, women with chronic pelvic pain were significantly more likely to have current major depression as well as lifetime histories of major depression, dysthymic disorder, somatization disorder, drug abuse, phobia, and sexual dysfunction, and significantly more medically unexplained physical symptoms across several organ systems despite no significant difference in objective laparoscopic findings.

Irritable Bowel Syndrome

Many patients with chronic abdominal pain are diagnosed with IBS. This disorder occurs in 10–20% of the general population, and can present either with or without pain complaints as the primary symptom. Very little is known about the patient with pain-predominant IBS in contrast to the diarrhea- and constipation-predominant forms; however, several studies of IBS suggest that, as with CPP, current and lifetime psychiatric disorders and somatization appear to play a part in the establishment and maintenance of the disorder.

In an investigation similar to the laparoscopy study for CPP, we administered structured psychiatric interviews and psychological self-report measures to 28 patients with IBS and 19 patients with inflammatory bowel disease (IBD) (8). Compared to the patients with IBD, the IBS patients were significantly more likely to have lifetime diagnoses of major depression, somatization disorder, generalized anxiety disorder, panic disorder and phobic disorder, as well as other pain syndromes (e.g., headache, low back pain). They had significantly more medically unexplained somatic symptoms and were likely to have suffered from a psychiatric disorder, particularly an anxiety disorder, prior to the onset of their IBS symptoms. While not all the IBS patients had chronic pain as part of their presentation, we are currently conducting a larger investigation of 71 IBS and 40 IBD patients in which we will analyze the pain-predominant group separately.

These investigations of IBS and CPP had similar methodologies, yet despite the different populations studied, found remarkably high rates of psychopathology in patients with either IBS or CPP. When analyzed using logistic regression (a statistical technique that controls for confounding and interactions between variables), both studies showed that the number of medically unexplained physical symptoms (i.e., somatization) was the best predictor of chronic abdominal pain (IBS or CPP).

Patients with Both CPP and IBS

Although CPP and IBS are common disorders in women, very little is known about their comorbidity. The high rates of psychiatric disorders in each syndrome suggest that some women may have both disorders and that some women may have been misdiagnosed. What is known of the prevalence of IBS in patients with CPP? What percentage of women with IBS also have CPP? Do women with both disorders have even greater severity of psychopathology and somatization than women with either disorder alone?

To study this overlap, we administered a CPP questionnaire to 651 women in two primary-care clinics. Two hundred fifty women (38%) reported some form of recurrent or chronic abdominal pain, with 91 (14%) reporting at least one prior episode of at least 6 months of continuous pelvic pain. Of these 250 women, 198 (79%) also met criteria for probable IBS. Patients meeting criteria for both CPP and IBS were more likely to have relatives with pain and to meet caseness criteria for psychiatric diagnosis on the General Hospital Questionnaire and had more associated pain symptoms when compared to women with CPP but without IBS (5).

In an ongoing study of the prevalence of CPP in IBS patients (9), a sequential sample of 55 women with IBS and 18 women with IBD in an urban GI clinic were evaluated by a medically trained interviewer using structured psychiatric, abuse, and GI-symptom interviews. We also used a structured interview to inquire about any lifetime history of CPP that was distinct from the history of bowel distress. We compared the rates of CPP and physical and sexual abuse, selected gynecological problems, dissociation, somatization, and lifetime psychiatric disorders among groups of women with IBD alone, IBS alone, and IBS+CPP.

CPP was reported in 38.9% of the IBS patients vs. 14.3% of the IBD group ($p < 0.05$). Compared with the IBD group, the IBS patients had significantly higher current and lifetime prevalence rates for several psychiatric disorders as well as higher rates of somatization, dissociation, and gynecological disorders, including dysmenorrhea and dyspareunia as well as higher rates of hysterectomy. However, the group with both CPP and IBS had prevalence rates that were even higher than those of patients with IBS alone. Logistic regression showed that number of somatization symptoms was the best predictor of comorbidity.

Taken together, these findings suggest that: 1) many women with IBS may have a history of CPP as well; 2) many women with CPP may also meet criteria for IBS; 3) the high rates of psychopathology associated with IBS and CPP independently are still higher in women with both disorders; 4) women who present with either IBS or CPP should probably be evaluated for both disorders; and 5) the number of somatization symptoms is a good predictor of psychopathology severity.

B. Sexual and Physical Abuse

In addition to significantly higher rates of current and lifetime psychiatric disorders and somatization, women with chronic abdominal pain may have higher rates of childhood and adult physical and sexual abuse.

Victimization in Women with CPP

In our previously cited study of women scheduled for diagnostic laparoscopy (10), we also administered structured sexual-abuse interviews. Compared to women who did not report abdominal pain, women with CPP reported significantly higher prevalence rates of all forms of childhood sexual abuse (58% vs. 30%), child rape or incest (24% vs. 4%), and adult sexual victimization (38% vs. 18%). The overall sexual-trauma rate of the nonpain group was close to the rate reported for the general population. Of the total sample of 100 patients, 14 women reported severe childhood sexual abuse; 12 of the 14 were in the CPP group.

Several studies have confirmed these findings in women with CPP. Reiter and Gambone (12) used a self-report questionnaire in 106 women attending a multidisciplinary clinic for evaluation of CPP. Compared to 96 pain-free patients, the women with pelvic pain had a significantly higher prevalence of overall sexual trauma (48% vs. 7%), including childhood sexual abuse (26% vs. 1%) and adult sexual assault (22% vs. 5%). Walling et al. (13) also found significantly higher rates of sexual victimization in women with CPP compared with women without pain as well as those in a non-pelvic-pain control group. However, one study, by Rapkin et al. (14), found no association between CPP and sexual victimization, but did find an association with physical abuse.

Victimization in Patients with IBS

Using a similar methodology, we have also found higher rates of sexual abuse in women with IBS compared with women with IBD (11). We administered structured sexual-trauma interviews to 28 patients with IBS and 19 patients with IBD and compared prevalence rates of sexual victimization between the two groups. Compared with patients diagnosed with IBD, patients with IBS had a significantly higher prevalence of severe lifetime sexual trauma (32% vs. 0%), severe childhood sexual abuse (11% vs. 0%), and any lifetime sexual victimization (54% vs. 5%). When patients (with either GI diagnosis) who had severe sexual trauma ($n = 9$) were compared with those having less severe sexual trauma or no trauma ($n = 38$), patients with severe lifetime victimization had significantly higher odds ratios for lifetime depression, panic disorder, phobia, somatization disorder, alcohol abuse, dyspareunia, and inhibited sexual desire. A logistic regression analysis showed that gender, the number of medically unexplained physical symptoms, and self-reported anxiety and hostility accounted for all of the variance in the victimized group.

Two recent reports have also suggested a possible association between a history of sexual and physical trauma and IBS. Drossman and colleagues (15) administered a self-report questionnaire to 206 patients in a university gastroenterology clinic and found that 44% of the patients reported a history of physical or sexual trauma in childhood or later life. The patients with functional GI disorders were significantly more likely to report histories of physical or sexual trauma compared with patients with organic disorders. In a second study, Felitti (16) reviewed the medical records of 131 members of a health maintenance organization who responded affirmatively to a screening question concerning a history of rape or sexual molestation. These patients were significantly more likely than a comparison group of patients who did not report such victimization to have had diagnoses of IBS or a benign course of nonspecific, recurrent GI symptoms such as cramping and diarrhea.

When examined together, these data suggest that psychological distress, history of prior sexual or physical abuse, and number of lifetime psychiatric disorders may be better discriminators of functional vs. organic abdominal pain, and may be significant factors in the development of chronicity through disability.

C. The Role of Disability

One of the more interesting recent findings in the area of chronic abdominal pain has been its relationship to disability. Studies of IBD have shown that the majority of patients continue to function remarkably well, despite the stress of repeated surgeries, parenteral nutrition, and recurrent episodes of diarrhea and pain (17,18). Despite the long-term discomfort and medical and surgical distress endured by IBD patients, they do not display rates of psychiatric disorder or abuse prevalence much higher than would be expected for medical clinical patients. On the other hand, IBS patients, who experience a much more benign course of illness and do not undergo such extreme treatments, show far greater levels of distress.

One of the important differences appears to be disability. People who are not disabled perceive themselves to be primarily healthy with occasional periods of illness. People with disability, on the other hand, perceive themselves as ill with occasional periods of health. This striking difference in world view is often found in people with somatization, and both somatization and disability can result in patients with early experiences of abuse or neglect. Thus, it is not surprising that patients with chronic abdominal pain, with their higher prevalence rates of psychiatric disorders and developmental stressors, should have increased risk for disability.

D. Can Patients Have Both Organic and Functional Disorders?

At least some patients with known organic abdominal pathology (e.g., IBD) appear to develop chronic abdominal pain and disability. As we have stated above, although a diagnosis of chronic abdominal pain is rarely considered in IBD patients, there is no reason that this cannot occur since the relatively benign pathophysiology of IBS (whatever that is) is likely to be distinct from the more severe organic pathology of IBD.

Our study of 71 IBS patients and 40 IBD patients found significant differences between the two groups with respect to the prevalence of lifetime and current psychiatric disorders, somatization, and abuse. However, there also appeared to be a subgroup of IBD patients who did less well than the majority of IBD patients in the study. These patients looked more like the IBS patients with respect to disability, lifetime psychiatric disorders, somatization, and prior episodes of abuse. This suggests that psychiatric disorders may significantly influence the expression of physical disease such as IBD and increase disability. This finding is in accord with several recent studies that have shown additive disability effects when psychiatric disorders are comorbid with physical disease (19).

Although it was possible in our previous study to clearly identify patients with comorbid IBS and CPP, the task of discriminating patients who might have both IBS and IBD is nearly impossible because of the common symptom set. Yet there are striking similarities between the IBS+CPP group and this putative IBS+IBD group, suggesting that the issue of simultaneous organic and functional disorders, or "double-dose" functional disorders, needs further investigation.

In summary, while the prospective definition of chronic abdominal pain using biomedical criteria remains (and probably will remain) elusive, current and lifetime psychiatric disorders, somatization and disability, and early sexual and physical victimization are important predictors of disease status, and may be more useful than physical symptom criteria to help discriminate between patients with organic disorders and those with functional disorders.

IV. AREAS FOR FUTURE RESEARCH

Previous studies of chronic abdominal pain have illuminated several opportunities for further research. More needs to be known about the natural history of this heterogeneous set of disorders, and how different comorbidity subtypes (i.e., abdominal discomfort referred to either GI or reproductive origins vary in onset and character. This may improve case definition as well as clarify subtle but important differences between patients with differing forms of abdominal pain. Studies of predictive psychosocial risk factors such as family history, prior victimization, and disability are essential to understand how chronic abdominal pain is established and maintained. This is particularly valuable since all patients with chronic abdominal pain started out being evaluated for acute pain. Identifying patients at the early part of their illness may avoid the destructive effects of prolonged disability on treatment outcome. Antidepressants, which have proven useful in the management of other forms of chronic pain, have not yet been thoroughly studied in patients with chronic abdominal pain, and may offer a convenient and effective therapy for these patients. Finally, multidisciplinary treatment approaches that have proven effective in other forms of chronic pain need to be tried in the more refractory patients with chronic abdominal pain for whom little else has proven effective.

V. EVALUATION AND TREATMENT

Evaluation of the patient with chronic abdominal pain begins long before the realization that the pain has become chronic (i.e., all chronic pain patients necessarily start out presumed to have acute pain). Unfortunately, we frequently inherit the patient at the time she has been labeled chronic, yet that declaration follows a long, expensive biomedical workup that has yielded little or no evidence of pathophysiology. This leaves us with two problems: 1) what to do when we receive an angry, frustrated patient who feels that she has been told "it's all in your head" and 2) how to teach our colleagues to modify the evaluation so that more psychosocial evaluation and treatment occur at the front end.

A. The Referred Chronic Patient

The chronic abdominal pain patient who is referred for psychosocial evaluation at the end of a long biomedical workup is understandably upset. Her doctor has found no explanation for this incessant pain. Not only is this intellectually unbelievable, it is emotionally unsatisfying. "What if they haven't looked far enough?" "Suppose I really have cancer!" "Why can't they give me something to take away the pain; don't they care?"

The first step is the difficult task of joining with the patient. Making her aware that you believe her pain to be real regardless of etiology is imperative. Use of the concept of stress as a common explanatory model may also assist the patient who is ambivalent about making links to depression, anxiety, and psychosocial vulnerabilities. Education about a "vicious cycle of pain" (i.e., pain leads to stress, which in turn leads to worsening pain) may help the patient see that stress is, indeed, a factor in worsening all forms of pain. Many patients will have already found that narcotic analgesics are of minimal value, and helping patients to understand the differences between operant and nociceptively derived pain may be useful.

Careful review of the medical history with the patient continues this bonding process. Were all common etiologies of abdominal pain considered? Is this a patient with multiple surgeries who was denied a laparoscopy when adhesions might be part of the ongoing pain pathophysiology? Is there a cyclic menstrual periodicity that suggests a process such as endometriosis? Be sure to let the patient know that you are interested in not only her psychosocial wellness but her medical history as well.

A comprehensive psychiatric interview, including detailed assessment of early developmental stressors, is essential. Pay particular attention to episodes of abuse, neglect, childhood experience of illness or sibling illness, and parental illness modeling (e.g., her mother solved problems through somatization). A thorough review of somatization symptoms may indicate that the patient not only has other pain syndromes but also may have broader patterns of somatization across many organ symptoms.

Generally, the treatment plan will focus on the reframing of somatization and pain as "stress" symptoms. Often these patients are not particularly psychologically minded, so techniques aimed at changing pain behavior rather than understanding it may be more effective. Focus on coping, and never promise a cure. Reduction of disability by restoration of adaptive coping skills is a far better endpoint than the possibly unreachable nirvana of freedom from pain.

Specifically, it is useful to employ the biopsychosocial model as a guide to care. This model can be conveniently divided into three components, as described below, each with a separate diagnostic and treatment formulation.

Patients can first be viewed from a biomedical perspective. Although much of this evaluation may have already been accomplished with little result, several aspects may have been overlooked. For example, many patients will be found to have physical deconditioning and pain behaviors that have caused splinting and limited range of motion. This suggests that physical therapy may have a place in treatment. Additionally, many patients will have developed narcotic dependence, requiring careful withdrawal. Although there have been very few controlled trials of antidepressants in chronic abdominal pain, their demonstrated efficacy in several other forms of chronic pain suggests that a trial is warranted. We have had considerable success with this approach, and a rationale may be found in our recent review (20).

Socially, patients may be in situations that reinforce or maintain their pain. Attention to support structures and family/work dynamics may suggest social and lifestyle interventions that provide similar benefits using pain-free behaviors. Finally, assessment of family of origin will bring to light psychodynamic forces that may need to be dealt with in psychotherapy. In many pain patients, these biological, social, and developmental forces have formed interlocking, mutually reinforcing maladaptive patterns that need to be modified together. Interventions that are not system-wide are likely to have limited effectiveness. This has been amply proved in the success of multidisciplinary pain-treatment centers, which emphasize integrated treatment strategies that are multimodal (21,22).

Thus, the treatment of "inherited" chronic abdominal pain requires a flexible multidisciplinary approach that combines physical therapy, antidepressants, individual and group therapy, and cognitive-behavioral and dynamic therapies as well as motivation toward wellness and positive lifestyle changes.

B. The "Acute" Chronic Abdominal Pain Patient

Every chronic pain patient starts out having an "acute" pain evaluation. Are there ways to identify patients at an earlier stage who are at risk for developing chronicity in order to avoid long, expensive workups with their attendant discomfort and possible iatrogenic harm?

Collaboration between primary-care physicians and consultation psychiatrists may be a profitable solution. Rather than expect an exhaustive biomedical evaluation followed by a psychosocial evaluation, the patient can be made aware that the primary-care physician believes in contemporaneous biomedical and psychosocial evaluation. During the initial visit, the patient is interviewed and examined thoroughly by the primary-care physician with an emphasis on increasing the therapeutic liaison through active listening and the "laying on of hands." Some further diagnostic testing may be scheduled at this time, but the patient is referred immediately for a "stress" evaluation to determine psychosocial factors that initiate and maintain pain.

Although many patients will resist accepting psychological factors as being causative of their pain, most will readily accept that their physical illness causes them stress, which in turn worsens their pain ("Doctor, if you had this pain, you'd be stressed too"). Although these "stress" factors may actually be *causal* in the development of pain, it is better not to press this point at the beginning. The acceptance that stress is also an object of treatment in pain reduction is enough. Open communication between the psychiatrist and family physician is essential in gradually moving the patient away from a disease-oriented model to one that includes treatment of disability and psychopathology as primary goals. The patient should identify both physicians as actively working together and should have strong therapeutic bonds to both. Psychiatrists with skills, experience, and interest in consultation-liaison psychiatry are likely to be best able to coordinate this process.

Hopefully, careful alternation between a graded, judicious biomedical investigation and a rational, progressive psychosocial evaluation will result in a treatment plan that is efficient, cost-conscious, and effective in these difficult patients. The rewards of collaborative interaction between the psychiatrist and primary-care physician will lead to a routine of earlier psychosocial evaluation and treatment as well as better outcomes for these highly distressed patients.

REFERENCES

1. Kroenke K. Symptoms in medical patients: an untended field. Am J Med 1991; 92(suppl 1A):3s–6s.
2. Walker EA, Katon WJ, Jemelka RP, Roy-Byrne PP. Comorbidity of gastrointestinal complaints, depression, and anxiety in the Epidemiologic Catchment Area Study. Am J Med 1991; 92(suppl 1A):26s–30s.
3. Drossman DA, Sandler RS, McKee DC, et al. Bowel patterns among subjects not seeking health care. Gastroenterology 1982; 83:529–534.
4. Manning AP, Thompson WG, Heaton KW, et al. Towards a positive diagnosis of the irritable bowel. Br Med J 1978; 2:653–654.

5. Walker EA, Katon WJ, Alfrey H, Bowers M, Stenchever MA. The prevalence of chronic pelvic pain and irritable bowel syndrome in two university clinics. J Psychosom Obstet Gynecol 1991; 12(suppl):65–75.
6. Walker E, Katon W, Harrop-Griffiths J, Holm L, Russo J, Hickok L. Chronic pelvic pain: The relationship to psychiatric diagnoses and childhood sexual abuse. Am J Psychiatry 1988; 145:75–80.
7. Walker EA, Katon WK, Hansom J, Harrop-Griffiths J, Holm L, Jones L, Hickok L, Jemelka RP. Psychiatric diagnoses and childhood sexual abuse in women with chronic pelvic pain. Psychosomatics 1995; 36:531–540.
8. Walker EA, Roy-Byrne PP, Katon WJ, Li L, Amos D, Jiranek G. Psychiatric illness and irritable bowel syndrome: a comparison with inflammatory bowel disease. Am J Psychiatry 1990; 147:1656–1661.
9. Walker EA, Gelfand A, Gelfand M, Green C, Katon WJ. Chronic pelvic pain in women with irritable bowel syndrome. Presented at 22nd annual meeting of the American Society for Psychosomatic Obstetrics and Gynecology, San Diego, CA, Feb 1994.
10. Walker EA, Katon WK, Hansom J, Harrop-Griffiths J, Holm L, Jones L, Hickock L, Jemelka RP. Medical and psychiatric symptoms in women with childhood sexual abuse. Psychosom Med 1992; 54:658–664.
11. Walker EA, Katon WJ, Roy-Byrne PP, Jemelka RP. Histories of sexual victimization in patients with irritable bowel syndrome or inflammatory bowel disease. Am J Psychiatry 1993; 150:1502–1506.
12. Reiter RC, Gambone JC. Demographic and historic variables in women with idiopathic chronic pelvic pain. Obstet Gynecol 1990; 75:428–432.
13. Walling MK, O'Hara MW, Reiter RC. Sexual abuse as a specific risk factor for chronic pelvic pain. Presented at 21st annual meeting of the American Society for Psychosomatic Obstetrics and Gynecology, Charleston SC, Feb 1993.
14. Rapkin AJ, Kames LD, Darke LL, Stampler FM, Naliboff BD. History of physical and sexual abuse in women with chronic pelvic pain. Obstet Gynecol 1990; 76:92–96.
15. Drossman DA, Leserman J, Nachman G, Li ZM, Gluck H, Toomey TC, Mitchell CM. Sexual and physical abuse in women with functional or organic gastrointestinal disorders. Ann Intern Med 1990, 113:828–833.
16. Felitti VJ. Long-term medical consequences of incest, rape and molestation. So Med J 1991; 84:328–331.
17. Helzer JE, Stillings WA, Chammas S, et al. A controlled study of the association between ulcerative colitis and psychiatric diagnosis. Digest Dis Sci 1982; 27:513–518.
18. Helzer JE, Chammas S, Norland C, et al. A study of the association between Crohn's disease and psychiatric illness. Gastroenterology 1984; 86:324–330.
19. Wells KB, Golding JM, Burnam MA. Psychiatric disorder and limitations in physical conditioning in a sample of the Los Angeles general population. Am J Psychiatry 1988; 145:712–717.
20. Walker EA, Sullivan MD, Stenchever M. The use of antidepressants in women with chronic pelvic pain. Obstet Gynecol Clin North Am, Dec 1993.
21. Peters AAW, van Dorst E, Jellis B, van Zuuren E, Trimbos JB. A randomized clinical

trial to compare two different approaches in women with chronic pelvic pain. Obstet Gynecol 1991; 77:740–744.
22. Kames LD, Rapkin AJ, Naliboff BD, Afifi S, Ferrer-Brechner T. Effectiveness of an interdisciplinary pain management program for the treatment of chronic pelvic pain. Pain 1990; 41:41–46.

13

Rational Medical Therapy of Functional GI Disorders

Richard M. Sperling
University of California, San Francisco
San Francisco, California

Kenneth R. McQuaid
University of California, San Francisco, and
Veterans Affairs Medical Center
San Francisco, California

I. INTRODUCTION

Alleviation of symptoms represents one of our primary goals in caring for patients. In no other gastrointestinal (GI) disease has this goal been more challenging and vexing to the practitioner than in the functional disorders. Rational management of these common disorders is made difficult by a lack of objective criteria with which to establish a definite diagnosis, a lack of understanding of their pathogenesis, and, consequently, a lack of specific, effective therapies.

The diagnosis of functional GI disorders has been hampered by the lack of positive objective criteria. By current definitions the functional GI disorders are a variable combination of chronic or recurrent GI symptoms *not explained by structural or biochemical abnormalities* (1). Several clinical entities may be subsumed under this broad rubric, including noncardiac chest pain, non-ulcer dyspepsia (NUD), irritable bowel syndrome (IBS), chronic abdominal pain, pelvic-floor dysfunction, and biliary dyskinesia (2). For each of these entities, there is no "gold standard" by which the diagnosis is established. Thus, the diagnosis is based on a the presence of a compatible symptom profile and the exclusion of other "organic" disorders. The limitations of this approach are obvious. The common symptoms that characterize these entities, such as chest and abdominal pain, constipation, diarrhea, nausea, and bloating may have multiple organic as well as functional etiologies. Some physicans may feel compelled to exclude these myriad organic diseases before treating the patient for functional illness. The extent of diagnostic workup required to exclude underlying disease may be unclear as there is always the small risk of an overlooked diagnosis. A variety of factors may influence the extent of workup, including the age of the patient, the duration of symptoms, previous medical history and evaluation, the presence of weight loss, abnormalities on physical examination, and results of screening blood tests, occult blood tests, or fecal cultures. Clinicians may also be driven by two other powerful forces: remuneration and fear of litigation.

A lack of understanding of the pathogenesis of functional disorders hampers efforts to develop specific effective therapies. Debate continues as to whether functional GI disorders are due primarily to disturbances in normal GI motility and physiology that interact with psychosocial factors that secondarily affect the GI tract (3–11). Although the etiopathogenesis of symptoms in most functional disorders is unproved, they are frequently attributed to dysfunction of the esophagus, stomach, small or large intestine, anorectum, or biliary tree. Alterations in motility can be demonstrated in some subsets of patients with functional disorders. In some, but not all, patients, there is a correlation between these motility abnormalities and symptom onset (12). Nevertheless, it is often unclear whether these motility disturbances cause the patient's symptoms or are merely a manometric marker of underlying psychological stress. Patients with functional disease have been shown to have a heightened sensitivity to a wide range of minor noxious stimuli, such as balloon distension, intraluminal infusions of acid, and neurohumoral agents (8,11,13). Whether this heightened visceral nocioception is due to a defect in visceral afferent sensation, abnormal central processing of afferent information, or psychosocial factors that alter the individual's perception and interpretation is undetermined.

A host of psychological abnormalities have been detected in subsets of patients with functional GI disorders, including depression, anxiety, somatization, phobia, and panic disorder (5,6,8,10,11,14–16). These psychological factors may profoundly influence symptom reporting, coping capabilities, and health-care-seeking behavior. For example, patients with IBS who seek medical attention tend to have more abnormal peronality profiles and psychological stress than

IBS nonpatients (17,18). Thus, patients with functional disease who seek medical evaluation may represent a self-selected group with psychosocial disturbances. Acute physical and emotional stress can trigger GI symptoms and alterations in GI motility in normal individuals as well as those with functional disorders; however, the effects of chronic psychosocial stress on the gut are only beginning to be undersood (4,6,19–22). Severe life stresses such as marital and financial difficulties precede the onset of symptoms in some patients. Finally, early-childhood reinforcement of illness behavior may generate a conditioned gut response to life stress in adulthood, as can a history of sexual abuse (5).

In view of the uncertainties that surround the pathogenesis of functional GI symptoms, it is difficult for clinicians to know how to approach therapy in a rational manner. Should they focus primarily on the patient's symptoms and attempt to afford relief with medications, biofeedback, or behavioral measures? In this regard, are pharmacological therapies targeted at observed disturbances in motility effective in providing symptom relief? Or should attention instead be focused on the patient's psychological profile and social situation? If so, identification and modification of the exacerbating psychosocial factors through behavioral or psychotherapeutic approaches may lead to diminished symptom severity and/or improved coping. The judicious use of psychopharmacological agents may also be helpful.

A hypothesis has been proffered by Drossman and Thompson (5) that ties together the manometric disturbances noted in many patients and the psychosocial abnormalities reported in patients who seek health care. They propose that, in certain susceptible individuals, environmental factors in early life may affect the susceptibility to developing symptoms of functional GI disease, such as painful gut contractions, and the ability to cope with them. Psychosocial factors such as personality, life stresses, social support, and coping mechanisms may influence how these symptoms are perceived (visceral nocioception), interpreted, and acted on (illness behavior). In other words, psychosocial factors may modify an underlying gut motor or sensory disturbance to determine the symptom severity and health care use. A person with GI symptoms with a normal psychological profile and good support structures may not seek attention or may be reassured easily by a limited medical evaluation. Conversely, a patient with a similar degree of motility disturbance and/or symptoms who has psychosocial problems, impaired coping, poor social support, or increased life stresses may become a chronic user of the health system.

In summary, a patient's symptoms may arise from a complex interaction of organic, psychological, and social factors. The circumspect clinician is advised to take an integrative treatment approach to the patient with functional GI symptoms. Rather than view the patient in the traditional dichotomous models of mind vs. body, organic vs. functional, or medical vs. psychiatric, the physican must attempt to understand the patient's psychological makeup and to consider the patient's symptoms in the context of the social and cultural milieu in which he or she lives. Only then can an appropriate therapeutic plan be applied.

This chapter describes a rational, integrated approach to the *medical* treatment of functional GI disorders from the perspective of the clinical gastroenterologist. Particular attention is given to the entities of noncardiac chest pain, NUD, and IBS. Other chapters in this book deal thoroughly with the approach to, the medical evaluation of, and the psychometric assessment of functional disorders. Additional chapters address the utility of psychotherapy, biofeedback, and psychopharmacological agents in the treatment of functional disorders. Thus, the thrust of this chapter is the *dietary* and *pharmacological* therapies of these diseases. In view of the foregoing discussion, it must be emphasized that such therapies should be employed in the context of the broader psychosocial perspective and in concert with other nonmedical therapies.

II. GENERAL APPROACH TO THERAPY

A. Reason for Seeking Medical Evaluation

In many cases, functional GI symptoms have been present for many years before the patient decides to seek medical attention. It therefore behooves the clinician to determine the factor(s) that precipitated the current medical consultation before embarking on an extensive—and possibly needless—diagnostic and therapeutic course. Careful inquiry into the patient's medical, social, and family history is time well spent. The reason for the visit may not be immediately forthcoming and, indeed, may not be apparent even to the patient. With persistent questioning, however, insights may be elicited (2,5,8,23,24).

A number of factors may precipitate a medical consultation for functional complaints. Serious illness in a family member or close associate may provoke personal concern in the patient that chronic GI symptoms could be indicative of undiagnosed disease (5). Although reassurance may suffice to allay anxiety in some patients, it may be far more "therapeutic"—and cost-effective—to address the patient's specific concerns early with a targeted diagnostic (especially radiologic or endoscopic) evaluation. Life stresses related to the patient's workplace, family, or living situation may cause a decompensation in a patient who was previously coping adequately with chronic symptoms (5,8,24). Recent changes in dietary intake or medications should be reviewed. GI complaints may represent a somatic symptom of serious underlying psychiatric disease such as depression, anxiety, or, rarely, psychosis. Finally, a small percentage of patients with chronic complaints may be seeking secondary gain such as narcotics, disability compensation, or involvement with physician and the medical system.

B. Importance of the Initial Evaluation

With the first visit, the physician should foster the trust and confidence of the patient by performing a careful, nonjudgmental history and thorough physical examination (5,23,24). Patients must feel that they have been completely heard. Therefore, the physician should allow sufficient time for the patient to relay his or her history in a calm, relaxed atmosphere. If time is running short, it is best to schedule a subsequent visit, so as not to appear rushed or impatient. A thorough, confident physical examination is also extremely important. Not only is it helpful in excluding organic causes of the patient's symptoms, but the "laying of the hands" often has palliative qualities. Patients who feel that their symptoms have been taken seriously by the physician are much more likely to trust in the physician's judgment and diagnostic plan.

After the history and physical examination, the physician may already have a high degree of suspicion that the patient suffers from a functional disorder. Nevertheless, a diagnostic evaluation is generally necessary to exclude obvious organic disorders. Prior to this investigation, it is important to inquire of patients what they believe or fear is causing their symptoms. It is also helpful to discuss the differential diagnosis—including functional disease—and explain why each entity is likely or unlikely. A reaonable, cost-effective, diagnostic workup is then proposed that addresses the needs of the physician and the concerns of the patient. The above has the effect of involving the patient in the diagnostic thought process. Once the diagnostic workup has been completed, it will be easier for the patient to accept a diagnosis of a functional disorder (4–6,8,24).

C. Education and Reassurance

Patients should be given a thorough description of their functional disorder, including what is known and unknown. It should be stressed that these conditions are extremely common but their cause in unknown. Patients should be told that everyone has an extraordinary number of nerves and hormones in the gut, which respond to a variety of poorly understood factors. Symptoms arise either from an increased sensitivity to minor pain or distension or from an increased reactivity to various factors, resulting in spasm or hypomotility. Although a variety of dietary, environmental, physiological, and psychological factors may trigger symptoms in some people, most patients are unable to identify specific inciting factors. The importance of the "mind–gut" interaction should be mentioned, but also that it is only beginning to be studied. Physicians should strive to avoid a "mind-versus-body" dualism, lest patients infer that the physician has concluded that they are "crazy" or that "it's all in my head." Patients should be reassured that the overwhelming majority of those with such disorders are otherwise perfectly normal people who lead productive lives. Fears that the symptoms will progress, require surgery, or degenerate into other illnesses should be allayed (5,23,24).

D. Setting Appropriate Goals and Limits

It is important for the physician to set reasonable goals and expectations early on with the patient. They must understand that symptoms tend to be chronic and characterized by periods of exacerbation and quiescence. It will be necessary for the patient to learn to adapt and cope with these symptoms through lifestyle adaptations (5,24). While physicians can assist in this regard, they cannot "cure" the illness. On the other hand, physicians should make it clear to the patient (and to themselves) that they will continue to follow and work with the patient as necessary.

As discussed below, the vast majority of patients will neither require nor benefit from drug therapy of their functional disease. Patients should be discouraged from looking to the physician for a pharmacological panacea. In selected patients with severe symptoms, drug treatment directed as a specific symptom may be helpful on an intermittent, short-term basis. However, chronic pharmacotherapy is not recommended in most patients.

E. The Importance of an Ongoing Relationship

Many patients may be reassured by the approach described above and require little or no ongoing care. A subset of functional patients will require ongoing care, either intermittently during periods of symptom exacerbation or on a regular basis. Over time, the life events that trigger symptom exacerbations may become more apparent. The importance of this ongoing therapeutic relationship cannot be overemphasized (5). In multiple controlled clinical trials, the symptomatic response to placebo therapy has been >50–65% (25). Although most primary practitioners are not psychotherapists, patients clearly derive great symptomatic relief from an ongoing relationship with a concerned, compassionate physician.

With some patients, it is helpful to have them keep a diary for several weeks in which they record their degree of symptoms, their diet, and associated events in their lives (8). By reviewing this diary with the patient, the physician may glean knowledge about dietary or psychosocial triggers. Such chronicles also provide greater insight into the patient's psychosocial situation.

Psychological difficulties that were not evident initially may become so with time. In some cases, referral to a psychologist or psychiatrist may be indicated (5,26). If a trusting physician–patient relationship has been established, most patients will acquiesce to such a referral. It is extremely important, however, that the medical physician continue to follow the patient so that he or she does not feel "abandoned."

III. TREATMENT OF SPECIFIC SYNDROMES

A. Chest Pain of Undetermined Etiology

Causes

Approximately 20% of patients who undergo cardiac catheterization for chest pain do not have evidence of ischemic coronary artery disease. Over half of these patient experience recurrent pain and are labeled as having "noncardiac" chest pain (9,27,28). Because a negative catheterization does not necessarily exclude all cardiac causes of chest pain, most investigators now prefer the term "chest pain of undetermined etiology" (CPUE). A host of problems related to the heart, the GI tract, and the chest wall may cause CPUE. In addition, a number of patients have underlying psychiatric abnormalities, discussed in detail elsewhere. Causes of CPUE include the following:

Musculoskeletal Causes Over 10% of patients with CPUE may have musculoskeletal causes of pain, including costochondritis, xyphoidalgia, rib tip syndrome, fibromyalgia, and cervical or thoracic spine disease (29). These are readily excluded with a careful physical examination.

Cardiac Causes Atypical chest pain occurs in up to 50% of patients with *mitral valve prolapse*, although this may be partially attributable to ascertainment bias (30). *Coronary spasm* can take place in patients with normal coronary arteries; this is characterized on EKG by ST-segment elevation during pain and may be provoked by an ergonovine challenge during coronary arteriography.

Recently, an entity known as *microvascular angina* or "syndrome X" has been characterized (31–33). Although the relative significance of this entity is unknown, it is diagnosed in >70% of patients referred to the National Institutes of Health (NIH) for CPUE. Patients have features of atypical or typical anginal pain, with relief by rest or nitrates. A variety of abnormalities may be noted on noninvasive cardiac testing. These include an abnormal exercise-tolerance test in up to 30%, an abnormal exercise nuclear cardiac ejection study in 40–70%, and the provocation of chest pain and ECG changes after a dipyridamole infusion. At cardiac catheterization, despite normal coronary arteries, >90% of patients develop chest pain during rapid atrial pacing followed by an ergonovine infusion. A defect in the vasodilatory response of the coronary microcirculation is postulated that results in increased vascular resistance and myocardial ischemia (33,34). It has been suggested that this is part of a more generalized defect that involves the esophagus, bronchioles, and systemic vasculature.

A full discussion of the diagnosis and treatment of microvascular anginal is beyond the scope of this chapter. The reader is referred to several excellent reviews (33).

Esophageal Motility Disorders Abnormalities in esophageal motility are evident on standard manometric testing in up to one-third of patients with CPUE (35,36); however, the importance of these findings as a cause per se of CPUE is unclear (9,20,37). Very few patients have serious abnormalities such as achalasia (<1%) or diffuse esophageal spasm (5%), which is characterized by the presence of simultaneous contraction on >10% of wet swallows. Almost half of the motility disorders are characterized by normal peristalsis but a marked increase in distal esophageal contraction amplitude, a condition known as "nutcracker esophagus." These high-amplitude contractions do not impair peristaltic function and are seldom associated with pain when noted during the manometry study (36). Furthermore, these "abnormalities" may be extremely labile and related to psychological stress. They resolve on repeat manometric study in almost half of patients over a 5-year period (38). An increase in esophageal peristaltic amplitude can be provoked in normal subjects as well as patients with nutcracker esophagus during laboratory-induced cognitive stress (39). Also, the finding of nutcracker esophagus is associated with a higher prevalence of hypochondriasis and somatic anxiety on psychological inventories (40).

Approximately 35% of patients have other nonspecific abnormalities such as intermittent nontransmitted contractions, abnormal wave morphology, or intermittent incomplete relaxation of the lower esophageal sphincter (35). As with nutcracker esophagus, the physiological significance of these nonspecific motility disorders is unclear. However, over 80% of patients with CPUE and nonspecific esophageal motility disorders have evidence of a major psychiatric diagnosis such as depression, somatization disorder, or anxiety disorder, in comparison with only 31% of CPUE patients with normal esophageal motility (41).

In summary, nutcracker esophagus and nonspecific motility disorders may represent a manometric *marker* of psychological distress rather than a bona fide physiological cause of chest pain (37). The relevance of these nonspecific motility disturbances to CPUE is dubious, making their detection of little clinical utility in most cases (36).

Stronger evidence of the importance of dysmotility as a cause of chest pain could be established by ambulatory motility studies. However, such studies suggest that motility disturbances are temporally correlated with episodes of chest pain in <14% of patients (42–47). Thus, esophageal dysmotility as a cause of CPUE appears to be important in only a small minority of patients.

Gastroesophageal Reflux Recently, gastroesophageal reflux has been promoted as a significant cause of CPUE (48). Up to 50% of patients with CPUE have a significant amount of acid reflux documented on an ambulatory prolonged pH study, i.e., have evidence of gastroesophageal-reflux diseases (49). In a number of studies, a correlation between chest pain and episodes of chest pain on ambulatory pH monitoring has been confirmed in 20–50% of patients (42–44,46–52).

Other GI causes of CPUE include peptic ulcer disease, biliary colic, and impaired belch reflex.

Abnormal Visceral Nocioception Many patients with CPUE have a heightened sensitivity to minor noxious visceral stimuli. Intraesophageal-balloon inflation provokes pain in 40–60% of patients, compared with only 20% of asymptomatic controls (53,54). Intraesophageal-acid infusion provokes pain in 20–30% of patients, only half of whom have significant gastroesophageal reflux on ambulatory pH monitoring (55,56). Nonspecific cholinergic stimulation with edrophonium provokes chest pain in 20–30% of patients, which is unrelated to any demonstrable changes in esophageal contractions (57–59). Finally, catheter manipulation in the right heart induces chest pain in up to 89% of CPUE patients but in only 5% of patients with coronary artery disease (60).

Psychological Abnormalities Approximately 80% of CPUE patients have been found on structured interview to have a psychiatric diagnosis (41). Overall, CPUE patients display a higher degree of neuroticism, poor coping strategies, somatic anxiety, clinical pain reporting, and GI symptom susceptibility on various psychological questionaires (15,16,61). Up to 35% of CPUE patients fulfill diagnostic criteria for a diagnosis of panic disorder (61,62). Patients with panic disorder may come first to the attention of internists, family physicians, or emergency physicians complaining of somatic symptoms such as chest pain. Compared with other patients with CPUE, these patients tend to have higher levels of anxiety and psychological distress and more functional impairment from their chest pain. It is helpful to identify these patients early in the evaluation of chest pain to avoid a costly and unnecessary evaluation. Panic disorder may be effectively treated with pharmacological therapies, including alprazolam (63). The psychometric assessment and treatment of psychological disorders in functional disease is discussed elsewhere.

Summary It has become increasingly apparent that a variety of cardiac, esophageal, and psychiatric abnormalities can be identified in a significant proportion of CPUE patients, as well as abnormalities in visceral nocioception. In investigating CPUE, cardiologists, gatroenterologists, and psychiatrists have tended to focus on tests and diseases related to their respective disciplines. It is increasingly apparent, however, that there is a large overlap among these problems and that a broader perspective is necessary. In a prospective study, patients with CPUE referred to the NIH for evaluation of CPUE underwent independent evaluation by cardiologists and gastroenterologists. Although a cardiac cause was found in 75% and an esophageal cause in 45%, a surprising 38% had evidence of both cardiac and esophageal causes (31). Psychiatric abnormalities have been found in 78% of CPUE patients with esophophageal dymotility compared with only 31% with normal motilities (41). Similarly, cognitive stress has been demonstrated to alter esophageal motility. Thus, abnormal motility may be a manometric marker of psychological stress rather than a cause per se of CPUE.

Evaluation

Before a diagnostic and therapeutic course is begun in a patient with CPUE, it is imperative that ischemic and valvular heart disease be excluded. History alone is notoriously unreliable in distinguishing cardiac from noncardiac causes. Hence, a workup is mandatory to exclude potentially lethal cardiac disease. The level of cardiac workup necessary will depend on the patient's age, family history, and risk factors for coronary artery disease. In most cases, an exercise or Persantine tolerance test (with or without thallium) is needed. Many patients with recurrent pain will undergo coronary angiography and echocardiography. Patients with abnormalities on noninvasive testing who have normal coronary angiography should be considered for evalution for micorvascular angina.

Patients referred for evaluation of CPUE should undergo a careful history and physical examination. Particular inquiry should be made into symptoms of esophageal diseases such as heartburn, regurgitation, dysphagia, and odynophagia. It should be remembered that symptoms of gastroesophageal reflux are common and do not necessarily confirm a causative relationship. Patients should be asked about the possible relationship between chest pain and eating, drinking hot or cold liquids and carbonated beverages, posture, physical activity, and psychosocial stress. In addition, the physician should look for symptoms of other functional disorders such as chronic dyspepsia or abdominal pain, or IBS. Finally, the physician should evaluate the patient for psychosocial factors that may be causing or exacerbating the patient's pain. Referral for formal psychological evaluation should be made as deemed appropriate.

Initial medical evaluation begins with a physical examination. It is important to examine the chest wall carefully, looking for evidence of "trigger points" that reproduce the patient's pain. An upper-GI series or upper endoscopy should be performed to look for structural causes of chest pain such as peptic ulcer disease, gastroesophageal-reflux disease, or achalasia. Abdominal ultrasonography is useful to screen for biliary disease. Subsequent evaluation should be tailored to the patient's symptoms and the clinical setting. Because it is common and readily treated, it is reasonable in most patients to look for evidence of gastroesophageal reflux with an ambulatory esophageal pH study or a Bernstein test.

Esophageal motility testing, pain provocation with edrophonium, and/or intraesophageal-balloon inflation may be useful in some patients. However, the presence or absence of abnormalities on these studies seldom influences the subsequent management of the patient. Hence, they are of limited utility in the routine evaluation of CPUE (36).

Finally, it must be recognized that in many patient who undergo extensive clinical testing, the cause of chest pain cannot be reliably determined.

Treatment of Esophageal Chest Pain

Non-Drug Management Patients with CPUE and normal coronary angiography have a 98% survival at 7 years, which is similar to that of an age-matched control population (64). Notwithstanding this favorable prognosis, up to 58% limit their activities, 25–45% continue to use antianginal medications, 10–44% continue to believe that they may have coronary artery disease, and 17% are rehospitalized per year. It would appear that the mere exclusion of coronary artery disease is not sufficient to allay patient anxiety (65). A major goal of therapy is to reassure patients that they do not have cardiac disease and to improve their functional status. The emphasis must gradually be shifted from the patient's (and physician's) desire to find the cause of the pain because a definite cause is seldom found and—except for acid reflux—does not lead to a specific, effective therapy. Asking the question only leads to patient frustration and anxiety, and often to repeated, unnecessary tests. It is far more productive to shift the emphasis to coping with the chronic pain.

Patients may benefit most from the reassurance of a steady relationship with a physician. Symptoms may fluctuate in intensity, but longitudinal studies suggest that chest-pain frequency and severity decline with time (9,66). Whether this reflects the natural history of the disease or the benefits of longitudinal care is unclear. Given the lack of specific effective therapies for most patients with CPUE, reassurance and constancy of care may be the most important therapy clinicians have to offer.

Treatment of Gastroesophageal Reflux Disease (GERD) GERD is a common medical condition that is readily treated with medical or surgical therapies (67–69). A full discussion of the treatment of GERD is beyond the scope of this chapter. Briefly, patients are generally treated in a stepwise fashion. Patients with occasional symptoms are instructed to use antacids as needed and to make certain dietary and lifestyle modification including adopting a low-fat diet; avoiding tomatoes, citrus, and alcohol; elevating the head of the bed; and avoiding snacks before bedtime. Patients with more frequent symptoms are treated twice daily with an H_2-receptor antagonist such as ranitidine 150 mg b.i.d. or famotidine 20 mg b.i.d. Finally, patients with severe disease and/or refractory symptoms are treated with a proton pump inhibitor such as omeprazole 20–40 mg q.d. or surgical fundoplication.

Given the strong association between acid reflux and CPUE that has been demonstrated in many studies, treatment of GERD in patients with CPUE has been recommended by a number of authorities. Indeed, *empirical* treatment is now endorsed in CPUE patients. It is therefore somewhat surprising—and troubling—that these recommendations are being made in the absence of any prospective, placebo-controlled trials. In an uncontrolled study, 12 patients with nutcracker esophagus and proven gastroesophageal reflux on ambulatory pH testing were given antisecretory therapy. These patients were treated in an unblinded fashion with either omeprazole 40 mg/day or high-dose ranitidine (300 mg q.i.d.) for 8 weeks with proven normalization of esophageal pH on repeat testing. A marked reduction in chest pain occurred in 10 of 12 (83%) of patients (70). In another uncontrolled, unblinded study, DeMeester and colleagues (71) reported symptom relief in 12 patients who had acid-induced chest pain demonstrated on pH monitoring who were treated with either surgical or medical antireflux therapy. In contrast, no improvement in chest pain was seen in 11 CPUE patients who had significant acid reflux but in whom no relationship could be demonstrated between episodes of acid reflux and chest-pain events. These studies—albeit promising—require confirmation by placebo-controlled trials.

Although acid reflux may play an important role in some patients with CPUE, there are reasons to suspect that its true importance has been exaggerated. First, although 25% of CPUE patients have at least some pain episodes associated with acid reflux, many other episodes are not (48). What causes these episodes of chest pain is unclear, but there is no reason to believe that antireflux therapy will relieve them. Second, approximately half of patients with acid-induced chest pain do not have abnormal *amounts* of acid reflux (49). That is, they seem to have a heightened sensitivity to normal physiological amounts of acid reflux (abnormal visceral nocioception). Whether these patients are best treated with antireflux measures versus other psychotropic medications or behavioral therapies is unknown.

Pending confirmation through controlled clinical trials, restraint is urged in treating patients with CPUE for acid reflux. The recommendation by some authorities for empirical antireflux therapy in CPUE is largely untested. Given the high placebo response that occurs in all trials of functional disease, symptomatic improvement cannot be accepted as "proof" that the chest pain is acid-induced. Long-term antireflux therapy, albeit safe, is expensive. Finally, it is a minority of CPUE patients who have a demonstrated relationship between reflux and chest pain on prolonged pH monitoring. At present, it is recommended that antireflux therapy be reserved for patients in whom an association between acid reflux and chest pain has been established by ambulatory pH testing. If pH monitoring is unavailable, an empirical, aggressive antireflux trial of omeprazole 20–40 mg/day should be given for 2 months to determine whether pain frequency diminishes.

Treatment of Esophageal Motility Abnormalities A number of medical and surgical measures have been used in the treatment of patients with CPUE and esophageal motility abnormalities. Unfortunately, their use is based almost solely on anecdotal recommendations. Very few have been submitted to any controlled clinical testing. The few studies that have been reported have suffered from a number of methodological problems, including small number of patients, lack of placebo controls, limited follow-up, vague or nonvalidated symptom assessment, and variable manometric diagnostic criteria. In reviewing these studies, it may be important to distinguish studies of diffuse esophageal spasm (DES) from those of nutcracker esophagus or nonspecific motility abnormalities. The treatment of achalasia is not addressed here.

Smooth-Muscle Relaxants: Theorizing that chest pain may arise from either esophageal spasm or increased contraction amplitude, smooth-muscle relaxants have been tried in patients with CPUE and esophageal motility abnormalities.

Nitrates and Anticholinergics: Nitrates and anticholinergic agents have been shown to cause a modest decrease in esophageal pressures in healthy adults, albeit transiently (72). There have been no controlled studies of these agents in patients with CPUE and esophageal dysmotility. Wide anecdotal experience suggests that nitrates may be effective in DES, though there is little published experience (73). In two uncontrolled studies of patients with DES, acute symptomatic and manometric improvement was seen in all patients given nitrates (74,75). Of note, patients placed on chronic therapy with long-acting nitrates became symptom-free. There are no published reports of the use of nitrates in patients with nutcracker or nonspecific motility disorders.

Calcium Channel Antagonists: Calcium channel blockers have been shown to decrease the amplitude of esophageal contraction, and the lower-esophageal-sphincter pressure in animals and normal controls (76,77). In small, open, uncontrolled studies of patients with DES, nifedipine has been reported to decrease the amplitude and frequency of simultaneous contractions and to decrease the frequency of chest-pain episodes (78–80). There are no controlled trials of calcium channel antagonists in patients with DES.

In patients with CPUE and nutcracker esophagus, a dose-dependent decrease in esophageal contraction pressure of 16–54% has been shown with both nifedipine (10–30 mg) and diltiazem (90–150 mg) (76,77). Two placebo-controlled studies of calcium channel antagonists in patients with nutcracker esophagus have had conflicting results. In a 14-week, double-blind, placebo-controlled crossover study of 20 patients, nifedipine significantly decreased distal esophageal contraction amplitude and lower sphincter pressure but was no better than placebo in the relief of severity or frequency of daily chest pain (81). Of interest, at follow-up a mean of 16 months after the study, chest pain had improved in the absence of specific therapy. In another double-blind, placebo-controlled crossover study of 22 nutcracker patients, diltiazem significantly lowered esophageal contraction amplitudes as well as mean chest-pain scores compared with placebo (82). This study is flawed, however, by the fact that only 14 patients completed the study and only nine of these fulfilled currently accepted manometric criteria for nutcracker esophagus.

Summary: Smooth-muscle relaxants have been shown to reduce esophageal contraction amplitude in normal controls and in patients with esophageal dysmotility. Anecdotal reports suggest that they may reduce the frequency of chest pain in patients with DES. Sublingual nitroglycerin 0.4 mg may be taken as needed for pain; patients with dysphagia may benefit from oral isosorbide dinitrate 10–30 mg taken 30 minutes before meals. Alternatively, nifedipine 10–30 mg t.i.d. may be given. There are no convincing data at this time that support the use of these agents in nutcracker esophagus. Because these agents may potentiate gastroesophageal reflux, their use could even *potentiate* chest pain in some patients. Given their cost, side effects (dizziness, headache, edema) and lack of proven efficacy, they cannot be recommended outside of controlled clinical trials.

Psychotropic and Psychological Therapies: The high prevalence of psychological abnormalities in CPUE, especially in those with esophageal dysmotility, suggests a role for psychotropic medications and/or psychotherapy. Anxiolytics and antidepressants have been used in the treatment of some CPUE patients. In a placebo-controlled trial of 29 CPUE patients with esophageal dysmotility, low doses of the antidepressant trazadone (50 mg t.i.d.) resulted in overall global symptom improvement without affecting esophageal pressures (83). Chest-pain frequency and severity improved in both treatment groups, corroborating the importance of placebo-controlled trials.

In contrast, in a recent, well-done, placebo-controlled study of 60 patients referred to the NIH with chest pain despite normal coronary angiograms, imipramine resulted in a 50% reduction in chest-pain episodes (84). In this study, patients underwent extensive cardiac assessment, including noninvasive standard treadmill exercise testing using a Bruce protocol and rest and exercise gated blood-pool technitium-99m radionuclide angiography. Twenty-one percent had abnormalities that were similar to those caused by ischemia during at least one of these tests despite normal epicardial arteries on catheterization, findings consistent with the diagnosis of "syndrome X." During cardiac catheterization, tests for heightened cardiac sensitivity were performed, including right ventricular pacing at a rate of 5 bpm faster than the resting heart rate and adenosine infusion into the left coronary artery. During these provocative maneuvers, 87% of patients reported pain that was typical of their usual chest pain, consistent with the presence of heightened visceral nociception. The majority of patients also underwent extensive esophageal testing. Forty-one percent met manometric criteria for an esophageal motility disorder (nutcracker, 22%; nonspecific abnormalities, 19%). Testing for heightened esophageal nociception included intravenous edrophium infusion, intraesophageal-acid instillation (Bernstein test), and esophageal-balloon insufflation. Forty-one percent of patients had their pain reproduced by one or more of these provocative maneuvers, consistent with heightened visceral nocioception. Finally, 63% of patients were found to fulfill DSM-III criteria for one or more psychiatric diagnoses (panic disorder, 43%; depression, 28%; somatization disorder, 18%).

Patients were treated in a single-blind fashion for 5 weeks and subsequently in double-blind fashion for 3 weeks with imipramine 50 mg at h.s., clonidine 0.1 mg b.i.d., or placebo. The frequency of chest pain during the double-blind trial was compared to that during the placebo lead-in phase. There was a reduction of 52% in the frequency of chest pain in patients treated with imipramine compared with 39% of clonidine-treated patients (NS) and 1% in those treated with placebo ($p < 0.05$). All 20 patients treated with imipramine had a reduction in pain frequency, compared with 14 of 20 treated with placebo. Improvement in the imipramine group did not depend on the results of baseline cardiac, esophageal, or psychiatric testing or on whether patients had evidence of heightened cardiac or esophageal nocioception. However, repeat assessment of cardiac sensitivity during treatment demonstrated a reduction in the prevalence of chest pain provoked by right ventricular pacing in patients treated with imipramine but not with clonidine or placebo. Likewise, improvement occurred independent of any change in psychiatric profile during the course of the study.

The authors of this important study postulated that the improvement noted with imipramine may have been mediated through a *visceral analgesic effect* rather than a psychotropic effect. Blockade of norepinephrine reuptake has been hypthesized to enhance the inhibitory action of pain-modulating neurons that descend from the brain stem to the spinal cord.

In addition to psychotropic medication, hebavioral and psychological therapies have also been reported to result in global symptom improvement. These therapies are reviewed in detail elsewhere.

Esophageal Dilation: Based on anecdotal clinical experience, passage of an esophageal dilator has sometimes been recommended for patients with dysphagia or chest pain and esophagel dysmotility. However, there are, no studies that support their use. In a small study, patients with nutcracker esophagus derived symptom relief after dilation with both a 54 Fr. bougie and a small 24 Fr. "placebo" bougie (85). Because bougienage is not without some risk and is of unproven efficacy, its use cannot be recommended. Rare patients with severe DES and impaired distal esophageal emptying are reported to benefit from pneumatic dilation of the LES, similar to patients with achalasia (86).

Surgical Therapy: Surgical treatment of esophageal motility disorders in patients with CPUE has never been tested in any controlled trial (87). A long esophagomyotomy has been used rarely for patients with severe esophageal dysmotility. In a review of 186 operations for diffuse spasm reported in the literature, improvement was observed in 77% (88). In another series of 34 DES patients, 30 patients were free of pain and dysphagia after surgery (89). It is recommended that surgical therapy be reserved for the small subset of patients with severe DES that results in dysphagia, documented weight loss, and/or intractable pain.

Surgery should seldom, if ever, be considered in CPUE patients with nutcracker esophagus. Although there have been two reports of symptomatic improvement following myotomy in small numbers of nutcracker patients (90,91), restraint is strongly advised. Given the high prevalence of psychological abnormalities associated with this diagnosis, surgery should be considered only if the pain is felt to be unequivocally related to the motility abnormality and is incapacitating and if the patient undergoes a thorough psychological evaluation. It may be desirable to refer the patient to a center where an ambulatory motility study can be performed.

Summary

Recurrent chest pain is an important clinical problem that causes great distress for patients and physicians. Coronary artery disease must be excluded before pursuing other causes because it is potentially life-threatening and is treatable. Microvascular angina should also be considered in patients with abnormalities on noninvasive cardiac testing. Rheumatological causes of chest pain are readily diagnosed and treated but easily overlooked. Other entities associated with CPUE include gastroesophageal reflux, esophageal dysmotility, psychological disorders, and heightened visceral nocioception. There appears to be a great deal of overlap between these abnormalities, and their cause-and-effect relationship to CPUE requires further elucidation.

Patients with CPUE and normal coronary angiography should be reassured that their prognosis is excellent. Diagnostic efforts should be limited to those entities for which we have reasonably effective therapies. Gastroesophageal reflux may cause or exacerbate CPUE in a significant number of patients. Because reflux can be effectively treated, efforts should be made to diagnose reflux-induced chest pain with ambulatory pH monitoring. CPUE patients should be observed closely for evidence of psychological abnormalities, including panic disorder. The development of simple questionnaires may aid in this regard. Referral for formal evaluation may be important. Psychotropic medications and/or behavioral therapy may prove to be the most helpful treatment modalities for many CPUE patients.

Formal esophageal testing with motility and provocative tests is of little utility in most circumstances. Indeed, a recent recommendation from the Patient Care Committee of the American Gastroenterological Association has recommended against its routine use for the initial evaluation of CPUE (92). The relationship between esophageal motility abnormalities and chest pain is doubtful. The association between manometric abnormalities and psychological disorders further confounds the issue. Finally, no therapies directed at esophageal dysmotility have proven effective in reducing chest pain. Positive provocative tests with edrophonium injection, esophageal-balloon inflation, or acid infusion point to increased visceral nocioception, although the significance and treatment of this entity are unclear. At present, no specific therapies exist to dampen this altered nocioception.

To develop specific therapies for CPUE, we require a better understanding of the factors that affect pain perception, amplification, and propagation. Further research must be done into the factors that alter pain perception, such as abnormal afferent receptors, altered central nervous processing, disruption of descending pain-control mechanisms, and the psychosocial factors that modify the interpretation and reporting of pain. In the meantime, the successful treatment of these difficult patients will depend more on the physician's healing nature than on scientific knowledge.

B. Non-Ulcer Dyspepsia

Dyspepsia is present in up to one-fourth of the population and is a frequent cause of medical consultation. The term *dyspepsia* is vague and has been used by physicians variably to refer to a host of symptoms, including upper-abdominal pain, bloating, postprandial fullness, nausea, early satiety, heartburn, or regurgitation (8,10). More recently, it has been defined by a panel of clinical investigators as an episodic or persistent abdominal discomfort located in the upper abdomen or epigastrium (8,93). Dyspepsia may be caused by a host of "organic" factors, including peptic ulcer disease, gastroesophageal reflux, gastroparesis, biliary-tract disease, pancreatic disease, mediations, and various systemic conditions.

After evaluation, there remain a large number (>50%) of patients with dyspepsia in whom no obvious organic cause can be found (94,95). These patients are often labeled as having NUD. A variety of other terms have been used more or less synonymously, such as nonorganic, functional, and essential dyspepsia. However, the term *non-ulcer dyspepsia* remains entrenched in the literature. In most recent discussions, NUD is defined as dyspepsia of several weeks' duration for which no focal or structural lesion can be found on upper endoscopy and that cannot be explained by other obvious structural or biochemical abnormalities (10,93).

Causes

The causes of NUD appear to be heterogeneous and are poorly understood. A number of physiological and psychological abnormalities have been identified in patients with NUD, but their relative importance is disputed (8,10,24,96).

Dietary Factors Intolerance to a number of foods is often cited by patients, but the results of double-blind food challenges cannot confirm it.

Endoscopic Duodenitis The prevalence of endoscopic duodenitis is greater in NUD than in matched controls. The etiology is unclear, but it does not appear to progress to peptic ulcer disease. Patients with erosive duodenitis may respond more favorably to antisecretory therapy.

H. pylori*–Associated Gastritis* The role of *Helicobacter pylori* (HP) gastric infection in NUD is controversial. Both HP infection and NUD are common entities, and a definite cause-and-effect relationship is difficult to establish. On the basis of several studies (97,98), it is clear that acute HP infection causes transient nausea, vomiting, and abdominal pain. Symptom resolution occurs in virtually all acute cases, however, despite ongoing chronic active gastric inflammation. The importance of chronic HP as an etiological agent in NUD is less clear. Two well-controlled epidemiological trials (99,100) do not convincingly show a higher prevalence of NUD among HP-positive patients. However, further large, well-matched, case-controlled studies are needed before the role of HP in NUD can be adequately assessed.

The importance of HP in NUD may also be studied by evaluating symptoms after therapy designed to eradicate HP. A number of such studies have been published. Regrettably, most trials to date have used only a single-agent therapy with bismuth or a single antibiotic; these regimens result in HP eradication in less than 30% of patients. Hence, the correlation between symptom improvement and HP eradication has not been adequately tested. Although several trials have reported symptomatic improvement compared with placebo-treated patients (101,102), serious deficiencies in the study design preclude any valid conclusions.

Recent studies by Patchett et al. (103,104) have corrected many of the problems with earlier studies. HP-positive patients with NUD were treated with one of three anti-HP regimens; symptoms were assessed by validated questionnaire before treatment, 4 weeks after eradication therapy, and at 1 year. Endoscopy with biopsy was performed after therapy to determine whether HP had been eradicated. The mean symptom scores at 4 weeks decreased in all treatment groups with or without HP eradication; however, at 1 year, the scores in patients in whom HP had been eradicated remained low whereas symptoms in those in whom HP infection persisted returned to pretreatment levels. Conflicting results were reported recently in another well-done study (105). In this study, 53 HP-positive patients were randomized to either placebo or HP-eradication therapy with a combination of three drugs (bismuth subsalicylate, amoxicillin, and metronidazole). The patients' symptoms were assessed 4 weeks and 6 months after completing therapy. Symptoms improved over time in both treatment groups, with no detectable difference between the groups. Further well-designed, long-term trials of anti-HP therapy in NUD are needed to determine whether HP eradication ameliorates symptoms in some patients.

Atypical Gastroesophageal Reflux Distinguishing between gastroesophageal reflux and functional dyspepsia can be difficult. The majority of patients with gastroesophageal-reflux disease have a normal-appearing esophagus at endoscopy; hence, a normal endoscopy does not exclude reflux disease. Nonerosive gastroesophageal reflux may contribute to symptoms in a subset of NUD patients, but the true importance is unknown. Neither the clinical history nor endoscopy reliably excludes GERD in patients with chronic dyspepsia. The presence of predominant symptoms of substernal burning with regurgitation is highly specific but relatively insensitive for a diagnosis of GERD. Indeed, many—perhaps most—patients with GERD also have some dyspeptic symptoms. Nevertheless, the overall sensitivity and specificity of the clinical diagnosis of GERD are 78% and 60%, respectively, compared with ambulatory pH monitoring (106). Up to one-half of patients with presumptive functional dyspepsia also have some degree of heartburn and regurgitation (suggestive of GERD) and may be labeled as having "reflux-like dyspepsia" (107,108). Likewise, over half of patients with proven GERD on endoscopy have associated dyspeptic symptoms (in addition to reflux symptoms), and almost 15% have dyspepsia alone (108). Whether these upper-abdominal symptoms are due to acid reflux or to concomitant NUD is unclear.

A recent study of ambulatory pH measurements in 100 patients with chronic dyspepsia and normal endoscopy demonstrated abnormal amounts of gastroesophageal reflux in 20% of patients, establishing a diagnosis of gastroesophageal-reflux disease. An additional 44% of patients had reflux-like symptoms with a normal amount of total acid reflux. In these patients, there was a higher correlation between acid-reflux events and dyspeptic symptoms than in patients without reflux-like symptoms (109). This suggests that, in these patients, physiological amounts of reflux may contribute to at least some dyspeptic symptoms, suggestive of heightened visceral nocioception.

In summary, many patients with GERD also report dyspepsia, and many patients with a diagnosis of NUD also report some degree of reflux-like symptoms. The honest, experienced clinician will realize that a clinical distinction between these entities is often problematic. Consideration may be given to an empirical trial of antireflux therapy or to a diagnostic ambulatory pH study in difficult patients.

Irritable Bowel Syndrome There appears to be a large overlap between various functional disorders, making the distinction between them a bit arbitrary in some patients. One-third of patients with NUD fulfill diagnostic criteria of IBS. A similar proportion of IBS patients also have dyspeptic symptoms (110).

Gastric-Acid Hypersecretion There is no evidence that gastric-acid hypersecretion is an important factor in NUD. Basal and peak acid outputs are equivalent between control subjects and NUD patients, including those with erosive duodenitis (111).

Abnormal Gastric Motor Function Evidence of gastroparesis is present in up to 60% of NUD patients as demonstrated by scintigraphic emptying studies or antral manometry (112–114). However, the cause-and-effect relationship between these abnormalities and NUD is unclear. There is a poor temporal relationship between these findings and the development of symptoms. The presence of "dysmotility-like" symptoms such as bloating or early satiety is not predictive of which patients have actual gastroparesis. Furthermore, the presence or absence of gastric-emptying delay is not necessarily predictive of which NUD patients will have a symptomatic response to promotility agents.

The etiology of gastroparesis in NUD is unclear. In most studies, the motor defect appears to be confined to the stomach and is not part of a more generalized visceral dysmotility. One group of invstigators at the Mayo Clinic, however, has reported evidence of autonomic denervation (both sympathetic and vagal) in NUD patients with dysmotility; the applicability of these findings to patients with NUD seen in nontertiary settings is unclear (115). Acute painful somatic stimuli such as electrical shock or hand immersion in cold water suppresses gastric motility in normal subjects and in NUD patients with normal baseline motility (21,22). Whether acute or chronic life stresses or psychological abnormalities can result in gastroparesis in NUD is unknown.

Heightened Visceral Nocioception Some NUD patients have a heightened sensitivity to a number of minor noxious stimuli. During intragastric-balloon inflation, NUD patients report pain at a lower balloon volume than do control subjects, despite normal gastric-wall tone and compliance and a normal sensation threshold (116–119). Somatic pain sensation is normal; i.e., the defect appears to be confined to visceral sensation. In a recent study, Coffin et al. (118) demonstrated a defect in the duodenogastric reflex in NUD patients. Under normal circumstances, duodenal distension with food (or a balloon) results in relaxation (accommodation) of the stomach, which slows further gastric emptying. In this study, the amount of gastric relaxation in response to balloon distension of the duodenum was significantly less in NUD subjects than in controls. They hypothesize that altered gut reflex activity leads to defective gastric accommodation to a meal, which in turn precipitates increased postcibal symptomatology in these patients with intrinsic heightened visceral nocioception.

Sensitivity to other stimuli is also reported. Pain during blinded intragastic infusions of 0.1 NHCl, saline, and pancreaticobiliary secretions has been reported (120). Some NUD patients also experience pain after an intravenous injection of pentagastrin—even when an H_2-antagonist is given to block the stimulated acid secretion (121). This may be analagous to the provocation of pain after edrophonium in patients with noncardiac chest pain.

Psychosocial Stress Psychosocial factors have undergone insufficient study in NUD. The personality profiles are similar to those of other patients with functional disorders (14,122). NUD patients score slightly higher in standardized inventories in areas of anxiety, neuroticism, hypochondriasis, and depression. Compared with matched controls, the number of major life stress events in NUD patients is no different (123,124). However, the perceived *magnitude* of the impact of negative events may be greater for NUD patients (125).

Evaluation

In evaluating the patient with dyspepsia, the physician endeavors to find an organic cause of the symptoms in order to direct therapy. To this end, the clinician is confronted by a cornucopia of expensive laboratory, endoscopic, and radiologic tests. The level of "appropriate" evaluation may depend on a number of medical and social factors and no rigid algorithm can be given. Tentative recommendations have been proffered by several expert panels. It must be emphasized that in over half of patients with dyspepsia, a cause will not be identified.

All patients should undergo a complete history and physical examination, including fecal occult blood testing. Routine hematology and biochemistry values should be obtained. In patients younger than 45 years, an empirical trial of antisecretory therapy should be considered. Young patients who fail to respond to empirical therapy or who have a relapse of symptoms after discontinuation of therapy should undergo endoscopy. In patients older than 45 years with new-onset dyspepsia, in any patient with "warning signs" of organic disease (such as weight loss, anemia, hemeoccult-positive stool, organomegaly, or palpable abdominal mass), and in patients from regions endemic for gastric cancer, endoscopy is warranted. Endoscopy may also be beneficial in relieving anxiety and symptoms in patients who are extremely concerned about their symptoms.

Given the importance of *H. pylori* as an etiological agent in peptic ulcer disease, some have advocated that a noninvasive test (serologic test or breath test) be performed to detect this infection in patients with acute or chronic dyspepsia. Patients who have evidence of *H. pylori* infection could be treated with empirical antibiotic therapy to eradicate the infection, which might lead to resolution of dyspeptic symptoms. In this algorithm, endoscopy would be reserved for patients in whom symptoms persisted despite *H. pylori* therapy. The impact on health care costs and patient satisfaction with this proposed algorithm have not been tested. It must be recognized that less than 25% of patients with dyspepsia have peptic ulcer disease. In the remaining 75% there is no convincing evidence that *H. pylori* is more common, or that eradication of the organism improves symptoms. Outcome-analysis trials are needed before empirical treatment of *H. pylori* can be recommended in patients with dyspepsia.

In patients with endoscopy-negative dyspepsia, abdominal sonography is commonly ordered to screen for pancreaticobiliary disease. Computed tomography or magnetic resonance imaging should be obtained only when there is a strong suspicion of intra-abdominal disease. Scintigraphic gastric-emptying studies and/or gastric motility do not influence clinical management and should be utilized only in a research setting. Similarly, provocation studies with intragastric balloon or infusions have no current utility.

Treatment

Non-Drug Management NUD can be extremely difficult to manage. Because a definitive cause cannot be pinpointed, patients may express frustration with the physician, and concern that an organic cause has been overlooked. A trial-and-error approach to pharmacological therapy is often required, further testing the patient's confidence. Retrospective studies suggest that dyspeptic symptoms continue in more than two-thirds of patients over several years (10). Nevertheless, it is apparent from the extraordinarily high placebo-response rates in NUD trials that the physician–patient relationship is salutary. Patience, a sympathetic ear, and confident reassurance of the part of the physician may be much more important in the long run than myriad tests and pharmacological interventions.

NUD patients should be encouraged to eat a balanced, regular diet and to avoid tobacco, excessive alcohol, and coffee, although none of these factors has been convincingly shown to induce dyspepsia in most studies (126,127). Beyond these common-sense admonitions, there is little evidence that diet plays a major role in NUD (10). Some patients are convinced of an association between particular foods and symptom provocation (128). In these cases, a food diary may be illustrative.

Drug Therapy of NUD Drugs have been disappointing in the treatment of NUD. The large number of therapeutic trials that have been conducted have produced a hodgepodge of conflicting results, making it difficult to draw firm conclusions. Methodological differences between these studies must be kept in mind when analyzing the disparate data (129–132). Difficulties in study design have included the following:

Symptom definition—the definition of NUD or of subsets of NUD has varied among the study groups.

Symptom assessment—validated symptom-assessment measurements have been lacking in many studies.

Study population—some investigators have attempted to exclude patients with IBS or a typical gastroesophageal reflux; others have not. If patients with GERD are included, greater therapeutic benefit may be demonstrated with antisecretory agents.

Placebo response—must studies have shown a 30–60% improvement in placebo-treated patients. Such a high placebo response makes it much more difficult to distinguish a statistically significant benefit for an active agent in individual studies. The follow-up in most studies is only 3–4 weeks, and the long-term response to therapy is seldom provided. A multicrossover study design, in which patients alternate between placebo and active therapy, may be a superior design for NUD trials (133).

Dyspeptic patients who seek medical attention are a self-referred subset of subjects with NUD. It is possible that patients who derive relief from nonproprietary treatment such as antacids may be disinclined to consult a physician. Thus, self-referred patients could be skewed toward nonresponse to medication.

Antisecretory Therapy: The utility of antisecretory agents in NUD is questionable. A number of placebo-controlled trials with H_2-antagonists or pirenzipine have yielded varying results. These have been compiled and analyzed in recent reviews (129,130,134). There have been no trials to date of proton pump inhibitors such as omeprazole in the treatment of NUD. Overall, the response rates have ranged from 35 to 80% with H_2-antagonists versus 30 to 60% with placebo. Approximately half of these studies have demonstrated a stastically significant advantage to active therapy, while the others have not. A meta-analysis of these trials detected a 20% therapeutic gain of antisecretory agents over placebo (134). In some studies, the greatest benefit was detected in patients with reflux-like dyspepsia, suggesting that some of the responders may be those with nonerosive GERD (135–137).

A recent double-blind placebo-controlled multicrossover trial was performed in NUD patients comparing cimetidine versus placebo taken "on demand" (as needed) for acute episodes of pain. Cimetidine provided superior symptomatic relief in 52% of patients (133).

Antisecretory agents seem to benefit a small subset of NUD patients. Given their excellent safety profile, an empirical trial is warranted, particularly with patients in whom GERD is suspected. Therapy should be discontinued, however, in patients who fail to respond.

Promotility Agents: Several promotility agents have yielded promising results in the treatment of NUD. Bearing in mind the high frequency of gastric-emptying abnormalities in NUD, agents that enhance gastric motility are appealing therapeutic options. The primary agents that have undergone clinical testing have been metoclopramide, domperidone, and cisapride, whose promotility effects are mediated by somewhat different mechanisms (see Section III.C below) (138). All these agents have been shown to accelerate gastric emptying in patients with gastroparesis by enhancing the coordination of antroduodenal contractility. In addition, these agents have different effects on the central nervous system (CNS).

Metoclopramide 10 mg q.i.d. has proven superior to placebo in three controlled trials of NUD (129). The high incidence of CNS side effects, however, limits the long-term use of this agent. Domperidone has undergone much greater clinical testing, demonstrating superior symptomatic improvement in 10 of 11 placebo-controlled trials. Overall clinical improvement has been reported in 65–90% of patients compared with 13–42% in the placebo groups (129). Unfortunately, this drug is not yet available in the United States. Finally, cisapride has also shown convincing symptomatic improvement in 13 of 14 placebo-controlled trials in patients with NUD. Symptomatic improvement ranged from 63 to 94% in patients on cisapride compared with 15 to 60% on placebo (129,134,139,140). Cisapride has been compared with metoclopramide in a recent randomized double-blind trial of patients with NUD (141). Patients in both treatment groups had a significant improvement in dyspeptic symptoms compared with baseline. Although no statistical difference could be demonstrated between the two treatment groups, 87% of cisapride-treated patients improved versus 77% of patients treated with metoclopramide. Another recent large, multicenter, comparative trial confirmed superior symptomatic relief in patients treated with cisapride versus cimetidine (142). Interestingly, no difference was detectable in patients with reflux-like dyspepsia, further suggesting that the major benefit of H_2-antagonists may be confined to this subgroup.

Although criticisms have been rendered of many of these trials, the consistent superiority of different types of promotility agents compared with placebo in patients with NUD is persuasive. The mechanism by which these agents produce symptomatic improvement has not been clarified. In most studies, gastric emptying was not studied before and after therapy. In those studies in which a gastric-emptying assessment was performed, the correlation between symptom response and the presence or absence of abnormal gastric emptying was variable. Similarly, there was an inconsistent correlation between symptom improvement and improvement in gastric emptying. Thus, it does not appear that symptomatic improvement in NUD patients is restricted to the subset with abnormal gastric motor function.

Other Therapies: Other pharmacological agents offer potential benefit in the treatment of NUD but have not undergone sufficient clinical testing. The CCK antagonist loxiglumide was superior to placebo in a small prospective trial (143). Loxiglumide accelerated gastric emptying, but the clinical improvement was not correlated to improved gastric emptying. The antibiotic erythromycin is a motilin agonist that stimulates antroduodenal activity and has been demonstrated to improve gastric emptying in diabetic gastroparesis. Serotonin 5-HT_3 antagonists may modulate afferent visceral sensation (see below), which could be of benefit in dyspeptic patients.

Psychotropic medications and behavioral therapies have been used successfully in the treatment of other functional disorders such as noncardiac chest pain and IBS but have not undergone sufficient clinical testing in NUD. It may nevertheless be appropriate to consider a trial of these therapies in NUD patients with psychological dysfunction.

Summary

Patients whose dyspepsia is unexplained after a thorough medical evaluation, upper endoscopy, and abdominal sonogram pose a difficult management problem. In the majority of instances, a specific cause of the patient's symptoms will not be identified; hence, further medical workup is seldom indicated. Finding a "cause" of the symptoms should be de-emphasized. Instead, attention should be focused on improved coping strategies and lifestyle modifications. Patients will require long-term follow-up for this problem. The physician and patient should endeavor to determine environmental, psychological, or social factors that trigger or exacerbate symptoms. Pharmacological modalities may provide some therapeutic benefit, but yield greatest benefit when used in an adjunctive capacity in the context of a therapeutic relationship.

It is apparent from the conflicting pharmacological trials that no single pharmacological agent can be expected to provide symptomatic improvement in all—or even most—NUD patients. This is hardly surprising, given the probable heterogeneous etiologies. Prokinetic agents and H_2-receptor antagonists are clearly beneficial in some patients and are worthy of an empirical trial. However, guidelines on selecting an antisecretory agent versus a promotility agent have not been established. Some investigators have tried to sort NUD patients into symptom subgroups according to how closely their dyspepsia resembled ulcer disease ("ulcer-like"), reflux disease ("reflux-like"), or dysmotility ("dysmotility-like") (93). It was hypothesized that these distinctions might be helpful in predicting response to diagnostic tests (pH monitoring, gastric-emptying studies, etc.) and in guiding medical therapy (antisecretory therapy versus promotility agents).

The clinical value of these symptom subgroups, however, has not been confirmed. Most therapeutic trials have not prospectively stratified patients into symptom subgroups. There is also enough overlap between subgroups to make assigning a patient to a particular group arbitrary (107). These clinical subgroups do not reliably distinguish functional from organic disease (108). In addition, the incidence of abnormalities of gastric motility has not been shown to differ among the various subgroups; however, further studies are needed. A patient with reflux-like symptoms may be as likely as a patient with dysmotility-like symptoms to have impaired gastric emptying.

Given the excellent safety profile of H_2-antagonists, an empirical trial would appear to be a reasonable first choice in most refractory NUD patients, particularly those with some symptoms of reflux. In the 35–80% who experience improvement, it is impossible to know whether this represents a placebo response. The physician is then in the difficult position of having to decide whether to withdraw a drug that the patient feels is beneficial or to continue something that may be nothing more than a costly placebo. A trial off drug therapy may be warranted. Patients who fail to improve on H_2-antagonists may benefit from a trial of a promotility agent. Cisapride is the preferred agent because of its lack of side effects and excellent safety profile. Metoclopramide is less expensive, but the higher incidence of side effects limits its utility. Therapy directed at *H. pylori* eradication cannot be recommended at this time outside of clinical trials.

C. Irritable Bowel Syndrome

Causes IBS is a functional disorder attributed to the intestine that is characterized by abdominal pain, alterations in bowel habits, and symptoms of abdominal distension. As with other functional disorders, the pathogenesis is not understood but appears to be heterogeneous. A number of pathophysiological mechanisms may be important, but their relative importance may vary among individuals.

Dietary Factors Intolerance to a number of foods is commonly reported by IBS patients; however, its importance remains unknown. In a carefully conducted study (144), 50% of IBS patients had symptomatic improvement during a strict exclusionary diet. As foods were gradually introduced, over 80% of these patients could identify at least one dietary trigger. When these patients were followed, 80% of these patients derived long-term symptomatic improvement by excluding these dietary triggers. Of patients in whom no dietary intolerance could be identified, virtually all patients remained symptomatic. Food sensitivity may be due to carbohydrate malabsorption, toxic effects of foods (monosodium glutamate, vasoactive amines, etc.), immediate hypersensitivy, and delayed immune reactions (145).

It is virtually everyone's experience that the ingestion of certain foods (e.g., legumes) results in increased gas production and bloating. Malabsorption of some sugars such as lactose, sorbitol, and fructose can be detected in many IBS patients and may provoke symptoms in some cases (146,147). Although the prevalence of carbohydrate malabsorption appears to be *similar* to that in asymptomatic controls, IBS patients may have increased sensitivity to the secondary effects of this malabsorption, i.e., gas production.

Ileal malabsorption of bile acids induces cholerrhcic diarrhea. Idiopathic bile-salt malabsorption has been detected in patients with functional diarrhea, although its exact importance is unclear (148,149).

Abnormal Intestinal Motility A variety of abnormal myoelectrical and motor abnormalities have been identified in the small intestine and colon of many patients with IBS. Whether these represent a primary motility disorder or are secondary to psychosocial stress and/or psychological abnormalities is debated. A full discussion of these abnormalities is beyond the scope of this chapter. In brief, abnormalities seen in some IBS patients include:

An increase in colonic, three-cycles-per -minute (cpm), slow-wave basal electric activity is present, compared with the six cpm activity that predominates in normal individuals (150). This activity does not correlate with symptoms and is also present in normal individuals and neurotic patients without IBS.

Differences between patients with constipation- and diarrhea-predominant IBS have been reported in some studies. Constipation-predominant IBS patients have increased non-propagating short-spike bursts (SSBs) and decreased high-amplitude propagating contractions; conversely, diarrhea-predominant patients have decreased SSBs and fast contractions. Intestinal transit time is accelerated in some patients with diarrhea-predominant IBS and delayed in patients with constipation.

In normal volunteers, ingestion of a meal induces increased rectosigmoid myoelectric and contractile activity (the gastrocolic reflex). This activity may be blocked by anticholinergic agents. The fat content of the meal is a major determinant of the magnitude of the reflex. In some IBS patients, increased, prolonged rectosigmoid activity occurs after a meal, contributing to postprandial urgency.

Abnormal jejunal, ileal, and colonic activity is temporally correlated with abdominal pain in some (but not all) IBS patients (12).

Progesterone has been shown to slow small-bowel transit (151) and alter jejunal MMCs (152); increased functional bowel symptoms in women after ovulation, with subsequent resolution at the onset of menstruation, may be due in part to the rise and fall in progesterone levels during these periods.

Acute emotional, psychological, or physical stress induces alterations in motility in the colon and small intestine of normal individuals as well as patients with IBS (3).

Heightened Visceral Nociception As in other functional disorders, such as NCCP and NUD, a variety of minor noxious stimuli provoke pain in some IBS patients. Balloon distension in the ileum, colon, and rectum induces pain in some IBS patients at lower volumes than in controls, and is accompanied by increased motor activity. Although many IBS patients complain of excessive gas and bloating, washout studies have shown that the absolute volume of intestinal gas is normal. Nevertheless, symptomatic patients complain of distension and discomfort at lower volumes of gas insufflation than do controls, suggesting heightened sensitivity. Finally, hormonal stimulation of intestinal motor activity with cholinergic agonists, serotonin, and CCK can also be associated with pain.

Patients with IBS often report "constipation" or "diarrhea" despite normal stool frequencies and intestinal transit. Patients often report urgency despite small volumes of formal stool, or straining despite loose stools. This suggests an alteration in the perception of feces in the rectum. In some patients, a sense of rectal urgency is detected at lower volumes of balloon distension than in controls.

Psychological Abnormalities Psychological symptoms are common in IBS patients. More than 50% of IBS patients who seek medical attention meet diagnostic criteria for a psychiatric disorder, such as depression, anxiety, and somatization. By contrast, people with IBS who do not seek medical attention are similar psychologically to normals. IBS patients display abnormal illness behavior manifested by excessive somatic focusing, increased health-related worries, and a greater sense that their illness interferes with their lives than IBS nonpatients or controls have.

Summary A variety of factors may be important in the pathophysiology of IBS but none is well understood. The relative importance of these various factors may vary among patients. Furthermore, the pathophysiology may be different in various symptom subgroups. There is evidence that intestinal dysmotility, abnormal visceral nocioception, luminal factors, and psychosocial factors all may play a role, but the *primary* defect is debated. It appears that psychosocial factors may modify an underlying intestinal motility or sensory abnormality, determining how a patient perceives and reacts to symptoms and interacts with the health care system.

Evaluation

The diagnosis of IBS is established in the presence of certain symptom criteria and after the exclusion of organic disease. A full discussion of the evaluation of patients with possible IBS appears elsewhere. The most recent diagnostic criteria put forth by an international committee are the presence of continuous or recurrent symptoms for at least 3 months characterized by (1):

1. Abdominal pain or discomfort, relieved with defecation or associated with a change in the frequency or consistency of stool
2. An irregular (varying) pattern of defecation at least 25% of the time that is associated with at least three of the following:
    a. Altered stool frequency
    b. Altered stool form (hard or loose and watery)
    c. Altered stool passage (straining, urgency, or feeling of incomplete evacuation)
    d. Passage of mucus
    e. Bloating or feeling of abdominal distension

When these clinical features are present in a patient 20–50 years of age, the picture is highly suggestive of IBS. The onset of symptoms above age 50, nocturnal diarrhea, hematochezia, rapidly progressive symptoms, or systemic symptoms such as weight loss or fever should suggest an underlying organic disease.

In a patient with a presumptive clinical diagnosis of IBS, a limited series of investigations is warranted to exclude organic disease. In all patients, a careful physical examination, including evaluation of stool for fecal occult blood and ova and parasites, and screening blood work (CBC, serum chemistries, ESR), is indicated. In patients under age 40, a flexible sigmoidoscopy should be obtained. In patients over age 40, consideration should be given to a complete colonic evaluation with colonoscopy versus barium enema.

The decision to pursue further studies depends on the clinical situation. In most cases it is reasonable to observe the patient's response to a trial of empirical medical management. In the majority of these patients, no further workup will be needed. The development of objective findings such as weight loss, anemia, hypoalbuminemia, or a change in the nature of the patient's complaints will necessitate further investigation. In some patients with diarrhea, further investigation will be warranted with a stool laxative screen, a colonic biopsy (to exclude collagenous colitis), an upper-GI series (to look for evidence of Crohn's disease), a breath-bile-salt test, or a breath-hydrogen test for carbohydrate malabsorption. Rarely, patients with predominant constipation may require investigation with a radioopaque marker colonic transit study, anorectal manometry, or defecography.

Treatment

General Measures As with other functional disorders, the most important therapies the clinician has to offer are reassurance and a confident explanation of the functional nature of IBS. Patients should be told that IBS is a chronic, relapsing disorder but that the condition does not deteriorate or progress to more serious disorders. Physicians will earn the confidence of their patients by being attentive to their complaints and vigilant for the development of organic disease. Nevertheless, they must resist the temptation to chase chronic or new complaints with new or repeated diagnostic studies. These studies will only lead to greater expense, and will reinforce the patient's fears that "something has been missed." The patient's (and physician's) emphasis should shift from finding the cause of the symptoms to finding productive ways to cope with a chronic disease.

Dietary Therapy Although the role of dietary triggers in IBS is disputed, many patients believe that certain foods exacerbate their symptoms. Such relationships are difficult to prove because of the complexity of most diets and the strong placebo effect of dietary exclusions. Notwithstanding the uncertainties that prevail, physicians should be open-minded to the idea that dietary manipulations—for whatever reason—may provide symptomatic benefit.

The patients most likely to benefit from dietary exclusions are those with complaints of excess gas and bloating and/or those with predominant diarrhea. A variety of foods may be extremely flatulogenic for some normal individuals as well as patients with IBS. Indeed, observant flatus producers (and their family members) can readily list the offending foods. These include: brown or black beans, brussel sprouts, cabbage, cauliflower, fresh onions, grapes, raisins, plums, apricots, coffee, red wine, beer, and other carbonated beverages. While these foods do not "cause" IBS, they can clearly lead to increased distension and discomfort in susceptible individuals. Patients with IBS may complain initially of increased flatus and distension after being placed on a high-fiber diet. In time, physiological adaptation usually occurs; however, some patients simply find a high-fiber diet intolerable. Caffeine is poorly tolerated in most IBS patients because of its direct effects on the bowel and its psychological effects.

Malabsorption of lactose, sorbitol, and fructose has been implicated in some IBS patients. Because lactase deficiency is common in adults with and without IBS, a lactose-exclusion trial should be performed. Bear in mind, however, that milk products can be an important source of calcium. Before restricting milk products permanently, patients who note apparent symptomatic improvement should undergo a formal breath-hydrogen study. Sorbitol is used as a sweetener in a number of sugar-free candies, syrups, gums, and medications. Fructose malabsorption may be a problem in patients ingesting excessive amounts of fruit and certain soft drinks.

In some cases, the use of a symptom diary for several weeks (described previously) may be of benefit in identifying possible dietary or environment triggers. If certain potentially offending foods are identified, an elimination trial can be performed. Later, patients can rechallenge themselves to see if the symptoms recur. As discussed above, some studies have shown that strict exclusion diets lead to symptomatic improvement in up to half of patients. By the gradual introduction of foods, triggering agents can be identified. In clinical practice, such trials are laborious for the patient and physician and are seldom used.

Drug Therapy A variety of pharmacological agents are available for the treatment of IBS. Despite their widespread use, it has been difficult to demonstrate their efficacy in controlled clinical trials. Indeed, after an erudite review of 43 randomized, double-blind, placebo-controlled IBS treatment trials published from 1966 to 1988, Klein (25) concluded that "the majority of published IBS trials fail to meet even simple criteria for acceptability." He concludes that "not a single study offers convincing evidence that any therapy is effective in treating the IBS symptom complex." There are a number of problems in the design of IBS trials that make any valid conclusions difficult and render any comparisons of trials almost impossible (25,153).

Disease definition—studies employ differing and vague definitions of IBS with unclear or different entry criteria. Hence, the patient population of one study may not be comparable to another.

Symptom subsets—IBS is a heterogeneous disease, with patients complaining of different presenting symptoms. Patients with diarrhea-predominant symptoms may respond differently to certain agents than patients with constipation- or pain/bloating-predominant symptoms. For example, an antispasmodic may relieve pain and bloating but exacerbate constipation. It may be important to either study specific symptom subsets or stratify IBS patients before randomization into symptom subsets. The use of "mean" symptom scores for the entire study population rather than for specific symptom subsets dilutes the ability to detect beneficial drug therapies.

Lack of objective assessments—there are no truly objective markers that can be used to assess drug efficacy in IBS trials. Hence, assessment is based on subjective symptom-scoring systems and global physician assessment. Validated measurements with clear symptom definitions and well-defined scales for grading symptom response have been lacking in most studies.

Variable placebo response—the placebo response has ranged from <20% to 70% in IBS trials. Such a wide range may reflect different patient populations, different means of assessing patient response, and variable degrees of physician–patient interaction. High placebo-response rates make it much more difficult to distinguish a statistically significant benefit to an active agent. To obviate this, many studies have employed a crossover design. Unfortunately, many of these studies have had an inadequate baseline symptom assessment and an inadequate washout period. Furthermore, it is difficult to maintain patient blinding in many crossover trials because of drug side effects.

Inadequate study periods—IBS is characterized by fluctuating periods of symptom intensity in most patients. Given this natural variability as well as the high placebo response, study periods should be a minimum of 8–12 weeks.

Inadequate sample size—many "negative" trials have suffered from inadequate study sizes and are therefore susceptible to type II error. Studies that include a number of symptom subsets require large sample sizes for a valid subset analysis.

Patient selection for nonresponse—people with IBS who seek medical attention already represent a small, selected subset of the overall IBS population. Those IBS patients who respond readily to conservative measures and/or to standard pharmacological interventions may not be disposed to enter pharmacological trials. Thus, patients who enter trials may be those with more severe or more refractory symptoms and/or psychological abnormalities. The results in these patients may not be extrapolated to the broader IBS population.

Impact of psychological profile—the impact of psychosocial stress on drug response in IBS needs clarification. Future trials should include standard psychological assessments.Invalid statistical measurements—at least one-third of trials have used invalid statistical techniques.

In light of the overwhelming deficiencies in IBS trials, one is inclined to conclude that drug therapy has no role in the treatment of IBS. However, such a conclusion would be spurious. While it is true that no drug is of proven benefit for IBS, the lack of demonstrable drug efficacy may reflect more on the inadequacy of the clinical trials than on the drug itself. Future trials should endeavor to overcome these shortcomings by careful attention to the study population, the study design, the measurements of efficacy, and the statistical analysis.

In the meantime, what can be said about the role of drug therapy in IBS? The majority of patients have mild symptoms and respond readily to reassurance, education, and, perhaps, dietary modifications, as noted above (5,6). Drug therapy should be reserved for patients with more severe symptoms that do not respond to conservative measures and that impair the patient's quality of life. No single agent can be expected to provide relief in all or even most IBS patients. Therapy directed at a specific bothersome symptom may be most beneficial. Furthermore, drug therapy should be viewed as only one part of a therapeutic arsenal that includes psychotherapy and behavioral therapy. That is, it is an *adjunctive* agent that is part of a larger therapeutic package. It should not be viewed by either the patient or the physician as a "cure" or an end unto itself. Medications should be given at the lowest effective dose and, where possible, for circumscribed periods of symptom exacerbation rather than on a chronic basis. Finally, it should be recognized that symptomatic improvement may be attributable to placebo effects rather than specific effects of the pharmacological agent.

Patients with IBS often have a variety of symptoms, such as diarrhea, constipation, abdominal pain, or bloating. In approaching the medical treatment of IBS, however, it is often helpful to focus on the *predominant* complaint (4). For most patients, this will be abdominal pain, constipation, or diarrhea. For the purposes of this discussion, the pharmacological treatment of each of these predominant symptoms is reviewed.

Treatment of Pain-Predominant Symptoms: A variety of agents are purported to relieve pain in IBS patients. These include anticholinergic agents, antispasmodic agents, analgesics, and psychotropic medications.

Anticholinergic agents are frequently prescribed for the treatment of patients with IBS, despite a paucity of data demonstrating their efficacy. They are believed to work by blocking the acetylcholine-medicated depolarization of intestinal smooth muscle, resulting in a decrease in colonic motor activity. As such, they are a type of "antispasmodic," of which there are several classes of agents. The anticholinergic agent clidinium reduces the postprandial increase in colonic myoelectrical and motor activity (154). Similarly, the agent cimetropium blocks the postprandial increase in rectosigmoid motility in patients with painful, constipation-predominant IBS (155). Thus, anticholinergic agents may be of potential benefit in pain-predominant IBS, especially those with postprandial symptoms that are ascribed to the gastrocolic reflex.

A variety of anticholinergic agents have been clinically tested, most of which are unavailable in the United States. These medications should be administered 30 to 60 minutes before meals. Side effects such as urinary retention, tachycardia, and dry eyes are common. To minimize side effects, one should begin with a small dose and titrate upward slowly. Table 1 lists the agents that are clinically available.

Despite their widespread use in IBS, there are no well-controlled trials that demonstrate the efficacy of anticholinergic agents in IBS. In extensive reviews by Klein (25) and Ivey (156), both authors concluded that the benefit of these agents in IBS was unproven. However, a more recent meta-analysis by Poynard et al. (177) does detect a benefit of these agents in the relief of pain (see next section).

A number of controlled trials have suggested benefit for some subsets of patients or specific symptoms. Dicyclomine 40 mg q.i.d. was superior to placebo in a 2-week trial in improving patients' overall sense of well-being and abdominal pain (157). However, anticholinergic side effects occurred in 69%, necessitating a dose reduction or withdrawal of medication in over half of these patients. Given the high incidence of side effects, the ability of the investigators

TABLE 1 Anticholinergic Agents

Medication	Dosage	Available in U.S.
Dicyclomine (Bentyl)	20–40 mg p.o. q.i.d., p.r.n.[a]	Yes
Hyoscyamine, atropine scopolamine, and phenobarb (Donnatal)	1–2 tabs/capsules t.i.d.-q.i.d., p.r.n.	Yes
Hyoscyamine (Levsin)	0.125 mg s.l. or p.o. q 4 hr, p.r.n.	Yes
Probantheline (Pro-Banthine)	15 mg p.o. t.i.d. or 30 mg h.s., p.r.n.	Yes
Prifinium	30 mg p.o. t.i.d., p.r.n.	No
Cimetroprium	50 mg p.o. t.i.d., p.r.n.	No

[a]As needed.

to remain blinded is suspect. In a smaller dose of 20 mg t.i.d., dicyclomine had no effect on abdominal pain, distension, or altered bowel movements (158). A 6-week double-blind crossover study of prifinium demonstrated a significant improvement over placebo in global symptoms (159). However, this study has been criticized for its inadequate assessment of treatment response, as well as poor study design (25). Two Italian studies looking at cimetroprium, a "gut-selective" antimuscarinic agent, deserve comment. In the first study, of 48 patients treated for 6 months, significant improvement compared with placebo was noted in the intensity and frequency of abdominal pain and in overall level of symptoms (160). In a second placebo-controlled trial, of 70 patients treated for 12 weeks, significant improvement in the frequency and severity of abdominal pain as well as in the overall assessment of treatment was noted in the cimetroprium group (161). In the two studies, 48% and 17% of patients, respectively, experienced anticholinergic side effects, although none required a dose reduction or study withdrawal.

There is little evidence from controlled clinical trials that anticholinergic agents benefit the majority of IBS patients. Nevertheless, it is the experience of many clinicians that these agents may be effective in some patients. Specifically, by reducing the cholinergically mediated gastrocolic reflex, these agents may reduce symptoms in patients with frequent postprandial pain when given before meals (see next section). Their use in patients with other symptoms, such as diarrhea, is of little utility. The use of combination agents is mentioned only to be discouraged.

Antispasmodic agents have been used in the treatment of IBS. They are believed to work by causing direct relaxation of the smooth muscle of the GI tract, thus decreasing colonic motor activity. Hence, the rationale supporting their use in IBS is similar to that for anticholinergic agents. The agents that have undergone the most clinical testing include mebeverine, trimebutine, ocylonium (none of which is available in the United States), and, more recently, calcium channel blockers. Mebeverine is a potent smooth-muscle relaxant that is similar in action to papaverine (an agent approved for the treatment of vascular and ureteral spasm) and devoid of anticholinergic action. Trimebutine is another spasmolytic agent with complex actions of the GI tract. It causes increased small-bowel motility through stimulation of peripheral opioid receptors but inhibition of colonic motility through a naloxone-sensitive pathway (162). Octylonium is an antispasmodic that is thought to work through inhibition of calcium mobilization. It has been shown to decrease postprandial colonic motility in patients with IBS (163).

The effects of various calcium channel blockers on the GI tract have been assessed, including those of pinaverium, nicardipine, and nifedipine. These agents have been shown to inhibit postprandial spike potentials in the colon and to abolish the postprandial gastrocolic reflex (164–167). They have also been shown to inhibit the number and amplitude of rectosigmoid contractions and distension-induced rectosigmoid contractions (165,166). Pinaverium has poor GI absorption and marked hepatobiliary excretion; hence, it appears to have limited cardiovascular side effects at doses that effectively relieve GI spasm.

Limited placebo-controlled trials of antispasmodics in the treatment of IBS have been performed, most of which suffer from such severe methodological flaws that no valid conclusions can be drawn. Mebeverine was reported to be superior to placebo in controlling symptoms in one study of 40 IBS patients (168), while another study reported significant improvement in 10 patients in bowel function, abdominal pain, and overall assessment (169). However, both studies used inappropriate statistical analysis, rendering all conclusions unreliable (25,156). In a 16-week, double-blind crossover study of 12 patients, Kruis et al. (170) was unable to show any significant improvement with mebeverine.

Controlled trials looking at trimebutine have also yielded mixed results. In a double-blind crossover trial in 39 patients of only 7 days' duration, more patients preferred the trimebutine treatment period, and improvement in pain, distension, and flatulence was reported (171). Symptomatic improvement in constipation and pain was reported in 20 patients with constipation-predominant IBS treated for 8 weeks in a placebo-controlled crossover study (172); however, this study suffers from faulty statistical analysis (25). In contrast, another placebo-controlled trial of 60 IBS patients failed to demonstrate any symptomatic benefit in patients treated with trimebutine for 6 months (173).

Octylonium has been shown to decrease postprandial colonic motility in IBS patients (163). In one study of 30 patients, octylonium significantly improved the weekly frequency of pain episodes (174), but this study has been criticized for patient selection because the majority of patients did not fulfill diagnostic criteria for IBS (25). Two recent large Italian studies have demonstrated a positive effect of octylonium. In a 12-month study of 114 patients (175), those treated with octylonium had a significant improvement in abdominal pain and distension compared with patients given fiber supplementation. In a 4-week placebo-controlled study of 72 pain-predominant IBS patients (176), improvement in pain and bloating was demonstrated with octylonium therapy. Octylonium has also been shown to significantly increase the pain threshold and reduce sigmoid motility during balloon distension (176).

In a recent meta-analysis, Poynard et al. (177) analyzed 25 randomized, double-blind, placebo-controlled trials that assessed the efficacy of eight smooth-muscle relaxants and anticholinergic agents in the treatment of IBS. A total of eight drugs were analyzed in these trials: cimetropium bromide (four trials), dicyclomine hydrochloride (two trials,) hyoscine butyl bromide (three trials), mebeverine (five trials), octylonium (two trials), pinaverium bromide (two trials), trimebutine (four trials), and peppermint oil (four trials). A statistically significant improvement in global improvement was detected in 62% of patients treated with active drug versus 32% with placebo. When analyzed separately, all drugs still demonstrated global improvement versus placebo. Pain improvement occurred in 64% of patients treated with myorelaxants compared with 45% of placebo-treated patients—a modest 19% improvement, which was statistically significant. However, when the drugs were analyzed separately, only three demonstrated significant efficacy versus placebo: cimetropium bromide, octylonium, and dicylomine bromide. No significant differences were detected in constipation or abdominal distension in the active treatment groups compared with placebo when the drugs were analyzed collectively or separately. The statistical power of meta-analyses provides strong evidence that anticholinergics and smooth-muscle relaxants do benefit a subset of patients with IBD, namely, those with pain-predominant symptoms.

More recently, attention has been focused on the calcium channel blockers in IBS therapy. Calcium channel blockers have been shown to decrease postprandial colonic motility and neostigmine-induced spasm in IBS patients (164,165,178,179). Unfortunately, there are insufficient trial data pertaining to the utility of these agents in treating patients with IBS. A single-blind crossover trial of pinaverium versus octylonium in 40 IBS patients demonstrated improvement in the number of pain attacks during both treatment periods (180). However, a double-blind trial of 18 IBS patients showed no significant improvement in patients treated with nifedipine compared with placebo (181).

Antispasmodics clearly inhibit colonic motility, including the postprandial gastrocolonic response in patients with IBS. However, they have not demonstrated convincing efficacy in the treatment of most patients with IBS. As with anticholinergic agents, the antispasmodics seem to benefit those patients in whom postprandial pain is problematic. The only agents clinically available in the United States are the calcium channel blockers, which have undergone very little clinical testing. In general, potential cardiovascular side effects hamper enthusiasm for the use of these agents, and their tendency to constipate may exacerbate this problem in patients with constipation-predominant IBS. Nevertheless, in patients with IBS who also have hypertension, a calcium channel blocker may be a reasonable therapeutic choice.

Peppermint oil is a naturally occurring carminative (antiflatulant), which causes relaxation of GI smooth muscle by blocking potential-dependent calcium channels (182). Several trials have looked at the effect of peppermint oil in the treatment of IBS (177). Two placebo-controlled crossover trials demonstrating improvement were both of short duration and criticized for using invalid statistics (183,184), and a third study showed no benefit (185). Thus, there is no good evidence that peppermint oil is active in IBS.

Analgesics and psychopharmacological agents—narcotic analgesics should seldom, if ever, be used in the treatment of abdominal pain in IBS patients due to the chronic nature of the illness and the consequent addictive potential. Similarly, anxiolytics, such as benzodiazepines, do not relieve pain and may lead to dependence. Antidepressants are used in a number of chronic pain syndromes, often in low doses. Their use in IBS is reviewed elsewhere.

Activated charcoal has been touted as a useful agent in IBS to absorb fecal hydrogen and carbon dioxide, thereby reducing distension and flatus (186). Levitt and coworkers (187), however, found that in vitro charcoal suspensions do not absorb these gases effectively. Two double-blind placebo-controlled studies of charcoal in healthy subjects have yielded opposite results. Jain et al. (188) reported that charcoal reduced breath-hydrogen excretion and symptoms of bloating after lactulose administration. In contrast, Levitt et al. (187) could detect no difference in breath-hydrogen excretion after bean ingestion. There have been no studies of activated charcoal in IBS, and its use cannot be recommended at this time.

Gonadotropin-releasing hormone (GnRH) agonists—the observations by women that functional GI symptoms often begin or are worsened at the time of ovulation and that they tend to improve after the onset of menstruation suggest a hormonal influence. Support for this hypothesis comes from the fact that elevated progesterone levels during both pregnancy and the luteal phase of the normal human menstrual cycle have been shown to slow small-bowel transit (189,190) and alter jejunal MMCs (191). Other ovarian hormones, such as relaxin, act as uterine smooth-muscle relaxants and may have as yet unknown effects on smooth muscle (192).

Understanding the role of GnRH agonists as possible therapeutic agents in IBS requires a brief review of reproductive endocrinology. *Endogenous* GnRH stimulates the release of follicle-stimulating hormone (FSH) and luteinizing hormone (LH) from the anterior pituitary. FSH triggers the ovary to secrete estrogen, while LH initiates a cascade of events that ends with progesterone secretion from the corpus luteum. However, continuous administration of GnRH reduces ovarian hormone release through "desensitization" (193). It is through this potential mechanism that GnRH agonists may benefit women with functional bowel symptoms.

Symptomatic improvement in five women with functional GI disease treated with leuprolide, a potent GnRH analog, in an uncontrolled, open-label trial was initially reported by Mathias et al. (192). The improvement was associated with a significant decrease in progesterone and LH levels, and the readministration of progesterone resulted in the prompt return of symptoms. More recently, Mathias et al. (194) randomized 30 women with functional bowel disease, all with abnormal UGI manometry, to receive a depot form of leuprolide or placebo in a double-blind study for 12 weeks. There was a significant improvement in symptom scores and global assessments in patients receiving leuprolide. Twenty-five of these patients continued on open-label, daily, subcutaneous leuprolide for an additional 40 weeks (195). There was a more striking improvement in individual and total symptom scores, as well as overall assessment scores in all patients. This improvement was associated with a significant decrease in progesterone, estradiol, and FSH levels in the first study, and LH levels in the follow-up study. There were few side effects, consisting of bone pain and edema most commonly, as well as headaches and hot flashes (the latter were usually controlled with estrogen replacement). While these data support the concept that GnRH acts through its effects on ovarian hormones, they would not explain the benefit from GnRH agonists seen in postmenopausal women (natural or surgical). Other theories include the existence of a direct action on neural elements of the enteric nervous system or an effect of GnRH agonists on neurons in the brain or spinal cord (196,197). Clearly, electrophysiological studies of the effects of leuprolide on the enteric nervous system are needed.

In summary, while there are not enough data to support its routine use at this time, preliminary data suggest that GnRH agonists hold promise in the management of patients with pain-predominant IBS, particularly those whose symptoms fluctuate with the menstrual cycle.

Serotonin 5-HT_3 antagonists may reduce visceral afferent sensation (198). Hence, they may offer a therapeutic benefit in IBS patients who have heightened visceral nocioception. The potential use of these agents is reviewed below.

Summary—Pharmacotherapy should be reserved for the minority of IBS patients with pain that does not respond to conservative measures and that interferes significantly with quality of life and daily function. Anticholinergic agents are available clinically in the United States and may be of benefit when given before meals in patients with predominant postprandial pain. The antispasmodic agents are not yet available in the United States and do not appear to offer any great therapeutic advantage over the anticholinergic agents. 5-HT_3 antagonists offer promise for the future but require further clinical testing before they can be recommended. Analgesics should be avoided. In unresponsive patients, nonphamamacological approaches should be considered, such as hypnosis, relaxation training, biofeedback, and psychotherapy. Finally, psychotropic agents may also be of benefit in selected patients. These alternative therapies are discussed elsewhere.

Treatment of Constipation-Predominant Symptoms: A trial of increased dietary fiber or fiber supplements is generally tried in most IBS patients with constipation. In patients who do not respond to this simple maneuver, several pharmacological agents may be considered.

Although variably defined, the term *dietary fiber* generally referes to a heterogeneous group of complex carbohydrates that includes plant cell-wall material and other polysaccharides that are resistant to hydrolysis by human digestive enzymes. Dietary fiber comprises a number of different substances—including cellulose, hemicellulose pectins, and lignins—which have different physical and physiological properties. In general, dietary fiber leads to an increase in stool weight through three mechanisms: by directly providing nondigestible bulk, by their hydrophilic potential for retaining water, and by serving as a substrate for microbial growth in the colon. The hydrophilic properties help prevent stool dehydration as well as excess stool liquidity (199). In addition to increasing stool weight, dietary fiber decreases colonic transit time in normal and constipated subjects (200). The mechanism for this action is unknown but may be attributable to increased stool bulk and weight, to the action of fermentation products derived from bacterial degradation of the nonabsorbed polysaccharides, or to direct irritant effects of fiber particles. Dietary fiber may also absorb bile salts.

Fiber may be important in the prevention as well as the treatment of IBS. It has been hypothesized that the apparent low prevalence of IBS in rural Africa may be the result of high dietary-fiber intake. The use of fiber supplements in patients with abnormal patterns of defecation is supported by studies in animals and humans. Altered colonic motility has been demonstrated by myoelectric studies in animals fed diets of varying fiber content (201). Pigs fed a high-fiber diet have an increase in the electrical activity leading to propulsive activity and fecal elimination and a decrease in the segmental contractions that slow transit and dehydrate stool. Thus, bulking agents may have a role in the treatment of *some* patients with constipation-predominant IBS.

The optimal daily intake of dietary fiber in normal subjects is unknown. However, a panel has recommended an intake of 25–35 g/day. Many patients ingest much less daily fiber, and it may be difficult for them to modify their dietary habits to achieve this goal. For this reason, fiber supplements are commonly recommended. A variety of supplements are available. Because these agents are derived from different chemical classes with somewhat different properties, they may not be entirely "equivalent" in efficacy or in patient acceptance.

Wheat bran or "Miller's bran" is an inexpensive form of fiber supplement. The recommended dose is 5–20 g (one to four tablespoons) per day, which may be mixed with water or juice or sprinkled on other foods. Psyllium mucilloid (Metamucil) is extracted from the seed husk of psyllium seed. Available in a variety of flavored and unflavored powders and wafers, it is administered at a dose of 3.4 g of fiber one to three times daily. Methylcellulose (Citrucel), another natural fiber, is recommended at a dose of 2 g one to three times daily. Ispaghula (Regulan) is a partially fermentable polysaccharide derived from flea-seed husks. Although not available in the United States, it has been used at a dose of 3.6 g t.i.d. Finally, polycarbophil (Fiberall, Fiebercon) is a synthetic fiber that is recommended at a dose of 1 g one to four times daily. It appears to promote less flatulence and bloating than other fiber supplements (202).

There has been no convincing evidence to date that bulking agents are effective in the treatment of most patients with IBS. Although many reports have suggested that patients with IBS benefit, most have been subject to faulty study design and analaysis. In a meta-analysis of studies that assessed the effects of wheat bran on colonic function, an increase in stool weight as well as a decrease in transit time is evident in normal subjects and patients with IBS (200). Nevertheless, it is not clear that fiber supplementation results in improvement in most IBS symptoms. Eight randomized, double-blind placebo-controlled trials of fiber supplementation have been published. Given the placebo response rate of 53–71% observed in these trials, the importance of the placebo-controlled design is apparent (25). Longstreth, Lucey, and Cook and their colleagues (203–205) all demonstrated an improvement in altered defecation, a decrease in pain severity, and overall subjective improvement in IBS patients treated with psyllium, bran, and corn fiber. However, there was no difference compared with the placebo-treated groups. Arffmann and Soltoft and coworkers (206,207) found no effect of wheat bran on abdominal pain or the number or consistency of bowel movements, although an increased stool weight and decreased transit time could be measured. Similarly, Lucey et al. (204) observed no correlation between symptomatic response and the change in stool weight.

A major problem with these studies is the lack of information provided regarding the number of IBS patients treated with constipation-predominant symptoms. In fact, the mean number of bowel movements in the study by Longstreth et al. (203) was greater than three per week, and Lucey et al. (204) had few constipated patients. A controlled trial by Prior and Whorwell (208) reported overall symtomatic improvement in 82% of IBS patients treated with ispaghula compared with 53% treated with placebo. Of note, nearly half of these patients had constipation. A decreased number of days without bowel movements and a decrease in intestinal transit time occurred in treated patients; however, there was no effect of treatment on pain or distension. Most recently, in a 6-month, double-blind, crossover trial of polycarbophil in 23 IBS patients, 71% of patients preferred the fiber treatment periods (202). Polycarbophil was preferred in 79% of patients with constipation, 87% of those with bloating, and 100% of patients with alternating diarrhea and constipation. However, when diary scores for individual symptoms were assessed, only ease of fecal passage was statistically better during treatment with polycarbophil. The scores for nausea, bloating, and pain did not change significantly. Thus, although target symptoms are not obviously improved, patients appear to derive some improved overall sense of well-being during fiber therapy (202).

In summary, it appears from the available data that bulking agents may increase stool weight and the number of bowel movements and decrease intestinal transit time in IBS patients. These effects may be beneficial to those IBS patients for whom constipation is a predominant problem. However, there are no data to support the use of fiber supplements to treat other symptoms of IBS, such as abdominal pain, distension, or diarrhea. Nevertheless, some patients may feel an overall sense of improvement with a higher fiber intake. Because fiber may have a number of salutary properties apart from its effects on IBS, its approprate dietary intake should be encouraged. However, it is not enough simply to tell patients to increase their fiber intake to 20–30 g/day. Many patients are ignorant of what constitutes a high-fiber diet and will require education. Others are simply unable to alter their dietary patterns. It should be recognized that for some patients a high-fiber diet may not be well tolerated because of complaints of bloating or flatulence or may not conform with their dietary preferences. In such patients, a judicious trial of fiber supplements may be attempted. Finally, dietary fiber may not improve constipation in many patients. In such cases, the physician should admit defeat and consider other approaches, rather than "pushing" the fiber to intolerable extremes.

A variety of pharmacological agents promote transit through the GI tract and are referred to as *prokinetic agents*. These agents are currently employed for a variety of disorders, including gastroesophageal reflux, diabetic gastroparesis, chronic intestinal pseudo-obstruction, and chronic constipation, as well as functional disorders such as NUD and IBS (138,198). Prokinetic agents act through a variety of mechanisms to enhance motility. These include: 1) directly or indirectly promoting cholinergic tone (cholinergic agonists or serotonin agonists), 2) antagonizing inhibitory neurotransmitters (serotonin or dopamine), 3) stimulating the release or mimicking the action of compounds that increase motility (motilin), and 4) stimulating the release of gut hormones (198,209–211). Prokinetic agents may be grouped into the following classes: cholinergic agonists (not discussed further), substituted benzamides, dopamine antagonists, opiate antagonists, and macrolide antibiotics.

1. Substituted benzamides and the gut serotonin system—the two substituted benzamides inclinical use in the United States are metoclopramide and cisapride. These agents have prokinetic effects throughout the GI tract. Although its mechanism of action has not been wholly worked out, cisapride has been shown to cause the release of acetylcholine from postganglionic nerves in the gut intramural plexus, resulting in smooth-muscle contraction (209,212). This effect may be mediated by a complex interaction involving serotonin receptors.

Found in the interneurons terminating in the myenteric and submucosal plexuses, serotonin can act as a neurotransmitter or local hormone and appears to be important in modulating GI function (213,214). A number of serotonin receptor sites *(5-HT$_1$*, 5-HT$_2$, 5-HT$_3$, and 5-HT$_4$) have been identified in the gut, which are thought to be either in the enteric nervous system or on smooth muscle (198). Stimulation of these receptors may result in either stimulatory or inhibitory effects. The importance of 5-HY$_3$ receptors in gut function is discussed below. The serotonin 5-HT$_4$ receptors are located in the nerve terminals of both cholinergic interneurons and motor neurons (198). Stimulation of these receptors appears to indirectly stimulate cholinergic neurons and results in a variety of prokinetic effects including an increase in the lower-esophageal-sphincter pressure, acceleration of gastric emptying, and stimulation of colonic motor activity with accelerated transit (198,215).Cisapride and metoclopramide have been shown to be 5-HT_4 agonists, which explains at least in part some of their prokinetic effects (198). Cisapride is a more potent agonist than metoclopramide. In addition, at high doses they also appear to be 5-HT_3 antagonists, but this would not be explain their prokinetic effects (198). Unlike cisapride, metoclopramide has both peripheral and central dopamine blocking effects (see below). The central antidopaminergic actions result in significant side effects in up to 30% patients. Because of these side effects and a relative lack of effect on colonic motility, metoclopramide has little role in the treatment of IBS patients and is not discussed further here.

Cisapride has been demonstrated to enhance small- and large-bowel transit in healthy subjects (215–221). These effects translate into an increased frequency of bowel movements in normal subjects as well as those with constipation (217,218). Several early, prospective, double-blind controlled trials have shown an increase in stool frequency, decreased laxative use, and overall global improvement in patients with chronic constipation (215).

It remains to be determined whether cisapride may have utility in the treatment of constipation-predominant IBS. Passaretti et al. (222) showed a decreased whole-gut transit time after 6 weeks of therapy with cisapride 10 mg t.i.d., which correlated with an increase in stool frequency and a decrease in abdominal pain. To date, there has been only one placebo-controlled study of cisapride in IBS. Van Outryve et al. (223) initially evaluated 46 patients with abdominal pain and either constipation (31 patients), diarrhea, or alternating bowel habits with cisapride in an open trial for up to 8 weeks. Patients with constipation appeared to respond well, with a significant decrease in number of days without a bowel movement, an increase in days with normal stools, and improvement in abdominal pain and distension; patients with diarrhea-predominant IBS deteriorated. In a subsequent double-blind trial, 69 patients were randomized to 12 weeks of casapride 5 mg t.i.d. versus placebo (223). Significant improvement in stool frequency and consistency, abdominal pain and severity, and abdominal distension was reported in the cisapride-treated patients. Interestingly, patient global assessment showed no difference between the treatment groups, while the investigators noted improvement in 80% of the cisapride group and 55% of the placebo group. A flaw of this study is that symptoms and stool patterns were assessed by monthly interviews without the use of daily diaries, subjecting the results to recall bias. Nevertheless, this is an encouraging report which suggests a role for cisapride in patients with constipation-predominant IBS. Further clinical studies are awaited.

2. Dopamine-receptor antagonists—although the role of dopamine in the control of GI function is unclear, it appears to be an inhibitory neurotransmitter that prevents the release of acetylcholine. Domperidone and metoclopramide are dopaminergic receptor antagonists, but only the latter is clinically available in the United States. These agents enhance gastric emptying but appear to have

only limited effects on colonic motility and transit (224). Hence, they have found greatest utility in the treatment of gastroparesis. Unlike metoclopramide, domperidone does not appear to have effects on the gut serotonin system. Furthermore, domperidone has only limited ability to cross the blood–brain barrier and, unlike metoclopramide, is well tolerated. Three placebo-controlled trials (225–227) have failed to demonstrate any benefit of domperidone in IBS. With the advent of more effective colonic prokinetic agents such as cisapride, domperidone is unlikely to undergo further clinical testing in the United States.

3. Other prokinetic agents—other prokinetic agents have undergone little or no study in patients with IBS. Macrolides such as erythromycin have profound effects on GI motility that are mediated through motilin receptors (228). When taken during a meal, erythromycin induces powerful gastric contractions and phase III small-intestinal contractile activity (229). These agents may therefore be useful in treating gastric-emptying disorders. The effects of macrolides on colonic motility have undergone less study. However, the limited data available in normal subjects and patients with constipation suggest little, if any, effect on colonic motility. Hence, they are unlikely to be of use in IBS (228).

Opiates have well-recognized effects on GI motility. They cause a delay in colonic transit, often resulting in constipation. That endogenous opiates may play an inhibitory role in the regulation of human intestinal transit is evidenced by the ability of naloxone, an opiate antagonist, to counter the delay in colonic transit caused by morphine in human volunteers (230). Naloxone and related opiate antagonists are believed to exert their effects on the mu opiate receptors (see below) (231). Oral opioid antagonists have been administered to small groups of patients with idiopathic constipation with mixed results (232,233), but were no better than placebo in a small group of patients with IBS (233,234). To date, there has not been enough experience with this group of drugs to recommend their use in patients with chronic constipation or IBS.

As a general rule, *laxatives* should be reserved for severe constipation, and are best avoided in patients with alternating constipation and diarrhea for obvious reasons. When using these agents, the smallest dose for the shortest period of time is prudent. Hyperosmotic laxatives such as oral lactulose or glycerin suppositories are reasonable choices given their relatively quick onset of action. However, lactulose may worsen bloating and flatulence, and electrolyte imbalance may occur with chronic use. Stool-softeners are safe agents, but have a slower onset of action.

In summary, constipation is often defined differently by the patient and the physician. To the physician, it typically means a reduced frequency of bowel movements to fewer than two to three per week. The patient may define constipation as hard or scybalous stools, a decreased frequency of movements, or straining and difficulty with evacuation. The approach to each of these complaints may be somewhat different. Therefore, to appropriately treat the patient's complaint, it is imperative that the physician understand it.

Patients with constipation-predominant symptoms should have a careful review of their dietary intake. An adequate trial of a high-fiber diet and/or fiber supplements should be performed in most cases. Fiber often leads to improved stool consistency, improved ease of passage, and an increased frequency of bowel movements.

Patients who are unresponsive to dietary fiber can be extremely difficult to manage. In these cases, constipation may arise from one of two pathophysiological processes: colonic inertia or rectosigmoid outlet delay (235). Before proceeding with further therapeutic trials, it is helpful to distinguish between these. A radioopaque-marker colon transit study is helpful both to confirm that constipation is truly present and to document colonic inertia. Patients with colonic inertia may respond to a trial of an osmotic laxative or the prokinetic agent cisapride. The diagnosis of outlet delay is based on the clinical history and may be confirmed by defecography or anal motility. This entity may be better approached with nonpharmacological means such as biofeedback and pelvic-floor retraining. These are reviewed in detail elsewhere (236).

Treatment of diarrhea-predominant symptoms: Some IBS patients with diarrhea-predominant symptoms may benefit from symptomatic therapy with antidiarrheal agents. Several classes of agents are available.

Opioid agonists may be of benefit in patients with loose, frequent stools. The currently available synthetic opiates commonly prescribed for diarrhea are loperamide (Imodium), codeine, and diphenoxylate (with atropine: Lomotil). Loperamide and diphenoxylate are preferred because they have poor penetration of the CNS, so there is little potential for physical or psychological dependence with prolonged usage. At least five opioid receptors have been identified; however, the mu, delta, and kappa receptors predominate in the intestinal tract (237). All these receptors regulate smooth-muscle tone, and the delta receptor increases fluid and electrolyte absorption. The currently available opiates interact primarily with the mu receptors, thereby affecting gut motility. They appear to decrease propulsive activity by causing contraction of the circular smooth muscle (230,238). In turn, this leads to prolonged colonic transit time, which results in greater stool fluid resorption and improved stool consistency. These agents may also increase anal-sphincter tone.

On the basis of limited clinical trials, opioids may be beneficial in the treatment of diarrhea-predominant IBS. In two double-blind placebo-controlled trials of IBS patients with diarrhea, loperamide 2–8 mg at h.s. improved stool consistency and reduced stool frequency and rectal urgency in patients with diarrhea-predominant symptoms (239,240). An additional double-blind crossover trial of loperamide 2–12 mg per day also demonstrated improvement in stool frequency and rectal urgency (241). There have been no published controlled trials of diphenyoxylate.

The judicious use of loperamide can be recommended in diarrhea-predominant IBS and/or rectal urgency. Some patients appear to be quite sensitive to loperamide, developing constipation at higher doses; hence, the lowest effective dose should be used. Loperamide may be given chronically as a bedtime dose with some success. In most patients, however, it is best used as a "prophylactic" agent when diarrhea is either anticipated (such as in stressful situations) or would be inconvenient (social engagements, lack of proximity to restrooms).

Bile-salt binding agents—the role of bile-salt malabsorption in diarrhea-predominant IBS remains controversial (see above). The bile-salt binding agent cholestyramine may be effective in reducing diarrhea in patients with documented bile-salt malabsorption, such as those with partial ileal resections. In addition, cholestyramine may cause constipation in normal subjects, suggesting that it has nonspecific constipating actions. Experience with cholestyramine in IBS has been extremely limited. In a study of 17 patients with idiopathic diarrhea (14 of whom had some evidence of increased bile malabsorption), cholestyramine had no significant effect on stool weight (242). In another study (243), cholestyramine resulted in "improvement" in four of six patients with diarrhea-predominant IBS and evidence of bile-salt malabsorption on nuclear testing. There may be rare IBS patients who experience symptomatic improvement with cholestyramine, but most patients find the agent unpalatable.

Serotonin 5-HT_3 receptor antagonists—As discussed above, the development of highly specific serotonin-receptor antagonists has helped elucidate some of the mechanisms through which serotonin affects the GI tract. 5-HT_3 receptors appear to facilitate the release of acetylcholine in the enteric nervous system, resulting in gut smooth-muscle contraction (198); highly specific 5-HT_3-receptor antagonists have been developed that appear to slow colonic transit in normal subjects (244). 5-HT_3 receptors may also modulate visceral afferent sensation; antagonists to these receptors have been demonstrated to reduce the visceral pain response in both animals and humans (198,245). Finally, 5-HT_3 receptors are present in the limbic and cortical areas of the brain (where they are important in controlling memory and mood) and in the area postrema; 5-HT_3 antagonists such as ondansetron have potent antiemetic action in patients receiving chemotherapy (198). With these properties in mind, the utility of serotonin 5-HT_3 antagonists has been studies in patients with diarrhea-predominant IBS both to reduce diarrhea and to dampen the heightened visceral nocioception that is commonly noted in IBS patients.

The only 5-HT_3 antagonists currently available in the United States are ondansetron and granisetron, which are approved as an antiemetic for patients receiving chemotherapy. However, similar agents have been developed and are in various phases of clinical testing, including tropisetron, renzapride, and zacopride. Ondansetron has been shown to have no effect on small-intestinal transit but significantly slows colonic transit, especially in the left and rectosigmoid colon, in healthy controls (244). Two studies to date have looked at the role of 5-HT_3 antagonists in diarrhea-predominant IBS. In a double-blind crossover study of ondansetron 4 mg t.i.d., Maxton et al. (246) demonstrated a significant improvement in stool consistency and a decreased number of bowel movements. Abdominal pain and distension, however, were not improved. In another randomized, double-blind, placebo-controlled crossover trial of ondansetron 16 mg t.i.d., Steadman et al. (247) demonstrated a significant improvement in stool consistency but no change in stool weight, stool frequency, or abdominal pain in 14 patients. Contrary to expectations, colonic transit time was not increased by ondansetron treatment.

The effects of 5-HT_3 antagonists on gut afferent sensation are only beginning to be studied. In a study of 12 patients (nine with diarrhea), Prior and Read (248) demonstrated significant increases in the mean threshold of latex-balloon-inflation volumes for perception of gas, stool urgency, and discomfort and a significant decrease in postprandial anorectal motility after administration of i.v. granisetron. However, in a slightly different study that employed barostats in the descending colon and rectum of 10 healthy volunteers and five diarrhea-predominant IBS patients, Camilleri et al. (249) could not detect a difference in rectal sensitivity or tone after ondansetron. Whether there are particular differences in efficacy between ondansetron and granisetron remains to be established.

The serotonin 5-HT_3 antagonists are another in a long line of drugs that have been touted as potential breakthroughs in the treatment of IBS. However, none of the other "magic bullets" has withstood the objective scrutiny of controlled clinical trial testing, and it is doubtful that these agents will be any different. At this time, the few available studies suggest that 5-HT_3 antagonists may play some role in treating the diarrhea associated with IBS. Whether they can be used to alter the perception of visceral pain remains to bedetermined. Further studies are needed before these agents can be recommended in routine clinical practice.

To summarize, while a discussion of the sundry causes of chronic diarrhea is beyond the scope of this chapter, it must be noted that diarrhea attributed to IBS must be distinguished from other organic causes of chronic diarrhea. These include parasitic infections, osmotic causes (lactose, sorbitol, magnesium), inflammatory conditions (collagenous colitis, Crohn's disease), malabsorptive states (sprue), secretory conditions, and laxative abuse. An extensive workup is not indicated initially in patients with mild diarrhea and a clinical history compatible with IBS. On the other hand, paticnts with worsening or severe diarrhea, weight loss, signs of dehydration or malabsorption, or abnormal laboratory values require an extensive evaluation. A 24-hour stool collection for fecal weight is an inexpensive means of assessing diarrhea. A total weight of >300 g suggests causes of diarrhea other than IBS.

Patients with diarrhea-predominant IBS should have a careful dietary screen for dietary factors, especially malabsorbed carbohydrates, that may be causative. Caffeine should be eliminated. A trial of increased dietary fiber is often given with the intention of "sopping up" the excess liquid. However, clinical trials and personal experience suggest that diarrheal symptoms do not respond well to this approach. Opioids may be extremely useful for some patients, particularly when used on an as-needed basis. Cholestyramine may be tried but is seldom of benefit. Further study of the utility of the serotonin 5-HT_3 antagonists in IBS is awaited before their use can be recommended.

IV. CONCLUSION

Functional GI symptoms are extremely common in the adult population, affecting 15–20% of people. Although a number of physiological and psychological abnormalities have been identified, their relative importance is uncertain and, indeed, may vary among individuals. GI motility disturbances (either primary or secondary to environmental or psychological stimuli), visceral hypersensitivity, dietary or environmental factors, and psychological abnormalities or stresses may interact to produce GI symptomatology. Initial diagnostic strategies should be directed at excluding obvious organic causes of the symptomatology. Specific patient concerns or fears should be determined and addressed. Once organic diseases have been excluded and a diagnosis of functional GI disease has been made, a careful, thorough discussion with the patient of the meaning, natural history, and pathophysiology of functional GI disease should take place. Efforts should shift from determination of symptom causation to symptom coping, dietary changes, and lifestyle modifications that involve stress reduction. The overwhelming majority of patients respond to education, reassurance, and a stable therapeutic relationship with the primary-care provider. Pharmacological therapies may be helpful on an intermittent or chronic basis in the treatment of a specific severe symptoms. However, both the physician and the patient need to avoid the search for "magic bullets," as they do not exist and the search for such will only bring frustration. Patients with obvious psychological problems or those who do not respond to conservative measures may benefit from referral to a psychologist or psychiatrist for behavioral treatments, psychotherapy, or pharmacological treatment.

REFERENCES

1. Drossman D, Funch-Jensen P, Janssens J, Talley HJ, Thompson WG, Whitehead WE. Identification of sub-groups of functional gastrointestinal disorders. Gastroenterol Int 1990; 3:159–172.
2. Drossman D, Richter J, Talley N, eds. The Functional Gastointestinal Disorders: Diagnosis, Pathophysiology, and Treatment—A Multinational Consensus. Boston: Little Brown, 1994.

3. Almy T. Management of the irritable bowel syndrome: different views of the same disease. Ann Intern Med 1992; 116:1027–1028.
4. Camilleri M, Prather C. The irritable bowel syndrome: mechanisms and a practical approach to management. Ann Intern Med 1992; 116(12 pt 1):1001–1008.
5. Drossman D, Thompson W. The irritable bowel syndrome: review and a graduated multicomponent treatment approach. Ann Intern Med 1992; 116(12 pt 1):1009– 1016.
6. Lynn R, Friedman L. Irritable bowel syndrome. N Engl J. Med 1993; 329:1940–1944.
7. McKee D, Quigley E. Intestinal motility in irritable bowel syndrome: is IBS a motility disorder? Dig Dis Sci 1993; 38:1761–1782.
8. McQuaid K. Dyspepsia and non-ulcer dyspepsia. In: Sleisenger M, Fordtran J, eds. Gastrointestinal Diseases—Update 10. Philadelphia: WB Saunders, 1993:1–13.
9. Richter J, Bradley L, Castell D. Esophageal chest pain: current controversies in pathogenesis, diagnosis and therapy. Ann Intern Med 1989; 110:66–78.
10. Talley N. Non-ulcer dyspepsia: myths and realities. Aliment Pharmacol Ther 1991; 5(suppl 1):145–162.
11. Zighelboim J, Talley N. What are functional bowel disorders? Gastoenterology 1993; 104:1196–1201.
12. Kellow J, Phillips S. Altered small bowel motility in irritable bowel syndrome is correlated with symptoms. Gastroenterology 1987; 92:1885.
13. Mayer E, Gebhart G. Basic and clinical aspects of visceral hyperalgesia. Gastoenterology 1994; 107:271–293.
14. Talley N, Phillips S, Bruce B, et al. Relation among personality and symptoms in nonulcer dyspepsia and the irritable bowel syndrome. Gastroenterology 1990; 99:327–333.
15. Clouse R. Psychiatric disorders in patients with esophageal disease. Med Clin North Am 1991; 75:1081–1097.
16. Bradley L, Richter J, Scarinci C, et al. Psychosocial and psychophysical assessments of patients with unexplained chest pain. Am J. Med 1992; 5A:65S–74S.
17. Drossman D, McKee D, Sandler R, et al. Psychosocial factors in the irritable bowel syndrome: A multivariate study of patients and nonpatients with irritable bowel syndrome. Gastroenterology 1988; 95:701–708.
18. Whitehead W, Bosmajian L, Zonderman A, et al. Symptoms of psychologic distress associated with irritable bowel syndrome: comparison of community and medical clinic samples. Gastroenterology 1988; 95:709–714.
19. Koch K. Facing up to the evanescent nutcracker. Am J Gastroenterol 1988; 83:661–662.
20. Cohen S. Noncardiac chest pain: The crumbling of the sphinx. Dig Dis Sci 1989; 34:1649–1650.
21. Camilleri M, Malagelada J, Kao P, Zinsmeister A. Gastric and autonomic responses to stress in functional dyspepsia. Dig Dis Sci 1986; 31:1169–1177.
22. Mearin F, Cucala M, Azpiroz F, Malagelada J. The origin of symptoms on the brain-gut axis in functional dyspepsia. Gastroenterology 1991; 101:999–1006.
23. Friedman G. GI drug column. Irritable bowel syndrome: I. A practical approach. Am J Gastroenterol 1989; 84:863–867.
24. Talley N. Nonulcer dyspepsia: current approaches to diagnosis and management. Am Fam Phys 1993; 47:1407–1416.

25. Klein KB. Controlled treatment trials in the irritable bowel syndrome: a critique. Gastroenterology 1988; 95:232–241.
26. Whitehead W. Behavioral medicine approaches to gastrointestinal disorders. J Consult Clin Psych 1992; 60:605–612.
27. Richter J, Castell D. Esophageal disease as a cause of noncardiac chest pain. Adv Intern Med 1988; 33:311–336.
28. Richter J. Practical approaches to the diagnosis of unexplained chest pain. Med Clin North Am 1991; 75:1203–1209.
29. Wise C, Semble E, Dalton C. Musculoskeletal chest wall syndromes in patients with noncardiac chest pain: a study of 100 patients. Arch Phys Med Rehabil 1992; 73:147–149.
30. Koch K, Davidson W, Day F, et al. Esophageal dysfunction and chest pain in patients with mitral valve prolapse: a prospective study utilizing provocative testing during esophageal manometry. Am J Med 1989; 86:32–38.
31. Cannon R, Cattau E, Yakshe P, et al. Coronary flow reserve, esophageal motility, and chest pain in patients with angiographically normal coronary arteries. Am J Med 1990; 88:217–222.
32. Cannon R, Schenke W, Quyyumi A, et al. Comparison of exercise testing with studies of coronary flow reserve in patients with microvascular angina. Circulation 1991; 83(suppl III):77–81.
33. Cannon R, Camici P, Epstein S. Pathophysiological dilemma of Syndrome X. Circulation 1992; 85:883–892.
34. Quyyumi A, Cannon R, Panza J, et al. Endothelial dysfunction in patients with chest pain and normal coronary arteries. Circulation 1992; 86:1864–1871.
35. Katz P, Dalton C, Richter J, et al. Esophageal testing of patients with noncardiac chest pain or dysphagia: Results of three years' experience with 1161 patients. Ann Intern Med 1987; 106:593–597.
36. Kahrilas P, Clouse RE, Hogan WJ. American Gastroenterological Association Technical Review on the Clinical Use of Esophageal Manometry. Gastroenterology 1994; 1994:1865–1884.
37. Valori R. Nutcracker, neurosis, or sampling bias? Gut 1990; 31:736–737.
38. Dalton C. Castell DO, Richter JE. The changing faces of nutcracker esophagus. Am J Gastroenterol 1988; 83:623–628.
39. Anderson K, Dalton DB, Bradley LA, Richter JE. Stress induces alteration of esophageal pressures in healthy volunteers and non-cardiac chest pain patients. Dig Dis Sci 1989; 34:83–91.
40. Richter J, Obrecht F, Bradley LA, Young LD, Anderson KO. Psychological comparisons of patients with nutcracker esophagus and irritable bowel syndrome. Dig Dis Sci 1986; 31:131–138.
41. Clause R, Lustman P. Psychiatric illness and contraction abnormalities of the esophagus. N Engl J Med 1983; 309:1337–1342.
42. Peters L, Maas L, Petty D, et al. Spontaneous noncardiac chest pain: Evaluation by 24-hour ambulatory esophageal motility and pH monitoring. Gastroenterology 1988; 94:878–886.
43. Lam H, Dekker W, Kan G, et al. Acute noncardiac chest pain in a coronary care

unit: Evaluation by 24-hour pressure and pH recording of the esophagus. Gastroenterology 1992; 102:453–460.
44. Hewson E, Dalton C, Richter J. Comparison of esophageal manometry, provocative testing, and ambulatory monitoring in patients with unexplained chest pain. Dig Dis Sci 1990; 35:302–309.
45. Hick D, Morrison J, Casey J, et al. Oesophageal motility, luminal pH, and electrocardiographic-ST segment analysis during spontaneous episodes of angina like chest pain. Gut 1991; 33:79–86.
46. Breumelhof R, Nadorp J, Akkermans L, Smout A. Analysis of 24-hour esophageal pressure and pH data in unselected patients with noncardiac chest pain. Gastroenterology 1990; 99:1257–1264.
47. Ghillebert G, Janssens J. Vantrappen G, et al. Ambulatory 24 hour intraoesophageal pH and pressure recordings v provocation tests in the diagnosis of chest pain of oesophageal origin. Gut 1990; 31:738–744.
48. Richter J. Gastroesophageal reflux disease as a cause of chest pain. Med Clin North Am 1991; 75:1065–1081.
49. Hewson E, Sinclair J, Dalton C. Richter J. Twenty-four hour esophageal pH monitoring: the most useful test for evaluating noncardiac chest pain. Am J Med 1991; 90:576–583.
50. Singh S, Richter J, Hewson E, et al. The contribution of gastroesophageal reflux to chest pain in patients with coronary artery disease. Ann Intern Med 1992; 117:824–830.
51. Soffer E, Scalabrini P, Wingate D. Spontaneous noncardiac chest pain: value of arbulatory esophageal pH and motility monitoring. Dig Dis Sci 1989; 34:1651–1655.
52. Hick D. Can esophagus be blamed for noncardiac chest pain? Gastroenterology 1992; 103:1698–1700.
53. Clause R, McCord G, Lustman P, Edmundowicz S. Clinical correlates of abnormal sensitivity to intraesophageal balloon distention. Dig Dis Sci 1991; 36:1040–1045.
54. Richter J, Barish C, Castell D. Abnormal sensory perception in patients with esophageal chest pain. Gastroenterology 1986; 91:845–852.
55. Richter J, Hewson E, Sinclair J, Dalton C. Acid perfusion test and 24-hour esophageal pH monitoring with symptom index: Comparison of tests for esophageal acid sensitivity. Dig Dis Sci 1991; 86:565–571.
56. Hewson E, Sinclair J, Dalton C, et al. Acid perfusion test: does it have a role in the assessment of noncardiac chest pain? Gut 1989; 30:305–310.
57. de Caestecker J, Pryde A, Heading R. Site and mechanism of pain perception with oesophageal balloon distention and intravenous edrophonium in patients with oesophageal chest pain. Gut 1992; 33:580–586.
58. Deschner W, Maher K, Cattau E, Benjamin S. Intraesophageal balloon distention versus drug provocation in thc evaluation of noncardiac chest pain. Am J Gastroenterol 1990; 85:938–943.
59. Dalton C, Hewson E, Castell D, Richter J. Edrophonium provocative test in noncardiac chest pain: Evaluation of testing techniques. Dig Dis Sci 1990; 35:1445–1451.
60. Cannon R, Quyyumi A, Wchenke W, et al. Abnormal cardiac sensitivity in patients with chest pain and normal coronary arteries. JACC 1990; 16:1359–1366.

61. Beitman B, Kushner M, Basha I, et al. Follow-up status of patients with angiographically normal coronary arteries and panic disorder. JAMA 1991; 265:1545–1549.
62. Beitman B, Mukerji V, Kushner M, et al. Validating studies for panic disorder in patients with angiographically normal coronary arteries. Med Clin North Am 1991; 75:1143–1155.
63. Beitman B. Panic disorder in patients with angiographically normal coronary arteries. Am J Med 1992; 92(5A):33S–40S.
64. Papanicolaou M, Califf R, Hlatky M, et al. Prognostic implications of angiographically normal and insignificantly narrowed coronary arteries. Am J Cardiol 1986; 58:1181–1187.
65. Ward B, Wu W, Richter J, et al. Long-term follow-up of symptomatic status of patients with noncardiac chest pain: Is diagnosis of esophageal etiology helpful? Am J Gastroenterol 1987; 82:215–218.
66. Achem S, Crettenden J, Kolts B, Burton L. Long-term clinical and manometric follow-up of patients with nonspecific esophageal motor disorders. Am J Gastroenterol 1992; 87:825–830.
67. Pope C II. Current concepts: Acid-reflux disorders. N Engl J Med 1994; 331:655–660.
68. DeVault K, Castell D. Current diagnosis and treatment of gastroesophageal reflux disease. May Clin Proc 1994; 69:867–876.
69. DeBoer W, Tytgat G. Review article: drug therapy for reflux oesophagitis. Aliment Pharmacol Ther 1994; 8:147–157.
70. Achem S, Kolts BE, Wears R, Burton L, Richter JE. Chest pain associated with nutcracker esophagus: a preliminary study of the role of gastroesophageal reflux. Am J Gastroenterol 1993; 88:187–192.
71. DeMeester T, et al. Esophageal function in patients with angina-type chest pain and normal coronary angiogram. Ann Surg 1982; 196:488–498.
72. Kikendall J, Mellow M. Effect of sublingual nitroglycerin and long-acting nitrate preparations on esophageal motility. Gastroenterology 1980; 79:703–706.
73. Parker W, MacKinnon G. Nitrites in the treatment of diffuse esophageal spasm. Drug Intell Clin Pharm 1981; 15:806.
74. Orlando R, Bozyinski. Clinical and manometric effects of nitroglycerin in diffuse esophageal spasm. N Engl J Med 1973; 289:23–25.
75 Swamy N. Esophageal spasm: Clinical and manometric response to nitroglycerine and long-acting nitrates. Gastroenterology 1977; 72:23–27.
76. Richter J, Spurling T, Cordova C, Castell D. Effects of oral calcium blocker, diltiazem, on esophageal contractions. Dig Dis Sci 1984; 29:649.
77. Richter J, Dalton C. Buice R, Castell D. Nifedipine: a potent inhibitor of contractions in the body of the human esophagus. Studies in healthy volunteers and patients with the nutcracker esophagus. Gastroenterology 1985; 89:549–554.
78. Blackwell J, et al. Effect of nifedipine on esophageal motility and gastric emptying. Digestion 1981; 21:50.
79. Alban Davies H, Lewis M, Rhodes J, et al. Trial of nifedipine for prevention of esophageal spasm. Digeston 1987; 36:81–83.

80. Nasrallah S. Nifedipine in the treatment of diffuse esophageal spasm. Lancet 1982; ii:1285.
81. Richter J, Dalton C, Bradley L, et al. Oral nifedipine in the treatment of noncardiac chest pain in patients with the nutcracker esophagus. Gastroenterology 1987; 93:21–28.
82. Cattau E, Castell D, Johnson D, et al. Diltiazem therapy for symptoms associated with nutcracker esophagus. Am J Gastroenterol 1991; 86:272–275.
83. Clouse R, Lustman P, Eckert T, et al. Low-dose trazodone for symptomatic patients with esophageal contraction abnormalities: A double-blind, placebo-controlled trial. Gastroenterology 1987; 92:1027–1036.
84. Cannon R, Quyyumi A, Mincemoyer R, et al. Imipramine in patients with chest pain despite normal coronary angiograms. N Engl J Med 1994; 330:1411–1417.
85. Winters C, Artnal E, Benjamin S, et al. Esophageal bougienage in symptomatic patients with the nutcracker esophagus. JAMA 1984; 252:363–366.
86. Ebert E, Ouyang A, Wright S, et al. Pneumatic dilatation in patients with symptomatic diffuse esophageal spasm and lower esophageal sphincter dysfunction. Dig Dis Sci 1983; 28:481–485.
87. McCord G, Stalano A, Clouse RE. Achalasia, diffuse esophageal spasm and nonspecific motility disorders. Baillieres Clin Gastroenterol 1991; 5:307–335.
88. De Meester T. Surgery for esophageal motor disorders. Ann Thorac Surg 1982; 34:225–229.
89. Henderson R, Ryder D, Marryatt G. Extended esophageal myotomy and short total fundoplication hernia repair in diffuse esophageal spasm: Five-year review in 34 patients. Ann Thorac Surg 1987; 43:25–31.
90. Traube M, Vijayaprasad T, Baue A, McCallum R. Surgical myotomy in patients with high-amplitude peristaltic esophageal contractions: Manometric and clinical effects. Dig Dis Sci 1987; 32:16–21.
91. Horton M, Goff J. Surgical treatment of nutcracker esophagus. Dig Dis Sci 1986; 31: 878–883.
92. Committee APC. An American Gastroenterological Association Medical Position Statement on the Clinical Use of Esophageal Manometry. Gastroenterology 1994; 107:1865.
93. Talley N, Colin-Jone D, Koch K, Cosk M, Myren OVS. Functional dyspepsia: a classification with guidlines for diagnosis and management. Gastroenterol Int 1991; 4:145–160.
94. Richter J. Dyspepsia: organic causes and differential characteristics from functional dyspepsia. Scand J. Gastroenterol 1991; 26(suppl 182):11.
95. Kagevi I, Lofstedt S, Persson L. Endoscopic findings and diagnoses in unselected dyspeptic patients at primary health care center. Scand J Gastroenterol 1989; 24:145.
96. Talley NJ. Non-ulcer dyspepsia: potential causes and pathophysiology. Ann Intern Med 1988; 108:865–879.
97. Talley N. The role of *Helicobacter pylori* in nonulcer dyspepsia: a debate against. Gastroenterol Clin North Am 1993; 22:153–168.
98. Laine L. *Helicobacter pylori* and non-ulcer dyspepsia. Gastroenterology 1992; 103:340–342.

99. Parsonnet J, Blaser M, Perez-Perez G, et al. Symptoms and risk factors of *Helicobacter pylori* infection in a cohort of epidemiologists. Gastroenterology 1992; 102:41–46.
100. Bernersen R, Johnsen R, Bostad L, et al. Is *Helicobacter pylori* the cause of dyspepsia? Br Med J 1992; 304:1276–1279.
101. Talley NJ. A critique of therapeutic trials in *Helicobacter pylori*–positive functional dyspepsia. Gastroenterology 1994; 106:1174–1183.
102. Veldhuyzen Van Zanten SJO. A systematic overview (meta-analysis) of outcome measures in *Helicobacter pylori* gastritis trials and functional dyspepsia. Scand J Gastroenterol 1993; 199(suppl 199):40–43.
103. Patchett S, Beattie S, Leen E, et al. Eradicating *Helicobacter pylori* and symptoms of non-ulcer dyspepsia. Br Med J 1991; 303:1238–1240.
104. McCarthy C, Patchett S, Collins R, Beattie S, Keane D, O'Morain D. Long term prospective study of *Helicobacter pylori* in nonulcer dyspepsia. Dig Dis Sci 1995; 40:114–119.
105. Veldhuyzen van Zanten S, Malatjalian D, Tanton R, et al. The effect of eradication of *Helicobacter pylori* on symptoms of non-ulcer dyspepsia: a randomized double-blind placebo controlled trial. Gastroenterology 1995; 108:A250.
106. Klauser AG, Schindlbeck NE, Muller-Lissner SA. Symptoms in gastroesophageal reflux disease. Lancet 1990; 335:205–208.
107. Talley N, Zinsmeister A, Schleck C, Melton L. Dyspepsia and dyspepsia subgroups: a population-based study. Gastroenterology 1992; 102:1259–1268.
108. Talley HJ, Weaver AL, Tesmer DL, Zinsmeister AR. Lack of discriminant value of dyspepsia subgroups in patients referred for upper endoscopy. Gastroenterology 1993; 105:1378–1386.
109. Small PK, Loudon MA, Waldron B, Smith D, Campbell FC. Importance of reflux symptoms in functional dyspepsia. Gut 1995; 36:189–192.
110. Talley NJ. Spectrum of chronic dyspepsia in the presence of irritable bowel syndrome. Scand J Gastroenterol 1991; 26(suppl 182):7.
111. Collen M, Lebenberg M. Basal gastric acid secretion in nonulcer dyspepsia with or without duodenitis. Dig Dis Sci 1989; 34:246.
112. Malagelada J. Gastrointestinal motor disturbances in functional dyspepsia. Scand J. Gastroenterol 1991; 26(suppl 182):29–32.
113. Waldron B, Cullen PT, Kumar R, et al. Evidence of hypomotility in non-ulcer dyspepsia: a prospective multifactorial study. Gut 1991; 32:246–251.
114. Stanghellini V, Ghidini C, Maccarini M, et al. Fasting and postprandial gastrointestinal motility in ulcer and non-ulcer dyspepsia. Gut 1992; 33:184–190.
115. Greydanus MP, Vassallo M, Camilleri M, Melson DK, Hanson RB, Thomforde GM. Neurohormonal factors in functional dyspepsia: insights on pathophysiological mechanisms. Gastroenterology 1991; 100:1311–1318.
116. Lemann M, Dedering J, Flourie B, Franchisseur C, Rambaud JC, Jian R. Abnormal perception of visceral pain in response to gastric distention in chronic idiopathic dyspepsia. Dig Dis Sci 1991; 36:52–58.
117. Bradette M, Pare P, Douville P, Morin A. Visceral perception in health and functional dyspepsia. Dig Dis Sci 1991; 36:1249–1254.

118. Coffin B, Azpiroz F, Guarner F, Malagelada JR. Selective gastric hypersensitivity and reflex hyporeactivity in functional dyspepsia. Gastroenterology 1994; 107:1345–1351.
119. Mittal RK, Hebbard G. An attempt to define the pathophysiological abnormality in patients with nonulcer dyspepsia using a gastric barostat. Gastoenterology 1994; 107:596–607.
120. George AA, Tsuchiyose M, Dooley C. Sensitivity of the gastric mucosa to acid and duodenal contents in patients with nonulcer dyspepsia. Gastroenterology 1991; 101:3–6.
121. Bates S, Sjoden PO, Fellenius J, Nyren O. Blocked and nonblocked acid secretion and reported pain in ulcer, nonulcer dyspepsia, and normal subjects. Gastoenterology 1989; 97:376–383.
122. Richter JE. Stress and psychologic and environmental factors in functional dyspepsia. Scand J Gastroenterol 1991; 26(suppl 182):40–46.
123. Talley NJ, Piper D. Major life event stress and dyspepsia of unknown cause: a case control study. Gut 1986; 27:127–134.
124. Talley NJ, Piper DW. A prospective study of social factors and major life event stress in patients with dyspepsia of unknown cause. Scand J Gastroenterol 1987; 22:268–272.
125. Hui WM, Ling PS, Lam SK. The perception of life events and daily stress in nonulcer dyspepsia. Am J Gastroenterol 1991; 86:292–296.
126. Elta GH, Behler EM, Colturi TJ. Comparison of coffee intake and coffee-induced symptoms in patients with duodenal ulcer, nonulcer dyspepsia, and normal controls. Am J Gastroenterol 1990; 85:1339–1342.
127. Talley NJ, Weaver AL, Zinsmeister AR. Smoking, alcohol, and nonsteroidal anti-inflammatory drugs in outpatients with functional dyspepsia and among dyspepsia subgroups. Am J Gastroenterol 1994; 89:524–528.
128. Kang JY, Tay HH, Guan R. Chronic upper abdominal pain: site and radiation in various structural and functional disorders and the effect of various foods. Gut 1992; 33:743–748.
129. Talley N. Drug treatment of functional dyspepsia. Scand J Gastroenterol 1991; 26(suppl 182):47–60.
130. Holtmann G, Telley NJ. Functional dyspepsia: Current treatment recommendations. Drugs 1993; 45:918–930.
131. Nyren O, Gustavsson S, Adami HO, Loof L. Methodological aspects of clinical trials in non-ulcer dyspepsia with special references to selectional factors. Scand J Gastroenterol 1985; 20 (suppl 109):159–162.
132. Veldhuyzen van Zanten SJ, Tytgat KM, Pollak PT, et al. Can severity of symptoms be used as an outcome measure in trials of non-ulcer dyspepsia and *Helicobacter pylori* associated gastritis? J Clin Epidemiol 1993; 46:273–279.
133. Johannessen T, Petersen H, Kristensen P, et al. Cimetidine on demand in dyspepsia: Experience with randomized controlled single-subject trials. Scand J Gastroenterol 1992; 27:188–195.
134. Dobrilla G, Comberlato M, Steele A, Vallaperta P. Drug treatment of functional dyspepsia: A meta analysis of randomized controlled clinical trials. J Clin Gastroenterol 1989; 11:169–177.

135. Johannessen T, Fjosne U, Kleveland P, et al. Cimetidine responders in non-ulcer dyspepsia. Scand J Gastroenterol 1988; 23:327–336.
136. Jebbink HH, Smout AJ, Van Berge-Henegouwen GP. Pathophysiology and treatment of functional dyspepsia. Scand J Gastroenterol 1993; 28(suppl 200):8–14.
137. Farup PG, Larsen S, Osnes M. Ranitidine for non-ulcer dyspepsia. Scand J Gastroenterol 1991; 26:1209–1216.
138. Reynolds JC. Prokinetic agents. Gastroenterol Clin North Am 1992; 21:567–596.
139. Rosch W. Efficacy of cisapride in the treatment of epigastric pain and concomitant symptoms in non-ulcer dyspepsia. Scand J Gastroenterol 1988; 24(suppl 165):54–58.
140. Hausken T, Berstand A. Cisapride treatment of patients with non-ulcer dyspepsia and erosive pre-pyloric chaanges. Scand J Gastroenterol 1992; 27:213–217.
141. Famagalli I, Hammer B. Cisapride versus metochlopramide in the treatment of functional dyspepsia. Scand J Gastroenterol 1994; 29:33–37.
142. Miazza B, Halter F, Brignoli R. A multicentric comparative trial in functional dyspepsia: cisapride versus cimetidine. Gastroenterology 1993; 104:A18.
143. Chua A, Bekkering M, Rovati L, Keeling P. Clinical efficacy and prokinetic effect of the CCK-A antagonist loxiglumide in non-ulcer dyspepsia. Gastroenterology 1993; 104:A491.
144. Nanda R, James R, Smith H, et al. Food intolerance and the irritable bowel syndrome. Gut 1989; 80:1099-1104.
145. Zwetchkenbaum JF, Burakoff R. Food allergy and the irritable bowel syndrome. Am J Gastroenterol 1988; 83:901–904.
146. Lisker R, Solomons NW, Briceno RP, Mata MR. Lactase and placebo in the management of the irritable bowel syndrome: a double-blind, cross-over study. Am J Gastroenterol 1989; 84:756–762.
147. Fernandez-Banares F, Esteve-Pardo M, de Leon R, et al. Sugar malabsorption in functional bowel disease: clinical implications. Am J Gastroenterol 1993; 88:2044–2050.
148. Sciarretta G, Fagioli G, Furno A, et al. 75SeHCAT test in the detection of bile acid malabsorption in functional diarrhea and its correlation with small bowel transit. Gut 1987; 28:970–975.
149. Merrick MV, Eastwood MA, Ford MJ. Is bile acid malabsorption underdiagnosed? An evaluation of accuracy of diagnosis by measurement of SeHCAT retention. Br Med J 1985; 290:665–668.
150. Snape WJ Jr, Carlson GM, Cohen S. Colonic myoelectric activity in the irritable bowel syndrome. Gastroenterology 1976; 70:326.
151. Wald A, VanThiel D, Hoechstetter L, et al. Gastrointestinal transit: the effect of the menstrual cycle. Gastroenterology 1981; 80:1497–1500.
152. Knanna R, Browne R, Heiner A, et al. Leuprolide acetate affects intestinal motility in female rats before and after ovariectomy. Am J Physiol 1992; 262:G185–G190.
153. Cann P. Approach to the design of therapeutic trials in IBS. Scand J Gastroenterol 1987; suppl 130: 67–76.
154. Sullivan M, Cohen S, Snape W. Colonic myoelectrical activity in irritable bowel syndrome: Effect of eating and anticholinergics. N Engl J Med 1978; 298:878.
155. Lanfranchi G, Bazzocchi G, Campiere M, et al. Reduction by cimetropium bromide

of the colonic motor response to eating in patients with the irritable bowel syndrome. Eur J Clin Pharm 1988; 33:571.
156. Ivey K. Are anticholinergics of use in the irritable colon syndrome? Gastroenterology 1975; 68:1300.
157. Page J, Dirnberger G. Treatment of the irritable bowel syndrome with Bentyl (dicyclomine hydrochloride). J Clin Gastroenterol 1981; 3:153.
158. Group GPR. Irritable colon syndrome treated with an antispasmodic drug. Practitioner 1976; 217:276.
159. Piai G, Mazzacca G. Prifinium bromide in the treatment of the irritable colon syndrome. Gastroenterology 1979; 77:500.
160. Centonze V, Imbimbo B, Campanozzi F, et al. Oral cimetropium bromide, a new antimuscarinic drug, for long-term treatment of irritable bowel syndrome. Am J Gastroenterol 1988; 83:1262.
161. Dobrilla G, Imbimbo B, Piazzi L, et al. Long term treatment of irritable bowel syndrome with cimetropium bromide: a double-blind placebo-controlled clinical trial. Gut 1990; 81:355.
162. Frexinos J, Fioramonti J. Bueno L. Effect of trimebutine on colonic myoelectrical activity in IBS patients. Eur J Clin Pharmacol 1985; 28:181.
163. Narducci F, Bassotti G, Granata M, et al. Colonic motility and gastric emptying in patients with irritable bowel syndrome. Dig Dis Sci 1986; 31:241.
164. Awad R, Dibildox M, Pietrasanta C. Randomized double-blind placebo-controlled trial of pinaverium bromide: rectoanal electromechanical response to food in irritable bowel syndrome. Gastroenterology 1992; 102:A419.
165. Sun WM, Edward CA, Prior A, et al. Effect of oral nicardipine on anorectal function in normal human volunteers and patients with irritable bowel syndrome. Dig Dis Sci 1990; 35:885–890.
166. Prior A, Harris SR, Whorwell PJ. Reduction of colonic motility by intravenous nicardipine in irritable bowel syndrome. Gut 1987; 28:1609.
167. Christen MO. Action of pinaverium bromide, a calcium-antagonist, on gastrointestinal motility disorders. Gen Pharm 1990; 21:821–825.
168. Connell A. Physiological and clinical assessment of the effect of the musculotropic agent mebeverine on the human colon. Br Med J 1965; 2:848.
169. Tasman-Jones C. Mebeverine in patients with the irritable colon syndrome: double blind study. NZ Med J 1973; 77:232.
170. Kruis W, Weinzierl M, Schussler P, et al. Comparison of the therapeutic effect of wheat bran, mebeverine and placebo in patients with irritable bowel syndrome. Digestion 1986; 34:196.
171. Luttecke K. A trial of trimebutine in spastic colon. J Intern Med Res 1978; 6:68.
172. Moshal M, Herron M. A clinical trial of trimebutine (Mebutin) in spastic colon. J Intern Med Res 1979; 7:231.
173. Fielding J. Double blind trial of trimebutine in the irritable bowel syndrome. Ir Med J 1980; 73:377.
174. Baldi F, Corinaldesi R, Ferrarini F, et al. Clinical and functional evaluation of octilonium bromide in the treatment of irritable bowel syndrome: a double-blind controlled trial. Clin Trials J 1983; 20:77.

175. Villagrasa M, Boix J, Humbert P, et al. Aleatory clinical study comparing otilonium bromide with a fiber-rich diet in the treatment of irritable bowel syndrome. Ital J Gastroenterol 1991; 23(suppl 1):67.
176. Baldi F, Longanesi A, Blasi A, et al. Octylonium bromide in the treatment of the irritable bowel syndrome: a clinical-functional study. Hepato-Gastroenterol 1992; 39:392.
177. Poynard T, Naveau S, Mory B, Chaput J. Meta-analysis of smooth muscle relaxants in the treatment of irritable bowel syndrome. Aliment Pharmacol Ther 1994; 8:499–510.
178. Maxton DG, Whorwell PJ. Effect of intra-colonic nicardipine on colonic motility in irritable bowel syndrome. Alim Pharm Ther 1990; 4:305–308.
179. Passaretti S, Sorghi M, Colombo E, et al. Motor effects of locally administered pinaverium bromide in the sigmoid tract of patients with irritable bowel syndrome. Int J Clin Pharm Ther Tox 1989; 27:47–50.
180. Defrance P, Casini A. A comparison of the action of otilonium bromide and pinaverium bromide: study conducted under clinical control. Ital J Gastroenterol 1991; 23:64–66.
181. Perez-Mateo M, Sillero C, Cuesta A, et al. Diltiazem in the treatment of the irritable bowel syndrome. Int J Clin Pharmacol Res 1986; 6:425.
182. Hills J, Aaronson P. The mechanism of action of pepperment oil on gastrointestinal smooth muscle. Gastroenterology 1991; 101:55–65.
183. Rees W, Evans B, Rhodes J. Treating irritable bowel syndrome with peppermint oil. Br Med J 1979; 2:835–836.
184. Dew M, Evans B, Rhodes J. Peppermint oil for the irritable bowel syndrome: a multicentre trial. Br J Clin Prac 1984; 38:394–398.
185. Nash P, Gould S, Barnardo D. Peppermint oil does not relieve the pain of irritable bowel syndrome. Br J Clin Pract 1986; 40:292–293.
186. Hall G, Thompson H, Strother A. Effects of orally administered activated charcoal on intestinal gas. Am J Gastroenterol 1981; 75:192–196.
187. Potter T, Ellis C, Levitt M. Activated charcoal: in vivo and in vitro studies of effect on gas formation. Gastoenterology 1985; 88:620–624.
188. Jain N, Patel V, Pitchumoni C. Efficacy of activated charcoal in reducing intestinal gas: a double-blind clinical trial. Am J Gastroenterol 1986; 81:532–535.
189. Wald A, Van Thiel DH, Hoechstetter L. et al. Gastointestinal transit: the effect of the menstrual cycle. Gastroenterology 1981; 30:1497–1500.
190. Wald A, Van Thiel DH, Hoechstetter L, et al. Effect of pregnancy on gastrointestinal transit. Dig Dis Sci 1982; 27:1015–1018.
191. Khanna R, Browne RM, Heiner AD, et al. Leuprolide acetate affects intestinal motility in female rats before and after ovariectomy. Am J Physiol 1992; 262:G185–90.
192. Mathias JR, Ferguson KL, Clench MH. Debilitating "functional" bowel disease controlled by leuprolide acetate, gonadotropin-releasing hormone (GnRH) analog. Dig Dis Sci 1989; 34:761–766.
193. Rabin D, McNeil LW. Pituitary and gonadal desensitization after continuous luteinizing hormone-releasing hormone infusion in normal females. J Clin Endocrinol Metab 1980; 51:873–876.

194. Mathias J, Clench M, Reeves-Darby V, et al. Effect of leuprolide acetate in patients with moderate to severe functional bowel disease: Double-blind, placebo-controlled study. Dig Dis Sci 1994; 39:1155–1162.
195. Mathias JR, Clench MH, Roberts PH, Reeves-Darby VG. Effect of leuprolide acetate in patients with functional bowel disease: long-term follow-up after double-blind, placebo-controlled study. Dig Dis Sci 1994; 39:1163–1170.
196. Wood J. Efficacy of leuprolide in treatment of the irritable bowel syndrome. Dig Dis Sci 1994; 39:1153–1154.
197. Heiner AM, Browne RM, Khanna P, et al. Effect of centrally administered leuprolide acetate on myoelectric activity of the small intestine in rats. Gastroenterology 1989; 96:A202.
198. Talley N. Review article. 5-hydroxytryptamine agonists and antagonists in the modulation of gastrointestinal motility and sensation: clinical implications. Aliment Pharmacol Ther 1992; 6:273.
199. Schuster M. Irritable bowel syndrome. In: Fordtran SA, ed. Gastrointestinal Disease: Pathophysiology, Diagnosis and Management. 6th ed. 1993; 917–933.
200. Muller-Lissner S. Effect of wheat bran on weight of stool and gastrointestinal transit time: a meta analysis. Br Med J 1988; 296:615.
201. Fioramonti J, Bueno L. Motor activity in the large intestine of the pig related to dietary fibre and retention time. Br J Nutr 1980; 43:155.
202. Toskes PP, Connery KL, Ritchey TW. Calcium polycarbophil compared with placebo in irritable bowel syndrome. Aliment Pharmacol Ther 1993; 7:87–92.
203. Longstreth G, Fox D, Youkeles L, et al. Psyllium therapy in the irritable bowel syndrome: A double-blind trial. Ann Intern Med 1981; 95:53.
204. Lucey M, Clark M, Lowndes J, et al. Is bran efficacious in irritable bowel syndrome? A double blind placebo controlled crossover study. Gut 1987; 28:221.
205. Cook I, Irvine E, Campbell D, et al. Effect of dietary fiber on symptoms and rectosigmoid motility in patients with irritable bowel syndrome. Gastroenterology 1990; 98:66–72.
206. Arffmann S, Andersen J, Hegnhoj J, et al. The effect of coarse wheat bran in the irritable bowel syndrome: A double-blind cross-over study. Scand J Gastroenterol 1986; 20:295.
207. Soltoft J, Gudmand-Hoyer E, Krag B, et al. A double-blind trial of the effect of wheat bran on symptoms of irritable bowel syndrome. Lancet 1976; i:270.
208. Prior A, Whorwell P. Double blind study of ispaghula in irritable bowel syndrome. Gut 1987; 28:1510.
209. Reyntjens A, Verlinden M, Schuurkes J, et al. New approach to gastrointestinal motor dysfunction: non-antidopaminergic, non-cholinergic stimulation with cisapride. Curr Ther Res 1984; 36:1029.
210. Koop H, Monnikes H, Koop I, et al. Effect of the prokinetic drug cisapride on gastrointestinal hormone release. Scand J Gastroenterol 1986; 21:907.
211. Janssens J, Peeters TL, Vantrappen G, et al. Improvement of gastric emptying in diabetic gastroparesis by erythromycin: preliminary studies. N Engl J Med 1990; 322:1028.
212. Van Nueten J, Schuurkes J. Stimulating effects of cisapride on isolated preparations

of stomach, small and large intestine of the guinea pig. Gastroenterology 1984; 86:1288.
213. Costall B, Naylor R. 5-hydroxytryptamine: new receptors and novel drugs for gastrointestinal motor disorders. Scand J Gastroenterol 1990; 25:769.
214. Gershon M, Wade P, Kirchgessner A, et al. 5-HT receptor subtypes outside the central nervous system: Roles in the physiology of the gut. Neuropsychopharmacology 1990; 3:385.
215. McCallum R, Prakash C, Campoli-Richards D, et al. Cisapride: A preliminary review of its pharmacodynamic and pharmacokinetic properties, and therapeutic use as a prokinetic agent in gastrointestinal motility disorders. Drugs 1988; 36:652.
216. Lee KY, Chey WY, You CH, et al. effect of cisapride on the motility of gut in dogs and colonic transit time in dogs and humans (abstr). Gastroenterology 1984; 86:1157.
217. Krevsky B, Malmud L, Maurer A, et al. The effect of oral cisapride on colonic transit. Alim Pharm Ther 1987; 1:293.
218. Lederer P, Ellermann A, Schmidt H, et al. Effect of cisapride on sigmoid motility in healthy subjects and in diabetic enteropathy with constipation. Digestion 1986; 34:155.
219. Baeyens R, Reyntjens A, Verlinden M. Cisapride accelerates gastric emptying and mouth-to-caecum transit of a barium meal. Eur J Clin Pharmacol 1984; 27:315.
220. Edwards C, Holden S, Brown C, et al. Effect of cisapride on the gastrointestinal transit of a solid meal in normal human subjects. Gut 1987; 28:13.
221. Van Wyk M, Sommers D, Steyn A. Evaluation of gastrointestinal motility using the hydrogen breath test. Brit J Clin Pharmacol 1985; 20:479.
222. Passaretti S, Tittobello A, Capozzi C, Verlinden M. Cisapride accelerates total intestinal transit in patients with irritable bowel syndrome-associated constipation. Progr Med 1987; 43(suppl 1):121–129.
223. Van Outryve M, Milo R, Toussaint J, et al. "Prokinetic" treatment of constipation-predominant irritable bowel syndrome: a placebo-controlled study of cisapride. J Clin Gastroenterol 1991; 13:49.
224. Longo W, Vernava A. Prokinetic agents for lower gastrointestinal motility disorders. Dis Colon Rectum 1993; 36:696.
225. Milo R. Use of the peripheral dopamine antagonist, domperidone, in the management of gastrointestinal symptoms in patients with irritable bowel syndrome. Curr Med Res Opin 1980; 6:577–584.
226. Fielding JF. Domperidone treatment in the irritable bowel syndrome. Digestion 1982; 23:125–127.
227. Cann PA, Read NW, Holdsworth CD. Oral domperidone: Double blind comparison with placebo in irritable bowel syndrome. Gut 1983; 24:1135–1140.
228. Peeters T, Matthijis G, Depoortere I, et al. Erythromycin is a motilin receptor agonist. Am J Physiol 1989; 257:G470–474.
229. Bailey LD Jr, Stewart WR Jr, McCallum RW. New directions in the irritable bowel syndrome. Gastrointest Clin North Am 1991; 20:335–349.
230. Kaufman PN, Krevsky B, Malmud LS, et al. Role of opiate receptors in the regulation of colonic transit. Gastroenterology 1988; 94:1351–1356.
231. Ruoff HJ, Fladung B, Demol P, Weihrauch TR. Gastrointestinal receptors and drugs in motility disorders. Digestion 1991; 48:1–17.

232. Fotherby KJ, Hunter JO. Idiopathic slow-transit constipation: whole gut transit times, measured by a new simplified method, are not shortened by opioid antagonists. Aliment Pharmacol Ther 1987; 1:331–338.
233. Kreek MJ, Paris P, Bartol MA, Mueller D. Effects of short term administration of the specific opioid antagonist naloxone on fecal evacuation in geriatric patients. Gastroenterology 1984; 86:1144A.
234. Rustgi VK, Maguire M, Wise TN, Cooper JN. Naltrexone use in the irritable bowel syndrome (abstr). Gastroenterology 1985; 88:1563.
235. Talley NJ, Weaver AL, Zinsmeister AR, Melton LJ. Functional constipation and outlet delay: a population-based study. Gastroenterology 1993; 105:781–790.
236. Camilleri M, Thompson WG, Fleshman JW, Pemberton JH. Clinical management of intractable constipation. Ann Intern Med 1994; 121:520–528.
237. Burks TF. Actions of drugs on gastrointestinal motility. In: Johnson LR, ed. Physiology of the Gastrointestinal Tract. Vol 1. New York: Raven Press, 1987:723–743.
238. Konturek SJ. Opiates and the gastrointestinal tract. Am J Gastoenterol 1980; 74:285–291.
239. Lavo B, Stenstam M, Nielsen A-L. Loperamide in treatment of irritable bowel syndrome—a double blind placebo controlled study. Scand J Gastroenterol 1987; 130(suppl):81.
240. Havdenak N. Loperamide treatment of the irritable bowel syndrome. Scand J Gastroenterol 1987; 130(suppl):81.
241. Cann PA, Read NW, Holdsworth CD, Barends D. Role of loperamide and placebo in management of irritable bowel syndrome (IBS). Dig Dis Sci 1984; 29:239–247.
242. Schiller LR, Hogan RB, Morawski SG, et al. Studies of the prevalence and significance of radiolabeled bile acid malabsorption in a group of patients with idiopathic chronic diarrhea. Gastroenterology 1987; 92:151–160.
243. Merrick MV, Eastwood MA, Ford MJ. Is bile acid malabsorption underdiagnosed? An evaluation of accuracy of diagnosis by measurement of SeHCAT retention. Br Med J 1985; 290:665–668.
244. Talley N, Phillips S, Haddad A, et al. GR 38032F (ondansetron), a selective 5-HT3 receptor antagonist, slows colonic transit in healthy man. Dig Dis Sci 1990; 35:477.
245. Moss HE, Sanger GJ. ICS 205-930 and ondansetron on the visceral pain reflex induced by duodenal distension. Br J Pharmacol 1990; 100:497–501.
246. Maxton D, Haigh C. Whorwell P. 5-HT3 antagonists: a role in irritable bowel syndrome and non-ulcer dyspepsia? (abstr). Gut 1991; 32:A1228.
247. Steadman C, Talley N, Phillips S, et al. Selective 5-hydroxytryptamine type 3 receptor antagonism with ondansetron as treatment for diarrhea-predominant irritable bowel syndrome: a pilot study. Mayo Clin Proc 1992; 67:732.
248. Prior A, Read N. Reduction of rectal sensitivity and post-prandial motility by granisetron, a 5HT3 receptor antagonist, in patients with irritable bowel syndrome (IBS). Gut 1993; 7:175.
249. Hammer J, Phillips SF, Talley NJ, Camilleri M. Effect of a 5HT3-antagonist (ondansetron) on rectal sensitivity and compliance in health and the irritable bowel syndrome. Aliment Pharmacol Ther 1993; 7:543–551.

14

Patient Advocacy and Self-Help Groups

Nancy J. Norton
International Foundation for Bowel Dysfunction
Milwaukee, Wisconsin

I. INTRODUCTION

Functional gastrointestinal (GI) disorders affect millions of people daily. The impact of these disorders is felt not only by the individual but also by his or her family, and by society as a whole. The rates of work and school absenteeism and visits to physicians are higher for those having a functional GI disorder. There is evidence that having a functional GI diagnosis will often lead to more physician visits than will a non-GI diagnosis (1).

Gastroenterologists report that more than 50% of their practice is devoted to patients with functional GI disorders. Functional bowel disorders, in particular, are very common and chronic, with irritable bowel syndrome (IBS) occurring in 10 to 20% of people (2). In the United States, IBS is two to five times more common in females. The disorder is found at all ages, but the highest rates occur between the ages of 45 and 64 years (3). Additionally, individuals who suffer from IBS will miss an average of 13.4 work days as opposed to the 4.9 national average (1), further contributing to higher health care costs and loss in productivity.

"I thought I was the only one." As the director and founder of the International Foundation for Bowel Dysfunction (IFBD), a nonprofit educational and research organization, I have heard these words over and over from people with bowel dysfunction or incontinence. They live in silence with their disorder, afraid or embarrassed to discuss it with family or friends. Feelings of shame may have kept them from discussing their symptoms with their own physician. Those who have talked about it, or sought help, may have been met with a lack of understanding or sensitivity. Perhaps they have been made to feel that their disorder is their own fault or told that they "just have to live with it."

Although millions of people suffer from these disorders, there is a lack of public information available through the media. Talking about a bowel problem often makes others uncomfortable, at the least. The general perception is that there is a psychosomatic association with these disorders. It is little wonder that otherwise healthy people with bowel dysfunction keep silent about it. Thinking that they suffer some unique disorder, they may remain unaware of what is causing their symptoms and what they can do about it.

In 1993, the IFBD began organizing public-education symposia and support and self-help groups for people interested in learning more about functional bowel disorders, particularly IBS and incontinence. Initially, we were uncertain of the response such an organization would receive from the public. Would people want to be actively involved in a self-help group? How close an association did people want with a group that was clearly labeled for those with bowel dysfunction?

We quickly found that those with a functional bowel problem were truly grateful for an opportunity to learn more about these disorders. For many, it was the first time they could talk to someone who understood exactly what they were experiencing. In Milwaukee alone, hundreds of people attend each of our public meetings. Requests for our programs come in from people around the United States. In this chapter I share some of what we have learned.

A. Why a Self-Help Organization?

Bowel dysfunction, disordered defecation, and incontinence are all topics that are extremely difficult for people to talk about. Many people who suffer from these disorders are reluctant to acknowledge their symptoms to anyone. They may be reluctant to discuss them even with their own physician. Personal, social, and economic relationships may be severely compromised by this condition. As a result, many people find themselves living in self-imposed isolation.

A stigma is associated with incontinence, in particular. Feelings of shame and embarrassment can be overwhelming for people. Rather than risk an embarrassing situation, many people limit their activities. Maintaining a job can be difficult. A feeling that their life is ruled by their bowel is predominant in the minds of many who live with these disorders. The constant uncertainty surrounding bowel control can cause anxiety, depression, and anger.

Functional bowel disorders result from a myriad of causes. The desire to resolve the symptoms can drive a person into a frustrating journey of physician visits, often with little or no result. Often, people are told that these disorders are something "you will just have to live with" or, worse, that it is "all in your head." Increasingly, medical professionals are working to change these viewpoints and find answers to the questions surrounding functional bowel disorders. Management and treatment options are available, and those who live daily with IBS, constipation, diarrhea, or incontinence need guidance to learn about them. Support is essential in learning to cope with the emotional roller coaster often caused by these disorders.

If a support network is not available, people can seek help through individual counseling. However, most therapists have not experienced a bowel disorder or incontinence. Although counseling can be helpful, those with severe functional disorders need to talk to someone who has experienced what they are going through. They need to find someone who knows exactly what is meant when they say that they feel like a prisoner in their own home, or that they fear going out because they are uncertain about having access to a bathroom. There is a need to talk to someone who truly understands that incontinence and irritable bowel can affect every aspect of a person's life, causing constant worry about losing bowel control. A person with a functional bowel disorder can easily feel that his or her life is as out of control as their bowel.

B. Community Education

IFBD's educational efforts have been focused on promoting awareness of the incidence of these disorders as well as treatment options for those affected. Most people are surprised to learn how common these disorders are. For example, the general perception regarding fecal incontinence is that it is exclusive to the older adult. The reality is that it affects a significant number of men, women, and children of all ages.

Awareness and education concerning IBS are especially challenging. IBS sufferers often hear the words "It's all in your head." Yet they experience very real physiological symptoms in their gut. The severity of the symptoms often triggers a psychological response that only adds to the complexity of the disorder.

Unfortunately, there is very little knowledge surrounding the pathogenesis of functional bowel disorders, and their classification is based solely on symptoms. Because of this, there historically has been a reluctance to legitimize these disorders, presenting a frustrating situation for both the patient and the physician. We are beginning to see an emergence of more research and validation of functional bowel disorders as awareness and education increase. It is important for a physician to recognize that patients with a functional bowel disorder may need more time devoted to them. The symptoms they experience are complex and need to be sorted through.

Addressing the social stigma associated with these disorders is a big challenge. Public information is essential. A major goal of the IFBD is to work toward a day when people will no longer feel compelled to hide these disorders.

II. SUPPORT GROUPS AND SELF-HELP GROUPS

A primary purpose in the development of the IFBD was to provide support for people affected by functional disorders. That support first took the form of a newsletter, *Participate*. Published quarterly, it serves as a forum in which people can express their concerns and voice their needs, and provides access to much needed information about these disorders.

The foundation evolved gradually. I attended two medical meetings with our first newsletter and a brochure describing the mission of the organization for distribution to medical professionals. As a result, nearly 100 physicians requested our newsletter to offer their patients. Word slowly began to spread of the existence of the IFBD. In the beginning we received only about 20 phone calls per week and about the same number of letters. We now receive at least that many per day from people asking about self-help and support groups. We did not expect the requests for such groups to happen as quickly as they have. In response to this need, we have developed a model for an IFBD support program.

I was fortunate enough to attend the first workshop on IBS sponsored by the National Institutes of Health in 1992. At that meeting I met Dr. Barry Blackwell, who was also from Milwaukee. We discussed the possibilities of developing a model for a support program and began working on it immediately—Dr. Blackwell and his colleagues in the University of Wisconsin GI department had already assessed the need for such a program.

With the support of Sinai Samaritan Medical Center in Milwaukee, we were able to sponsor the first public symposium on functional bowel disorders. The hospital covered the expenses for a meeting room, advertising, and printing the agenda. We were able to get a local home-health-care company to furnish refreshments. We offered a small exhibit space for vendors and the IFBD had a table filled with our publications. The program focused on IBS and fecal incontinence. The agenda included the following topics:

- Medical evaluation and treatment of IBS
  - Signs and symptoms
  - Anatomy and physiology of the digestive system
  - Medical evaluation of the bowel and treatment
- New developments in treatment of functional bowel disorders

Bowel incontinence: etiology, treatment and biofeedback
Emotional aspects and support groups

Our speakers included gastroenterologists, psychiatrists, psychologists, specialists in behavioral medicine, continence specialists with an expertise in biofeedback and bowel management, and a pharmacist.

Much to the surprise of everyone, nearly 300 people attended the first program. We now sponsor this type of educational program regularly and have incorporated it into our IFBD Support Program Guidelines. This program continues to draw several hundred people with every presentation.

We found that there was considerable interest beyond this educational program for a more personalized support group. We have put together a model for a support group that could be offered by any hospital or clinic interested in sponsoring an IFBD support program. The model was a collaborative effort by Dr. Barry Blackwell, Kathleen Traub, R.N., and me. The basis of the model was the personal experience we all brought, as well as what we felt were the key issues to be addressed in a group of this nature. We also developed and utilized a questionnaire at the public symposium to get more input about people's needs regarding a support group. The following issues were identified:

Information and a better understanding of functional bowel disorders
Help in coping with bowel disorders
How to control the stress, anxiety, depression, and fear that result from bowel dysfunction
How to deal with a functional disorder in the workplace and at home with family and friends
Feelings of frustration and lack of understanding from physicians

With a professional facilitator from behavioral medicine, we developed an 8-week support group. The participation and interest generated from the support group can lead to the formation of a self help chapter of the IFBD.

Historically, peer- and professionally led self-help groups have embraced a set of beliefs that include the following:

Group members experience feelings of shared identity and common concern.
The group process emphasizes mutual aid through discussion and sharing of experiences.
The group focuses on activities that help members achieve successful management or resolution of the concern.
Small fees collected from members are directed toward group maintenance.
Networking ensures that members stay in touch.

Groups are self-governing.
Groups are open without restrictions to those who share the concern.

An IFBD chapter becomes the self-help group. The group consists of those affected by functional bowel disorders and their family and friends. A self-help group can be led by an affected person. The chapter sponsors a monthly meeting for all those who are interested. Educational speakers, a question-and-answer period, or an open forum for discussion can be offered. The opportunity for socialization is also important for those in the group, because many have limited social activities because of their disorder.

III. DEVELOPING AN 8-WEEK SUPPORT GROUP: THE IFBD EXPERIENCE

Our support groups have a professional facilitator from mental health with a knowledge of GI disorders. It is also important that the facilitator be knowledgeable in the group process. I feel it is imperative to have this combination of skills to facilitate an IFBD support group.

The people attending the support group usually have overlapping symptoms ranging from motility disorders to extreme psychosocial issues. The facilitator needs to be a trained professional with an understanding of the complexities of these disorders.

The groups have approximately 15 people. The members are diverse, with different lifestyles, ages, and levels of coping with a functional bowel disorder. Initially, we expected that individuals would be reluctant or embarrassed to talk about what has historically been a socially unacceptable topic. Instead, we have discovered that people are so eager for a receptive, understanding, nonjudgmental, and tolerant audience that it is often difficult to follow a structured format in the first meeting. People want not only to relate their own story but also to feel validated, not alone, and, most of all, not "crazy." For some people, attending the first session is all they need.

Over the course of 8 weeks, we provide an opportunity for people to gain more insight into the complexities of functional bowel disorders. At the beginning of each session, every participant answers the questions "How are you feeling physically and how are you feeling emotionally?" Our goals include realizing the brain–gut connection, offering relaxation techniques, and providing supportive information about assertiveness and getting one's needs met. Topics of discussion include everyday living with a functional disorder that encompasses loss of control and dignity, altered body image, reduced physical activity, dietary restrictions, and social disruption.

It is important to be aware that each individual in the group will have a different presentation of symptoms and psychosocial history, and a different combination of levels of wellness, productivity, coping skills, and, most importantly, feeling in control of his or her life.

Frequently, questions are asked about the nature of functional disorders and their causes and effects. There is also often inquiry about medications—their effectiveness, how they work, and the side effects. We provide supporting educational material, including newsletters, fact sheets, and brochures, at every group meeting. People are eager to become more knowledgeable about their disorder. The more information they have, the more in control of the situation they feel. There is less of a tendency to feel that their life is ruled by their bowel.

The experience and outcome of being in an IFBD support group are different for each participant. Some people realize that they need more individualized therapy, one-on-one. The group offers a safe environment in which to bring out issues that many may never have spoken about. Some members will talk about abuse issues and sexual dysfunction; clearly these people may benefit from a more personalized form of therapy. For those who recognize they could benefit from further therapy, the group is a source of encouragement. The idea of seeking further treatment is less threatening and no longer a confirmation that "it's all in your head."

Many people undergo physiological tests that are unsettling. Other members who have been through the same tests can appreciate the sense of anxiousness that surrounds any diagnostic procedure.

As the weeks go by, the support group comes into its own. The members feel comfortable with one another, sharing information that they had initially been hesitant to voice. They begin to become aware of the factors that exacerbate their own bowel symptoms and can recognize them in other group members. The group experience is a powerful motivator for many people. They recognize how the bowel disorder influences them individually and in relationships with others. By sharing information, they begin to understand the kind of skills they need to develop for coping with their disorder.

The benefits gained are recognized by all the members. They have a better understanding of their disorder and seem to feel less anxious about symptoms. Many feel that they understand the brain–gut connection and that they are more in control. Often, people will begin to increase their social activities and be less reluctant to avoid situations that in the past had created feelings of uncertainty.

IV. GOALS AND DIRECTION OF THE IFBD

As a result of our experiences since 1992, we have developed a support program that works through the cosponsorship of a hospital, clinic, or other medical group coordinated with a medical advisor. A facility may provide any or all levels of sponsorship depending on the need and the desired outcome. The levels of sponsorship include the following:

Public symposium
Support group (8-week session)—professional facilitator
Self-help group (ongoing)—regional or local Chapter of IFBD

Progress is being made toward an important goal of the IFBD as our support programs are initiated; we are seeing more awareness of functional disorders. They are being written about in newspapers and magazines. People with the disorders have always been quietly among us, hoping for answers, unsure of where to look, or afraid to describe their symptoms. Now we have an organization, easily accessible to people, that can provide information and a source of support.

V. ENCOURAGEMENT AND HOPE

The nature of functional bowel disorders can lead to feelings of isolation. People often contact the IFBD with the comment, "I thought I was the only one." They are relieved and encouraged to discover that they are not. Knowing that they are not alone can be tremendously comforting. As they become better educated about their bowel, they often feel empowered, and able to take an active part in their own health care. By sharing experiences, people learn how others manage their bowel disorder and gain helpful insights and practical advice for everyday living with the disorders. When offered a nonjudgmental atmosphere for discussion, people with bowel disorders exhibit a genuine willingness to share experiences and to help one another.

Hopefully, future medical research will unravel some of the mysteries surrounding functional bowel disorders and incontinence. The International Foundation for Bowel Dysfunction remains committed to the millions of people affected by these disorders and the need for educational information and support services.

REFERENCES

1. Drossman DA, et al. U.S. householder survey of functional gastrointestinal disorders: prevalence, sociodemography and health impact. Dig Dis Sci 1993; 38:1569.
2. Drossman DA. The Functional Gastrointestinal Disorders. Boston: Little, Brown, 1994.
3. Everhart JE. Digestive Diseases in the United States: Epidemiology and Impact. Bethesda, MD: National Institutes of Health, 1994.

15

Psychopharmacological Interventions for Functional Bowel Disease

R. Bruce Lydiard
Medical University of South Carolina
Charleston, South Carolina

I. INTRODUCTION

The use of psychopharmacological agents in the treatment of functional gastrointestinal (GI) disorders arises, in part, from clinical observations that individuals presenting for treatment for these disorders appear to exhibit a high prevalence of concurrent psychiatric morbidity. Additionally, scientific data have accumulated over the years to support the concept that there is an intimate interaction between the central nervous system (CNS) and the enteric nervous system (ENS) on a more or less continuous basis, and that the brain and the gut can mutually influence each other. Since this association is a key aspect of evaluation of patients with functional GI disorders, this chapter reviews the association of functional GI disorders and psychiatric illness in treatment-seeking patient samples, and examines the prevalence of medically unexplained GI symptoms in a large community sample of individuals screened for psychiatric disorders. An overview of the brain–gut interaction is presented. Based on these data, a model is presented that suggests practical guidelines for the use of psychopharmacological agents in the treatment of functional GI disorders in patients with and without concomitant psychiatric disorders.

II. ASSOCIATION OF FUNCTIONAL GI DISORDERS AND PSYCHIATRIC DISORDERS

The prevalence of functional GI disorders in the general population is high. As many as 69% of a community sample met criteria for one of the 25 functional GI disorders in a 3-month period (1). The most information about the prevalence of psychiatric disorders in samples of patients with functional GI disorders is available from studies of irritable bowel syndrome (IBS), non-ulcer dyspepsia (NUD), esophageal motility disorders, and functional abdominal pain. These patients are often nonresponsive to standard treatments, and are consulting a specialist in a secondary or tertiary referral center. Accordingly, it is difficult to extrapolate this information to the general population of individuals who suffer from functional GI disorders (2). On the other hand, psychopharmacological treatment for patients with functional GI disorders is considered relatively often in the small population of individuals who are assessed in these secondary- or tertiary-care settings (1).

A. IBS and Psychiatric Illness

IBS is a common and often debilitating functional GI disorder, affecting 8–17% of the general population (1). Individuals suffering from IBS are defined as having continuous or recurrent symptoms for at least 3 months of abdominal pain or discomfort, relieved with defecation or associated with a change in frequency or consistency of stool, disturbed defecation, and at least three of the following: altered stool frequency or form, altered stool passage (straining or urgency, incomplete evacuation), passage of mucus, bloating, or feelings of abdominal distension. There are no physical findings or laboratory abnormalities indicative of an organic etiology. Diagnostic features are shown in Table 1. IBS is a chronic condition that commonly begins in early adulthood and affects females approximately twice as often as males (3).

IBS is associated with significant morbidity, and it is estimated that IBS ranks second only to the common cold as a cause of work absenteeism; the total cost in the United States for this disorder, including medical evaluation, treatment, and disability/lost work, is estimated to be as much as $1 billion per year (4). Drossman et al. (1) reported that over half of a sample of individuals in a nonpatient population who met criteria for a functional bowel disorder had never been to a doctor. Those not seeking health care had better coping patterns and

TABLE 1 Symptom Criteria for IBS

Recurrent symptoms (over at least 3 months):
Abdominal pain
Typically relieved with defecation
Change in frequency or consistency of stool
and/or
Disturbed defecation (three or more of the following at least 25% of the time):
Change in stool frequency
Change in stool form (hard or loose/watery)
Change in stool passage (straining or urgency, feeling of incomplete evacuation)
Passage of mucus
Bloating or sensation of abdominal distension

Additional laboratory investigation (e.g., complete blood count, erythrocyte sedimentation rate) and a sigmoidoscopy (fiber-optic) should be completed to ensure that inflammatory bowel or other pathology is not present. Additional tests, if any, are based on clinical indications (7).

fewer abnormal personality patterns, and experienced less disruption due to their symptoms. Several investigators have identified factors that may contribute to health-care-seeking behavior; these include psychological and psychosocial factors (5–11).

Of the published studies to date that assessed psychiatric diagnoses in patients with IBS utilizing standardized interview techniques, to date only three (12–14) have applied the DSM-IIIR criteria (15). Prior to the DSM-IIIR, there was a diagnostic hierarchy that excluded the mutual diagnoses of anxiety and depression. We reported several years ago the common occurrence of prominent GI symptoms in patients suffering from panic disorder (16) (see Table 2 for current diagnostic criteria (17), which are similar to those in DSM-III). In that report we noted an unusually high prevalence (42%) of anxiety-related discomfort, cramping, and diarrhea in patients with panic disorder. Five patients with panic disorder who were diagnosed and treated for IBS experienced apparent resolution of IBS and panic disorder symptoms with effective antipanic treatment. We subsequently conducted structured psychiatric interviews on a series of patients with IBS, utilizing a Structured Clinical Interview for DSM-IIIR (SCID) (18).

We found that 94% of the patients had a lifetime history of a major psychiatric illness. Over 80% were currently psychiatrically ill, primarily with anxiety and mood disorders; many of these patients were unaware of their psychiatric diagnosis. Walker and colleagues (14) reported findings in a blinded study compar-

TABLE 2 Panic Disorder

A discrete episode, usually lasting no longer than 30 minutes and peaking within 10 to 15 minutes, with intense fear/discomfort. At least four of the following symptoms occur (usually several are present):
Palpitations increase heart rate
Sweating
Tremulousness or shaking
Shortness of breath/air hunger
Choking or difficulty swallowing
Chest pain, tightness/discomfort
Nausea, abdominal discomfort/cramping, urgency to defecate
Dizziness, unsteady sensation, lightheadedness, or feeling faint
Feelings of unreality (derealization), being detached from oneself depersonalization)
Fear of loss of control of one's mind or body
Fear of dying or imminent catastrophe
Paresthesias
Hot flushes and/or chills
For at least 1 month after a panic attack, affected individuals experience fearful anticipation or its implications (e.g., fear of heart attacks, stroke, insanity) or alter their behavior because of these concerns (for example, repeated medical evaluations).

ing patients with inflammatory bowel disease (ulcerative colitis and Crohn's disease) with patients with IBS. Similar to our findings, in that sample over 90% of the patients with IBS had a lifetime prevalence of psychiatric disorder, predominantly mood and anxiety disorders. Interestingly, they found a 29% prevalence of panic disorder in that sample. In contrast, Blanchard and colleagues (12) found less psychopathology in a treatment-seeking group of IBS patients presenting to a psychology-based stress-management center. It appears, then, that treatment-seeking IBS patients who present to medical centers often suffer from concomitant psychiatric conditions, and that panic disorder is common in this population.

B. Post-Traumatic Stress Disorder

Recent reports indicate that there is a significant association between sexual and physical abuse and IBS, as well as other functional bowel disorders. Sexual and physical-assault history have been identified as a second potentially important determinant of health-care-seeking behavior in IBS patient samples. Drossman and colleagues (19) administered a self-report questinonaire to 206 patients at a

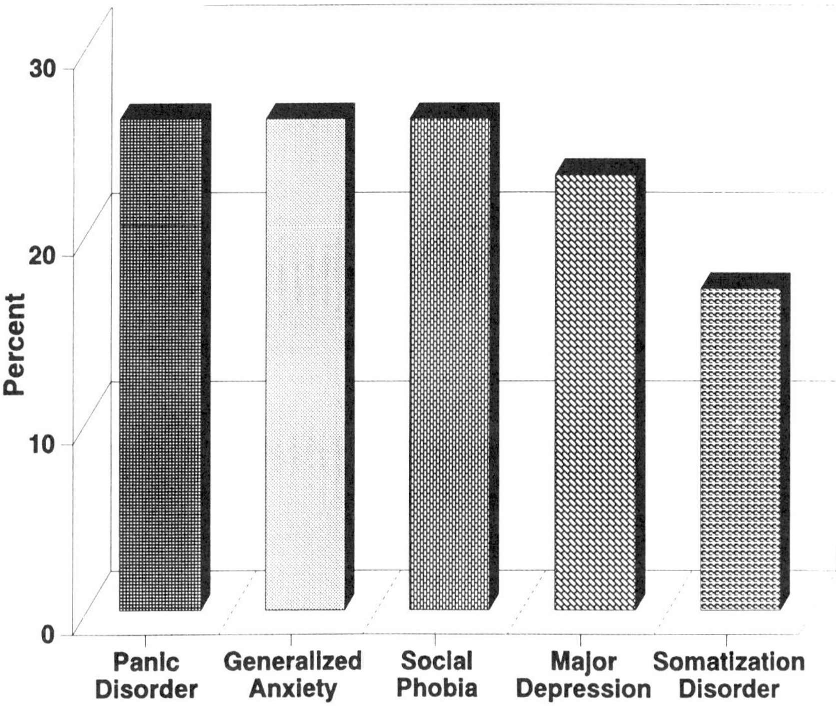

Figure 1 Prevalence of DSM-IIIR psychiatric disorders in IBS patients. (Some had more than one diagnosis.)

university-based gastroenterology clinic and found that patients with functional GI disorders, particularly IBS, had a significantly higher rate of physical and sexual trauma in childhood or later in life than a comparable sample with organic illness. A second report, by Felitti (20), reviewed records from a health maintenance organization. They found that individuals who had affirmatively answered a screening question about rape or sexual molestation were significantly more likely to have IBS than a comparison group who answered negatively to the question of sexual trauma. Walker and his colleagues (21) have also recently reported that prevalence of a history of sexual victimization was significantly higher in IBS patients (55%) than in a control group with inflammatory bowel disease (5%). Patients with IBS had more medically unexplained symptoms and psychiatric disorders than the control group with inflammatory bowel disease. Lechner et al. (22) reported increased rates of unexplained GI complaints in patients who acknowledged a history of abuse. In a group of patients receiving treatment at the Mayo Clinic, Talley and colleagues reported that females with GI symptoms were 2.8 times more likely to have a functional rather than structural bowel disorder if they had an abuse history. Finally, Scarinci et al. (23) reported rates of abuse history of 82% in patients with IBS.

Our group recently reported the prevalence of Post-Traumatic Stress Disorder (PTSD) in treatment-seeking patients with IBS (see Table 3) (24). That survey, which included structured interviews for major psychiatric disorders, revealed a 36% rate of PTSD. The most common histories included sexual (26%) and/or physical abuse (22%) as the identified stressors initiating the disorder. It is important to note that this is a conservative estimate of the abuse history of these patients, since only those who satisfied DSM-IIIR diagnostic criteria were included; those with a history of victimization who did not develop PTSD were not represented. Whether health-care-seeking is higher in PTSD victims than in those with victimization who do not meet diagnostic thresholds for PTSD is an important, but unanswered, question. It appears that a history of victimization may be an important determinant of health-care-seeking behavior. Individuals with a history of abuse were more likely to have surgery with normal findings, visit a physician, or be hospitalized (19–25). Because history of sexual or physical abuse is associated with health-care-seeking and utilization, as is suggested by these studies, the importance of recognizing

TABLE 3 Posttraumatic Stress Disorder

Exposure to a traumatic event that:
- The patient experienced, witnessed, or was confronted with that involved threat (real or believed to be real) to the physical safety of self or others
- Provoked intense fear, helplessness, or horror
- Is persistently reexperienced:
  - Recurrent and intrusive distressing recollections
  - Recurring distressing dreams
  - Acting or feeling as if the traumatic event were recurring
  - Intense distress at exposure cues that recreate, even in part, the traumatic event

Avoidance of stimuli associated with the trauma or numbing of general responsiveness; avoidance of thoughts, feelings, or conversations related to the trauma or activities, locations, or people that remind individual of the trauma; often unable to recall some important aspect of the trauma; loss of interest or participation in significant activities; detachment or estrangement; constricted range of affect; doesn't think or plan about the future

Persistent posttraumatic arousal: sleep disturbance, irritability or anger, has difficulty concentrating, notable hypervigilance, easily startled

Duration of symptoms of more than 1 month

Significant interference in social, occupational, or other roles patients with an abuse history is an important part of the evaluation of individuals with functional GI disorders. This would be particularly important in the evaluation of treatment-resistant patients for whom psychopharmacological intervention is being considered.

C. IBS in Psychiatric Patients

We surveyed 68 patients who met DSM-IIIR criteria for panic disorder with or without agoraphobia who were entering treatment studies in our Anxiety Disorders Program, applying the criteria noted in Table 1 for IBS (26). No additional laboratory or endoscopic evaluations that had not already been completed were obtained. Of these, 28 (41%) met diagnostic criteria for IBS. Improvement in GI symptoms closely paralleled improvement in panic symptoms. Similarly, Noyes and colleagues (27) recently reported that a group of patients with panic disorder exhibited a high frequency of IBS-like symptoms that abated in conjunction with effective treatment for panic. Tollefson and colleagues (28) recently described an unexpectedly high prevalence of IBS in patients with generalized anxiety disorder (37%) (see Table 4 for diagnostic criteria for generalized anxiety disorder) and in patients with major depression (29%) (see Table 5 for diagnostic criteria for major depression) relative to normals (11%). They also described improve-

Table 4 Generalized Anxiety Disorder

Excessive worry most days for at least 6 months, about a number of life circumstances
The worry persists, and is not well-controlled
Symptoms present most days: restlessness or feeling keyed up or on edge, fatigue, subjective complaints of concentrating and/or mind going blank, irritability, muscular tension, sleep disturbance

Table 5 Major Depression

Depressed mood or loss of interest or pleasure with a total of at least five symptoms:
Significant weight change
Significant sleep change
Psychomotor change
Loss of energy
Worthlessness or excessive or inappropriate guilt
Difficulty thinking or concentrating
Suicidal ideation
Nearly every day, most of the day for at least 2 weeks

ment in psychiatric symptoms in conjunction with IBS-like symptoms with effective treatment for the psychiatric disorder. Thus, in both treatment-seeking IBS patients and treatment-seeking psychiatric patients, particularly those with panic disorder, there appears to be a diagnostic overlap between GI symptoms and psychiatric illness. Importantly, the limited data suggest that when IBS and a psychiatric disorder coexist, treatment of the psychiatric disorder often results in relief of IBS-related symptoms. More recently, Olden and colleagues (29) reported, in a sample of patients with obsessive-compulsive disorder, a 44% prevalence of IBS (see Table 6). Finally, recent data from our Anxiety Disorders Program indicate that a significant percentage of patients with anxiety disorders have IBS (30). These included panic disorder (44%), generalized anxiety disorder (20%), social phobia (20%) (see Table 7 for diagnostic criteria for social phobia), and normal (8%).

TABLE 6 Obsessive-Compulsive Disorder

Obsessions

- Recurrent, persistent, intrusive thoughts, images, or impulses experienced as senseless, repulsive (e.g., fear of harming loved ones or others or fear of contamination or of leaving stove on, disturbing sexual thoughts or urges)
- The individual is unable to ignore or suppress them
- The individual clearly sees these as coming from his or her own mind

Compulsions

- Repetitive, ritualistic behaviors (e.g., washing, checking) or mental rituals (e.g., counting, repeating words)
- The rituals, even if they don't make sense to the individual, are intended to neutralize or prevent the feared consequence
- Obsessions and compulsions interfere with some aspect of functioning of the individual and/or cause marked distress.

TABLE 7 Social Phobia

Significant fear/avoidance of one or more social situations in which the individual is exposed to possible scrutiny by others.

- The socially phobic individual fears that he or she will behave in a way—or show symptoms of anxiety—that will be humiliating or embarrassing.
- The feared situation almost invariably provokes anxiety, which may take the form of a panic attack.
- The affected individual recognizes that the social fear is excessive or Phobic avoidance, fearful or anxious anticipation, or distress related to these social situation(s) interferes significantly with the person's occupational, family, or social activities.

D. Psychiatric Disorders and GI Symptoms in a Nonpatient Sample: Findings from the NIMH Epidemiological Catchment Area Project

Studies to date suggest that there is a tendency for individuals with psychological/psychiatric distress to seek treatment, while those with similar functional GI symptoms without psychological distress and better coping skills did not become patients (31). Since we had found a high rate of IBS in treatment-seeking patients with panic disorder, we were interested in finding out whether there was a similar association in a non-treatment-seeking sample of individuals with panic disorder compared with other psychiatric disorders (32). To assess medically unexplained GI symptoms in a nonpatient, community-based sample, we surveyed the prevalence of GI symptoms in individuals with panic disorder, other anxiety disorders, other psychiatric disorders, or no psychiatric disorders, using data obtained in a national community survey. At four sites of the NIMH Epidemiological Catchment Area (ECA) project, the prevalence of psychiatric diagnoses was determined using the Diagnostic Interview Schedule (DIS) for 13,537 respondents. GI symptoms were assessed from the somatization (30) disorder section of the DIS. Such an approach would allow for examination of this association without the potential confounding effect of "treatment-seeking bias," which has been thought to underlie the high prevalence rates of anxiety and other psychiatric disorders in treatment-seeking samples of IBS patients.

The ECA project is an epidemiological study of the rates and risks of psychiatric disorders conducted between 1980 and 1984. The DIS is a highly structured interview designed to be used by lay interviewers in epidemiological studies and generates DSM-III diagnoses of psychiatric disorders (33). Also included in the DIS are questions about the occurrence of several GI symptoms in the somatization disorder section; for example, "Have you ever had a lot of trouble with [nonmenstrual] abdominal or belly pain?" Similar questions were asked about frequent vomiting, nausea without vomiting, diarrhea, constipation, abdominal or stomach bloating, and becoming sick from certain foods.

In addition to the specific GI symptoms, the proportion of subjects who endorsed the combination of symptoms that approximated the diagnostic criteria for IBS (i.e., abdominal pain, diarrhea and/or constipation, abdominal bloating) was assessed. It should be noted that these symptoms may not necessarily have occurred concurrently in those individuals endorsing this IBS composite.

A total of 194 persons from the four sites had a lifetime DIS/DSM-III diagnosis of panic disorder, a weighted mean rate of 1.5%; 2438 persons had another anxiety disorder (phobia or obsessive-compulsive disorder), a weighted mean rate of 15.3%. A total of 1932 persons had another psychiatric disorder excluding panic, phobia, and obsessive-compulsive disorder (weighted prevalence, 15.8%), and 8973 persons had never had a psychiatric disorder (weighted prevalence, 67.4%).

The lifetime prevalence of the GI symptoms in the respondents was as follows: abdominal pain, 6.2%; vomiting, 1.8%; nausea, 4.2%; diarrhea, 3.5%; stomach bloating, 6.8%; sickness from certain foods, 2.8%; constipation, 6.9%; IBS-like symptoms, 0.8%. The general demographic profile of a person endorsing any unexplained GI item was a white, married woman aged 18–44, in the mid-socioeconomic range.

Persons with panic disorder had the highest rate of unexplained GI symptoms compared to those in the other diagnostic classifications (see Figure 2). The rates of unexplained GI symptoms in persons with panic disorder versus no panic disorder was statistically significant for all the GI symptoms except for "becoming sick from certain foods." Notably, there is a 4.7-fold increased risk

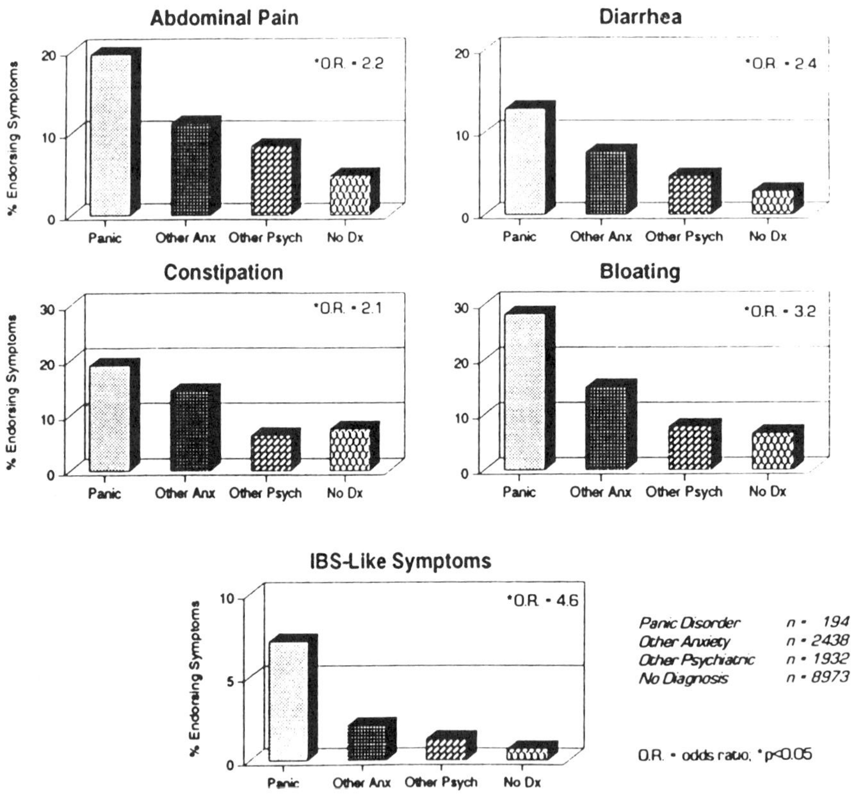

Figure 2 Prevalence of unexplained GI symptoms in a community sample of individuals with psychiatric disorder or no psychiatric disorder. OR = odds ratio; $p < .05$; panic disorder $n = 194$, other anxiety, $n = 2438$; other psychiatric disorder, $n = 1932$; no diagnosis, $n = 8973$.

for persons with panic disorder to report nausea without vomiting compared to persons without panic disorder; there is a 4.6-fold increased risk for persons with panic disorder to have the IBS-like composite of symptoms compared to persons without panic disorder.

We are aware of the numerous limitations to this study, most of which are obvious. Within these limitations, however, a survey of a large, well-selected, nonclinical sample of subjects suggests that GI symptoms are reported significantly more frequently by subjects with panic disorder. The analysis did not include specific examination of the other psychiatric disorders, but Figure 2 suggests that the lowest prevalence was in individuals who had never been psychiatrically ill, and the highest was in patients with anxiety disorders in general. Our data suggest that the coexistence of panic disorder and psychiatric IBS may represent true diagnostic overlap between these two disorders. The data also suggest that IBS-like symptoms are more common in individuals with psychiatric disorders than in those with no psychiatric disorder. There is evidence that treatment of a coexisting psychiatric disorder in individuals with IBS results in alleviation of both psychiatric and GI symptoms in many patients (see below). Therefore, discerning the presence of a psychiatric disorder in patients with IBS and other functional GI disorders may provide important clues for treatment planning.

E. Other Functional GI Disorders

While it is clear that there is a high prevalence rate in the general population of the 25 functional GI disorders (1), the literature regarding the association of psychiatric illness and other functional bowel disorders is considerably less rich than for IBS.

Esophageal Disorders

There are few data regarding the prevalence of psychiatric disorders in individuals with esophageal disorders. The most carefully conducted study to date was reported by Clouse and Lustman (34). They found that there was a considerable prevalence in individuals with documented esophageal dysmotility: major depression, 52%; generalized anxiety disorder, 36%; panic disorder, 4%; somatization disorder, 20%, social phobia, 4%. Eighty-four percent (84%) of the total sample had a current psychiatric disorder. Richter and colleagues (35) found that individuals with "nutcracker" esophagus exhibited more psychological distress than controls without esophageal complaints. Noncardiac chest pain, which often accompanies esophageal motility disorders, has been associated with psychiatric disorders. A significant body of work by Beitman and colleagues has indicated that a significant percentage of individuals with normal coronary arteries verified by angiography suffer from panic disorder (36,37), and that these individuals can respond to pharmacological intervention (38).

Non-Ulcer Dyspepsia

Investigations regarding the association of non-ulcer dyspepsia (NUD) have suggested that there is a significant prevalence of psychiatric disorders in these individuals. Using a self-rating method, Kane et al. (39) reported that individuals with NUD satisfied criteria for generalized anxiety disorder (70%), panic disorder (30%), and major depression (35%). The authors concluded that NUD symptoms in treatment-seekers was "strongly related to psychiatric diagnosis." Similar findings were reported by Magni and colleagues (40), who examined 30 patients with dyspepsia of unknown origin and 30 with known etiology for dyspeptic symptoms. They found that the individuals with dyspepsia of unknown origin had a significantly higher current prevalence of 86.7% of DSM-III psychiatric diagnoses (53.3% had generalized anxiety disorder) vs. a total of 25% of the patients with known etiology for dyspepsia ($p < 0.001$). Not all researchers, however, have concluded that NUD is associated with psychiatric disorders or stressful life events. Talley and colleagues (41–46) examined a variety of aspects of prior stressful life events, both retrospectively and prospectively, and found relatively few differences in the histories of patients and controls—in fact, in one study (41), controls had experienced more bereavement than NUD patients. This group also examined the psychological characteristics of individuals with NUD vs. various PUD and nondyspeptic control groups, and could not identify clinically meaningful differences in illness behavior, neuroticism, or other psychological characteristics. Minor increases in chronic anxiety, neuroticism, and depression were noted in patients with NUD and PUD vs. healthy community controls, but these were not felt to be of clinical significance (41–44). Finally, examination of the childhood experiences of individuals with NUD vs. controls did not provide any information that discriminated NUD patients from controls (45). It may be that cultural differences in the settings in which these various studies were carried out, as well as the methodology employed, could account for some of the differences in study results noted above. Clearly, additional examination of the psychiatric aspects of patients with NUD could shed further light on the question of whether there is clinically significant psychiatric morbidity in these patients and, if so, whether treatment would benefit thte symptoms of NUD.

Functional Abdominal Pain

It is clear that pain of various types, including functional abdominal pain, can be exacerbated by psychosocial factors. For some individuals, abdominal pain can be a symptom of depression or anxiety. Functional abdominal pain, if it coexists with a psychiatric disorder, may respond to treatment of the disorder to some extent. After ruling out physical causes, examination of psychosocial factors and assessment of the psychiatric disorder may provide clues for the most appropriate intervention (46). In one series of patients with functional abdominal pain, most of whom were female, hypochondriasis, depression, and histrionic personality disorder were identified (46). Many had symptoms associated with a significant loss in their lives. None had sought psychiatric help, although four eventually had psychiatric hospitalizations. Only one patient experienced resolution of symptoms, but half did show some improvement in psychosocial functioning. Treatment with psychotropic medication targeted at pain control (47) is indicated after more conservative treatments have been utilized. The prognosis for individuals with psychogenic abdominal pain is guarded (46). One recent report, however, documented improvement in a woman with functional abdominal pain in the absence of any apparent psychiatric disorder who was treated with fluoxetine (48).

III. BRAIN–GUT INTERACTIONS

As noted above, there may be a more fundamental relationship between functional GI disorders and certain psychiatric disorders than previously appreciated. There have been some interesting advances in our understanding of how the brain and gut communicate with respect to stress. Anxiety/stress responses are mediated in part via the septohippocampal area, the amygdala component of the limbic system, and midbrain central gray areas (49). The hypothalamus receives input from these areas, integrating the input and orchestrating the appropriate set of autonomic and somatic responses, including output to the gut via sympathetic and parasympathetic pathways (50,51).

The enteric nervous system (ENS), a rich neuronal network in the gut, is an elaborate neuronal structure that has been referred to as the "little brain" or the third division of the autonomic nervous system. The vast majority of the vagal fibers connecting the gut and central nervous system (CNS) are afferent fibers bringing information to the CNS (50). The ENS appears to function somewhat autonomously, and can maintain many important GI functions even when connections with the CNS have been severed, including reflex and other sophisticated activities (2,52). The ENS is similar to the CNS in several ways, including the presence of interneurons, a myenteric–blood barrier (analogous to the blood–brain barrier), the presence of glial cells instead of Schwann cells usually found on peripheral nerves, and numerous neurotransmitters and neuropeptides also found in the CNS (53). The recent description of the anxiogenic properties of cholecystokinin, a "gut" peptide, is of interest (54).

One recently described and potentially important link between the CNS and the GI system may be at the level of a pontine noradrenergic nucleus, the locus ceruleus, which has been postulated to mediate some aspects of fear and arousal states, including panic disorder (54,55). This nucleus receives afferent input from the gut such that perturbation of the bladder, bowel, or stomach may cause increased neuronal firing of this noradrenergic nucleus (55). This suggests a possible model for brain–gut interaction in which patients with anxiety disorders such as panic disorder may experience GI distress as part of the sympathetic discharge, with resultant afferent input back to the locus ceruleus (and/or other important brain areas), potentially creating a vicious positive-feedback circle. Patients with IBS or certain psychiatric conditions such as anxiety or depression also often complain of numerous autonomic symptoms, suggesting that there may be some common pathophysiology, perhaps in part at the level of this noradrenergic nucleus (15). Interestingly, many psychiatric medications (tricyclic and monoamine oxidase inhibitor antidepressants, benzodiazepines) that are effective in reducing panic attacks appear to reduce the firing rate and/or sensitivity of this nucleus to afferent input (56). This model may help explain why there appear to be significant anxiety symptoms in patients with unexplained GI symptoms (15,57). Disturbed CNS function (locus ceruleus or other areas) may affect the GI system via neuronal and neurohumoral pathways with resulting GI symptoms and distress; GI motility disturbance, via feedback to arousal centers at the CNS, may cause psychiatric symptoms such as anxiety; both may occur simultaneously and mutually exacerbate each other (15,57) (see Figure 3). Since the neuronal cells for both the ENS and CNS arise from the same embryonic source, it is not surprising that abnormal function of both the ENS and CNS would co-occur frequently. Clearly more study of the interplay between the gut/ENS and the CNS (in particular, the locus ceruleus) may be important in understanding the brain–gut interaction. However, based on this model, psychoactive agents that affect the sensitivity of the locus ceruleus to afferent input may have a place in treatment of individuals with IBS and psychiatric disorders, as well as of individuals with no psychiatric disorder.

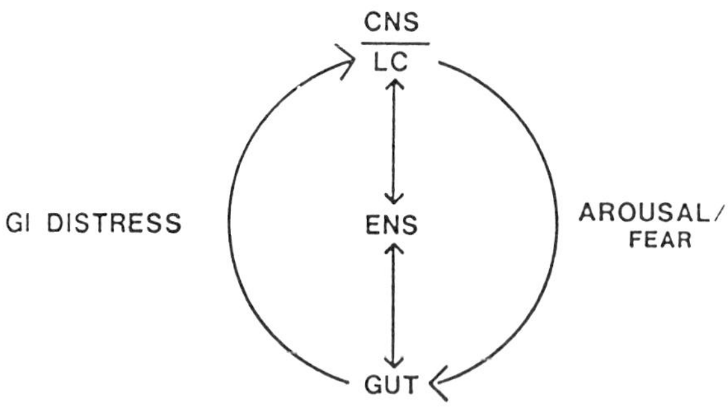

Figure 3 Brain–gut interaction. LC = locus cereleus; CNS = central nervous system.

IV. THEORETICAL AND PRACTICAL IMPLICATIONS OF BRAIN–GUT INTERACTION

Using the model described above, there are some potentially clinically useful strategies that may be suggested. For patients presenting to GI specialists with significant psychopathology, it appears from the limited data available that psychopharmacological treatment of the psychiatric disorder (most evidence is from patients with anxiety or mood disorders) may be associated with improvement in GI function as well.

A. Treatment of Functional GI Disorders: General Considerations

In general, nonpharmacological treatments are preferable. These include education, dietary discretion, stress-management techniques, and use of bulk/fiber products as the basis for conservative initial medical management (see Chapter 9). Drossman (8,31) has suggested several measures that may also be useful. Scheduling of regular appointments indicates interest on the part of the treating clinician as well as commitment for the long term. Education about the nature of the disorder being evaluated is important, especially about its being a chronic or intermittent condition that will probably require long-term management. In our experience, providing information about the nature of the illness and making a positive diagnosis can reassure patients that they do not have a structural lesion such as a cancer. Reorientation toward reasonable treatment goals—such as improvement in functioning rather than complete relief from all symptoms—may be useful. Psychotherapy may be indicated for some patients with severe psychosocial stressors (see Chapter 9). However, a substantial percentage of patients, particularly those with significant anxiety or mood symptoms, achieve only partial relief from these treatments. Treatment with psychopharmacological agents may be a useful adjunct in such patients. The use of psychoactive medications for GI disorders should be based on clinical judgment. The presence of a psychiatric disorder is an indication for treatment regardless of whether the specific GI symptoms will be improved. Thus, the decision to recommend treatment for a patient with a functional GI disorder with psychopharmacological agents is based on several observations. The majority of the available data are derived from a relatively small, scientifically controlled literature. In the sections below, the limited treatment literature is reviewed.

B. Esophageal Motility Disorders

Clouse (47) has recently reviewed the psychopharmacological treatment of patients with chest pain of presumed esophageal origin. The rationale for the use of psychotropic medications is based on the observations that 1) there are similarities between esophageal pain disorders and other functional pain disorders, including IBS, 2) there are recognized psychophysiological effects of psychotropic medications on esophageal motor mechanisms, and 3) that there are frequently (>70%) coexisting psychiatric disorders in patients with functional esophageal disorders. In a group of patients with documented esophageal motility disorders, Clouse and colleagues (58) treated a group of individuals with trazodone (100–150 mg/day). In this controlled study, motility patterns did not change, but there was a significant reduction in both GI and emotional symptoms reported by the subjects compared with placebo treatment.

Other psychopharmacological interventions may be useful, such as anxiolytics or antidepressants, based on the specific psychiatric symptoms present. It should be mentioned that benzodiazepines and antidepressants with anticholinergic effects may impair saliva secretion and reduce lower-esophageal-sphincter pressure and acid clearance (47). Since esophageal dysmotility can present as chest pain, patients may initially visit a cardiologist or internist for evaluation. A recent report by Cannon and colleagues at the NIH (59) indicated that in patients with chest pain but normal coronary arteriograms, treatment with imipramine (50 mg h.s.), but not clonidine or placebo, effected a statistically significant 50% reduction in chest-pain episodes. Patients included in this study also had concomitant esophageal motility disorders (41%), psychiatric disorders (63%), and abnormal electrocardiographic response to exercise (22%), but none of the above predicted response to treatment. The authors hypothesized that imipramine had a visceral analgesic effect rather than a psychotropic benefit in these patients with normal coronary arteries and chest pain.

C. Functional Abdominal Pain Syndromes

Psychoactive drugs have been utilized in a variety of pain syndromes, and often result in significant improvement in symptoms (60). Psychopharmacological approaches to pain in functional GI disorders may be indicated in a variety of situations (61). By extrapolation, for patients who have significant pain—a frequent concomitant of functional GI disorders—treatment for this component may be indicated. Most of the available literature on chronic pain includes reports of the effects of tricyclic antidepressants. These agents have known beneficial effects, but also have a significant side-effects burden, including significant anticholinergic effects. Trazodone, a second-generation antidepressant, has beneficial effects in pain syndromes and no significant anticholinergic effects. Newer agents that are selective and potent inhibitors of serotonin may also be beneficial in treatment of pain syndromes. One study (46) reported beneficial effects of fluoxetine in a patient with chronic abdominal pain. Agents that modify visceral afferent transmission include the tricyclic antidepressants (TCAs) (imipramine, amitriptyline, and others), selective serotonin reuptake inhibitors (SSRIs) such as fluoxetine, sertraline, paroxetine, fluvoxamine, and clomipramine (the last is both a tricyclic and serotonin-selective). Nefazodone, an atypical antidepressant with serotonin and norepinephrine reuptake inhibition and post-synaptic serotonin receptor (type 2) blockade, also may have clinical utility in pain syndromes.

D. IBS

A number of studies have employed neuroactive medications in patients with functional GI disorders, including various tricyclic and nontricyclic antidepressants and benzodiazepines. The majority of the treatment literature focuses on IBS. Unfortunately, almost all studies conducted to date have been methodologically flawed (62). Many of the studies suggest that these medications were helpful; however, the specific benefits reported in these studies varied. For example, Greenbaum et al. (63) noted that desipramine treatment of IBS patients was most effective for diarrhea-predominant IBS, but that these effects were not seen in the group as a whole and data were affected by the order of treatments used. Interestingly, the pain complaints of the patient group were significantly improved relative to those of the control subjects in that study. Similarly, the study by Clouse and colleagues (58) indicated improvement in esophageal pain complaints and sense of well-being, but no motility change was demonstrated. Treatment of IBS patients with benzodiazepines has occurred only in conjunction with other treatments. In one study (64), benefits from various combinations of benzodiazepines, bulk, and antispasmodics were reported. However, the placebo response rate was probably 0% in that study, leaving open questions about the study blind and other methodological factors. Despite the significant literature indicating that treatment-seeking patients with functional GI disorders commonly suffer from psychiatric disorders, attention to psychiatric diagnosis has been absent from almost all treatment studies published to date.

E. Non-Ulcer Dyspepsia

The prevalence of psychiatric disorders in treatment-seeking individuals with NUD appears to be high, as was mentioned earlier. There are no systematic studies utilizing psychotropic medications in NUD. Tricyclic antidepressants reduce baseline acid secretion, presumably via histamine receptor blockade. However, effects of TCAs, which also reduce esophageal-sphincter pressure, are difficult to predict on an individual patient basis. It would seem reasonable to complete a trial with a TCA in patients with NUD, particularly those with concomitant psychiatric disorders that would benefit from treatment, but, unfortunately, no controlled data are available. Similarly, the SSRIs, which could be helpful in treating concomitant psychiatric syndromes, can apparently cause dyspepsia in some patients as a side effect, particularly early in treatment. Again, individual psychopharmacological trials must be used to determine if a specific agent is helpful, but if a psychiatric disorder is present, it is strongly recommended that treatment for the disorder be given.

V. PSYCHOPHARMACOLOGICAL TREATMENT APPROACHES

Since the substantial majority of the information is from the literature on IBS, this syndrome will be used as a model for the use of psychopharmacological treatment of functional GI disorders. Recognition of the presence of a mood or anxiety disorder in a treatment-resistant IBS patient can be difficult. However, considering that the likelihood of a coexisting psychiatric disorder is, conservatively, 70%, the clinician should make every attempt to detect if one is present. The following section contains an admixture of information derived from the literature as well as my clinical experience.

A. IBS Patients with Panic Disorder

As reviewed above, there appears to be a significant percentage of treatment-seeking IBS patients with panic disorder. In particular, this group of patients may have significant avoidance behavior, often based on fear of loss of bowel control and anticipated embarrassment. It may be helpful for the clinician to inquire about patient concerns regarding limitations imposed by the IBS symptoms, and encourage patients who may be reluctant to take medication to comply with suggested interventions.

If conservative management strategies for patients with coexisting panic disorder provide inadequate control of symptoms, the traditional antipanic agents may be particularly useful. These include high-potency benzodiazepines such as alprazolam, which has been shown to be effective in panic disorder (65) and specifically in patients with IBS-like symptoms (27), or clonazepam, a long-acting potent benzodiazepine. Dosage requirements for alprazolam in panic disorder range from 0.5 mg t.i.d. to 8 mg per day; for clonazepam, 0.25 to 2 mg b.i.d. Of course, other benzodiazepines would also be likely to show similar benefit in these patients in equipotent doses. Because patients with panic disorder often experience concomitant depression, antidepressants are also useful—for example, for IBS patients with panic disorder with predominant diarrhea, imipramine or desipramine starting at dosages of 10 mg daily, increasing as tolerated. Because these patients are often quite activated by antidepressant agents, it is important to explain in advance that stimulation may occur, and to initiate treatment at very low dosages. It is sometimes necessary to use dosages in excess of 200 mg daily, but often patients will respond to lower dosages (see below).

For patients with sensitivity to anticholinergic effects (such as those with predominant constipation), agents such as fluoxetine, initiated at a low dose in the morning and increasing over several days or weeks to 20 per day, or sertraline, beginning at 25 mg in the morning and increasing to 50–100 mg over several days or weeks, may be a reasonable alternative. Paroxetine, which has some anticholinergic effects, may be useful for individuals with diarrhea-predominant or alternating constipation and diarrhea, beginning with 10 mg/day and rising to 30–50 mg/day. N efazodone, which has been clinically reported to have some antipanic effects, may also be a reasonable agent, beginning at 50 mg and increasing gradually to 300–500 mg given in two daily doses. The strategy for all patients is to initiate low dosages and increase as tolerated until the desired antipanic effect is achieved.

B. IBS Patients with Generalized Anxiety Disorder

Many IBS patients exhibit symptoms of generalized anxiety disorder (GAD) without panic attacks. For these patients, agents such as buspirone may be helpful, beginning in doses of 5 mg t.i.d., increasing to 30–60 mg daily as tolerated. To date there are no controlled data, but clinical experience suggests that it may be useful. Additionally, tricyclic antidepressants have been shown to be effective in GAD and may represent a useful alternative. Finally, for anxious patients with IBS and GI symptoms benzodiazepines have been shown in a recent open study to be effective in relieving both anxiety and GI symptoms in patients with combined GAD and IBS (66). Trazodone, which has been shown to be effective in treating GAD, and nefazodone, a newer antidepressant with anxiolytic properties, would also probably be useful, particularly since their effects on GI motility appear to be modest.

C. IBS Patients with Mood Disorders

Many patients in the treatment-seeking samples appear to exhibit major depression or depressive symptoms with significant frequency. As noted earlier, for patients with diarrhea-predominant IBS and panic, TCAs with anticholinergic properties, such as imipramine or desipramine, are particularly useful. Patients with constipation-predominant IBS may tolerate agents with less anticholinergic effects, such as fluoxetine, sertraline, paroxetine, or trazodone.

D. IBS Patients with PTSD

PTSD is a complex disorder with multiple symptoms. Pharmacological treatment represents only a part of the treatment plan (for review see Ref. 67). Treatment is aimed at: reduction of intermittent intrusive symptoms, improvement of avoidance behaviors, reduction of hyperarousal, relief of depression and anhedonia, and improved modulation of impulse control. Only a few double-blind, placebo-controlled studies have been complete din PTSD, and none detailed the presence or absence of IBS. To date, evidence suggests that the TCAs amitriptyline and imipramine are effective to some extent. These may be beneficial in patients with diarrhea-prone IBS. Fluoxetine has been shown to be effective in PTSD in reducing some symptoms, and may be useful in patients with constipation-predominant IBS, while clomipramine may be useful for those with diarrhea-predominant IBS.

E. IBS Patients with No Psychiatric Disorder

IBS patients without significant psychopathology may benefit from neuroactive agents, which may serve to attenuate the postulated positive-feedback circle between the gut and the brain that was outlined above. Using this schema, it is possible that agents that may reduce responsivity of the locus ceruleus may be useful. It should be mentioned that these agents, presumed to act primarily at the CNS level, may well have effects in the ENS, or "little brain." Clouse and colleagues (60) reported that in treatment-refractory IBS patients referred to a university-based gastroenterology practice, nearly half of whom had no psychiatric disorder, over 90% benefited from the addition of low-dose antidepressants or antianxiety agents. In this study, 92% of patients improved, 56% experienced complete remission of their IBS symptoms, and 44% experienced remission after the first medication trial. The reasons for a good response to psychotropic agents in individuals with IBS with no psychiatric illness are unclear. Attenuation of the "brain–gut" feedback loop or a reduction in afferent pain signals from the viscera distinct from this mechanism are both potential mechanisms. Finally, psychiatric syndromes (e.g., anxiety or mood disorders) that were "subdiagnostic" may have existed in some of these individuals and may also have been positively affected by treatment.

VI. CONCLUSIONS

It appears that treatment-seeking patients with functional GI disorders frequently present with concomitant psychiatric disorders. Findings to date suggest that knowledge about coexisting psychiatric illnesses in patients with IBS and other functional GI disorders may enable us to treat them more effectively. A model has been offered that suggests that in patients withou psychiatric disorders, neuroactive medications may be a useful tool in improving functioning in individuals with functional GI disorders who have not responded to standard, conservative treatments. Neuroactive medications may be useful in treating patients with IBS, particularly those with coexisting psychiatric illness. As more is learned about the interaction between the brain and the gut, additional helpful treatments will surely result.

REFERENCES

1. Drossman DA, Li Z, Andruzzi E, et al. U.S. Householder Survey of functional gastrointestinal disorders: Prevalence, sociodemography, and health impact. Dig Dis Sci 1993; 38:1569–1580.
2. Almy TP, Rothstein RI. Irritable bowel syndrome: classification and pathogenesis. Annu Rev Med 1987; 38:257–265.
3. Fielding JF. The irritable bowel syndrome. Part I: clinical spectrum. Clin Gastroenterol 1977; 6:607–622.
4. Whitehead WE, Schuster MM. Behavioral approaches to the treatment of gastrointestinal motility disorders. Med Clin North Am 1981; 65:1397–1411.
5. Sandler RS, Drossman DA, Nathan HP, et al. Symptom complaints and health care seeking behavior in subjects with bowel dysfunction. Gastroenterology 1984; 87:314–318.
6. Sandler RS, Drossman DA. Bowel habits in young adults not seeking health care. Dig Dis Sci 1987; 32:841–845.
7. Hislop IG. Psychological significance of the irritable colon syndrome. Gut 1971; 12:452–457.
8. Drossman DA. Psychosocial treatment of the refractory patient with irritable bowel syndrome (editorial). J Clin Gastroenterol 1987; 9:253–255.
9. Whitehead WE, Engel BT, Schuster MM. Irritable bowel syndrome: physiological and psychological differences between diarrhea-predominant and constipation-predominant patients. Dig Dis Sci 1980; 25:404–413.
10. Whitehead WE, Winget C, Fedoravicius AS, et al. Learned illness behavior in patients with irritable bowel syndrome and peptic ulcer. Dig Dis Sci 1982; 27:202–208.
11. Young SJ, Alpers DH, Norland CC, et al. Psychiatric illness and the irritable bowel syndrome: Practical implications for the primary physician. Gastroenterology 1976; 70:162–166.
12. Blanchard EB, Scharff L, Schwarz SP, et al. The role of anxiety and depression in the irritable bowel syndrome. Behav Res Ther 1990; 28:401–405.
13. Lydiard RB, Fossey MD, Marsh W, et al. Prevalence of psychiatric disorders in patients with irritable bowel syndrome. Psychosomatics 1993; 34:229–234.
14. Walker EA, Roy BP, Katon WJ, et al. Psychiatric illness and irritable bowel syndrome: a comparison with inflammatory bowel disease [see comments]. Am J Psychiatry 1990; 147:1656–1661.
15. Diagnostic and Statistical Manual for Mental Disorders. 3rd ed, revised. Washington, DC: American Psychiatric Press, 1987.
16. Lydiard RB, Laraia MT, Howell EF, et al. Can panic disorder present as irritable bowel syndrome? J Clin Psychiatry 1986; 47:470–473.
17. Diagnostic and Statistical Manual for Mental Disorders. 4th ed. Washington, DC: American Psychiatric Press, 1994.
18. Spitzer R, Williams J, Gibbon M, et al. Structured Clinical Interview for DSM-IIIR, 1990.
19. Drossman DA, Leserman J, Nachman G, et al. Sexual and physical abuse in women with functional or organic gastrointestinal disorders. Ann Intern Med 1990; 113:828–833.

20. Felitti V. Longterm medical consequences of incest, rape and molestation. South Med J 1991; 84:328–331.
21. Walker EA, Katon WJ, Roy BP, et al. Histories of sexual victimization in patients with irritable bowel syndrome or inflammatory bowel disease. Am J Psychiatry 1993; 150:1502–1506.
22. Lechner M, Vogel M, Garcia-Shelton L, et al. Self-reported medical problems of adult female survivors of childhood sexual abuse. J Fam Pract 1993; 36:633–638.
23. Scarinci I, Haile J, Bradley L, et al. Altered pain perception and psychosocial features among women with gastrointestinal disorders and history of abuse. Am J Med 1994; 97:108–118.
24. Irwin C, Lydiard R, Emmanuel N, et al. Comorbidity of post traumatic stress disorder and irritable bowel syndrome. Anxiety Disorders Association of America, Charleston, SC, March 1993.
25. Sedney M, Brooks B. Factors associated with a history of childhood sexual experience in a nonclinical female population. J Am Acad Child Adolesc Psychiatry 1984; 9:889–895.
26. Lydiard RB, Fossey MD, Ballenger JC. Irritable bowel syndrome in patients with panic disorder (letter; comment). Am J Psychiatry 1991; 148.
27. Noyes RJ, Cook B, Garvey M, et al. Reduction of gastrointestinal symptoms following treatment for panic disorder. Psychosomatics 1990; 31:75–79.
28. Tollefson G, Tollefson SL, Pederson M, et al. Comorbid irritable bowel syndrome in patients with generalized anxiety and major depression. Ann Clin Psychiatry 1991; 3:215–222.
29. Olden K, Jenike M, Baer L. Is irritable bowel related to OCD? Annual meeting of the American Psychiatric Association, May 1993.
30. Johnson M, Lydiard R, Mintzer O, et al. Prevalence of irritable bowel syndrome in anxiety. American Anxiety Disorders Association of America, March 17–20, 1994.
31. Drossman DA, McKee DC, Sandler RS, et al. Psychosocial factors in the irritable bowel syndrome: A multivariate study of patients and nonpatients with irritable bowel syndrome. Gastroenterology 1988; 95:701–708.
32. Lydiard RB, Greenwald S, Weissman MM, et al. Panic disorder and gastrointestinal symptoms: findings from the NIMH Epidemiologic Catchment Area project. Am J Psychiatry 1994; 151:64–70.
33. Robins L, Regier D. Psychiatric Disorders in America. New York: The Free Press, 1991.
34. Clouse RE, Lustman LP. Psychiatric illness and contraction abnormalities of the esophagus. N Engl J Med 1983; 309:1337–1342.
35. Richter JE, Or W, Bradley LF. Psychological comparison of patients with nutcracker esophagus and irritable bowel syndrome. Dig Dis Sci 1986; 31:131–138.
36. Beitman BD, Basha IM, Trombka LH, et al. Alprazolam in the treatment of cardiology patients with atypical chest pain and panic disorder. J Clin Psychopharmacol 1988; 8:127–130.
37. Beitman BD. Panic disorder in patients with angiographically normal coronary arteries. Am J Med 1992; 92.
38. Beitman BD, Mukerji V, Flaker G, et al. Panic disorder, cardiology patients, and atypical chest pain. Psychiatr Clin North Am 1988; 11:387–397.

39. Kane FJ, Strohlein J, Harper RG. Nonulcer dyspepsia associated with psychiatric disorder. South Med J 1993; 86:641–646.
40. Magni G, F, DM, G, B et al. DSM-III diagnoses associated with dyspepsia of unknown cause. Am J Psychiatry 1987; 144:1222–1223.
41. Talley NJ, Piper DW. Major life event stress and dyspepsia of unknown cause: a case control study. Gut 1986; 27:127–134.
42. Talley NJ, Fung LH, Gilligan IJ, et al. Association of anxiety, neuroticism, and depression with dyspepsia of unknown cause: A case-control study. Gastroenterology 1986; 90:886–892.
43. Talley NJ, Piper DW. Comparison of the clinical features and illness behaviour of patients presenting with dyspepsia of unknown cause (essential dyspepsia) and organic disease. Aust NZ J Med 1986; 16:352–359.
44. Talley NJ, Piper DW. A prospective study of social factors and major life event stress in patients with dyspepsia of unknown cause. Scand J Gastroenterol 1987; 22:268–272.
45. Talley NJ, Jones, Mand Piper DW. Psychosocial and childhood factors in essential dyspepsia: A case-control study. Scand J Gastroenterol 1988; 23:341–346.
46. Drossman DA. Patients with psychogenic abdominal pain: six years' observation in the medical setting. Am J Psychiatry 1982; 139:1549–1557.
47. Clouse RE. Psychopharmacologic approaches to therapy for chest pain of presumed esophageal origin. Am J Med 1992; 92.
48. Eisendrath SJ, K, KT. Fluoxetine management of chronic abdominal pain. Psychosomatics 1992; 33:227–229.
49. Gray J. The neuropsychological basis of anxiety. In: Last CG, ed. Handbook of Anxiety Disorders. New York: Pergamon Press, 1988.
50. Nauta W, Fiertag M. Functional Neuroanatomy. New York: WH Freeman, 1986.
51. Kuperman I. Hypothalamus and limbic system. I. Peptidergic neurons, homeostasis and emotional behavior. In: Kandel SJ, ed. Principles of Neural Science. 2nd ed. New York: Elsevier Science Publishers, 1985.
52. Kelly J. Principles of the functional and anatomical organization of the central nervous system. In: Kandel SJ, ed. Principles of Neural Science. 2nd ed. New York: Elsevier Science Publishers, 1985.
53. Gershon MD. The enteric nervous system. Annu Rev Neurosci 1981; 4:227–272.
54. Bradwejn J, Koszycki, Dand Shriqui C. Enhanced sensitivity to cholecystokinin tetrapeptide in panic disorder: Clinical and behavioral findings. Arch Gen Psychhiatry 1991; 48:603–610.
55. Elam M, ST, Thoren P. Locus ceruleus in sympathetic nerves: activation by visceral afferents. Brain Res 1986; 375:117–125.
56. Uhde TW, Boulenger JP, Post RM, et al. Fear and anxiety: relationship to noradrenergic function. Psychopathology 1984; 3:8–23.
57. Fossey MD, Lydiard RB. Anxiety and the gastrointestinal system. Psychiatr Med 1990; 8:175–186.
58. Clouse RE, Lustman PJ, Eckert TC, et al. Low-dose trazodone for symptomatic patients with esophageal contraction abnormalities: A double-blind, placebo-controlled trial. Gastroenterology 1987; 92:1027–1036.

59. Cannon R, Quyyumi AA, Mincemoyer R, et al. Imipramine in patients with chest pain despite normal coronary angiograms. N Engl J Med 1994; 330:1411–1417.
60. Clouse RE, Lustman PJ, Geisman RA, Alpers DH. Antidepressant therapy in 138 patients with irritable bowel syndrome: a five-year clinical experience. Aliment Pharmacol Ther (England), Aug 1994; 8:409–416.
61. Egbunike I, Chaffee B. Antidepressants in the management of chronic pain syndromes. Pharmacotherapy 1990; 10:262–270.
62. Klein KB. Controlled treatment trials in the irritable bowel syndrome: a critique. Gastroenterology 1988; 95:232–241.
63. Greenbaum DS, Mayle JE, Vanegeren LE, et al. Effects of desipramine on irritable bowel syndrome compared with atropine and placebo. Dig Dis Sci 1987; 32:257–266.
64. Ritchie JA, Truelove SC. Treatment of irritable bowel syndrome with lorazepam, hyoscine butylbromide, and isphagula husk. Br Med J 1979; 1:376–378.
65. Ballenger JC, Burrows GD Jr, DR et al. Alprazolam in panic disorder and agoraphobia: results from a multicenter trial. I. Efficacy in short-term treatment. Arch Gen Psychiatry 1988; 45:413–422.
66. Tollefson GD, Luxenberg M, Valentine R, et al. An open label trial of alprazolam in comorbid irritable bowel syndrome and generalized anxiety disorder. J Clin Psychiatry 1991; 52:502–508.
67. Vargas M, Davidson J. Post-traumatic stress disorder. Psychiatric Clin North Am 1993; 16:737–748.

16

Biofeedback, Relaxation Training, and Cognitive Behavior Modification: Treatments for Functional GI Disorders

Ann L. Davidoff
Johns Hopkins University School of Medicine
Baltimore, Maryland

William E. Whitehead
University of North Carolina at Chapel Hill
Chapel Hill, North Carolina

I. INTRODUCTION

The purpose of this chapter is to review the research literature on biofeedback, relaxation training, and cognitive behavior modification treatment approaches for a range of functional gastrointestinal (GI) disorders. Only functional disorders whose treatment has been researched were selected for review. Biofeedback, relaxation training, and cognitive behavior modification are all plausible treatment strategies for functional GI disorders in which stress plays an important role in inducing or exacerbating symptoms. Biofeedback is appropriate when specific pathophysiological mechanisms are known and the control of relevant responses can be achieved by systematic information about a function that is not usually monitored consciously. This review does not cover hypnotherapy and psychotherapy, both of which are covered in Chapter 17.

II. IRRITABLE BOWEL SYNDROME

A. Description

Irritable bowel syndrome (IBS) is a disorder characterized by abdominal pain and altered bowel habits, either constipation or diarrhea—or both in alternation—in the absence of any structural or metabolic lesion that can explain the symptoms (1). IBS is very common; it affects 8–19% of the general population (2–4) and accounts for 20–50% of consultations to gastroenterologists (5,6).

IBS is an attractive candidate for psychological treatment for several reasons: 1) roughly 70–100% of medical clinic patients with IBS have significant psychological symptoms (7) [the kinds of psychological symptoms, and psychiatric diagnoses, most frequently seen are somatization disorder, depression, and anxiety (7)]; 2) approximately 85% (3) of IBS patients report that stress exacerbates their bowel symptoms; and 3) medical treatments often produce disappointing results (8).

B. Relaxation Training and Cognitive Behavior Modification, Including Nonspecific Biofeedback Training

Bennett and Wilkinson (9) compared behavioral stress-management training alone with medical management in 24 newly diagnosed IBS patients. The behavioral intervention had three major components: education about normal variations in bowel function, stress-management training based on progressive relaxation exercises, and training in self-instruction techniques to cope with stress. Medical management consisted of a bulking agent, an anticholinergic, and a drug with both anxiolytic and antidepressant properties. Pain and diarrhea improved in both groups to a similar extent; psychological symptoms decreased significantly more in the relaxation group, however.

In a similar study, Voirol and Hipolito (10) compared relaxation training with conventional medical treatment and found relaxation training to be associated with significantly greater reductions in number of pain episodes and number of medical consultations, results that were maintained during 40 months of follow-up. Likewise, Rumsey (11) found an advantage for a 6-week group intervention with cognitive behavioral stress management (emphasizing information about IBS, progressive muscle relaxation, diet, fitness, problem-solving, and long-term management) as compared to 6 weeks of conventional pharmacological treatment with phenothiazine and tricyclic antidepressents in 45 consecutive patients randomly assigned to one of the two conditions. Assessments were completed at the end of the treatment and at 6-month follow-up. Pharmacotherapy and cognitive behavioral stress-management training reduced pain, bloating, anxiety, depression, and subjective stress measurements to a similar degree by the end of treatment; but at follow-up, the psychological approach had a substantial advantage.

A controlled study by Guthrie et al. (12) compared six sessions of brief psychotherapy (relaxation being a prominent component) combined with medical therapy to medical therapy alone for 102 patients with IBS. Greater short- and long-term improvements were reported for the group receiving psychotherapy. The relative contribution of relaxation to the superior outcome of psychotherapy and medical therapy combined was unclear; the fact that patients under periodic stress improved differentially suggests that relaxation may well have made an important contribution to the therapy outcome. On balance, the available research literature suggests that relaxation training is effective for reducing pain and diarrhea associated with IBS.

Other studies have used biofeedback as an adjunct to teaching relaxation in combination with cognitive therapy techniques. One such multicomponent treatment program, developed by Blanchard's laboratory (13–15) emphasized four components: 1) education about the relationship between psychological stress and exacerbations of bowel symptoms, 2) progressive muscle-relaxation training via audiotaped instructions, 3) relaxation training using thermal biofeedback, and 4) cognitive coping-skills training to replace self-defeating thoughts with more positive thinking. In the earlies two studies, outcomes in patients treated with this protocol were compared to changes observed in patients awaiting treatment. (Since patients awaiting treatment have negative expectations about improvement, this experimental design maximizes the probability that placebo effects contribute to differences between experimental and control groups.) For 21 patients treated individually in the initial study, Neff and Blanchard (13) reported that symptom severity was reduced by at least 50% in 11 patients (52%). At follow-up 1 year later, 57% of the patients met the same criterion for clinical improvement (16). In a second study of treatment in groups (13), nine of 14 patients (64%) improved by at least 50%.

A similar multicomponent treatment strategy was studied by Lynch and Zamble (17). These investigators, however, used assertiveness training instead of thermal biofeedback training in addition to patient education, progressive muscle-relaxation training, and cognitive coping-strategies training. Although patients were recruited from a gastroenterology clinic, only 37.5% agreed to participate, limiting the generalizability of the findings. Bowel symptoms improved significantly more in the treated group than in a control group awaiting treatment, and this difference was maintained at follow-up 5 months later.

In a third study by Blanchard and his colleagues (15), IBS patients were randomized to three groups: 1) the multicomponent behavioral treatment group, described above, 2) a waiting-list control group, and 3) an active placebo group whose members received a bogus treatment intended to elicit positive expectations without providing effective treatment. The placebo involved two components paralleling progressive muscle relaxation and biofeedback in the active treatment: pseudomeditation (instructions to attend to muscle tension, but not to relax) and biofeedback to *decrease* alpha EEG activity. Although members of the active treatment group improved more than the controls on the waiting list, the members of the placebo and treatment groups were indistinguishable. Blanchard speculated that patients in the placebo group may have converted the placebo treatment procedures into active treatment strategies. There is also the possibility that expectancy effects may have contributed to positive outcomes in previous studies. Thus, definitive support for the efficacy of this multicomponent cognitive behavior-modification treatment program in IBS is lacking, although earlier studies (9–12) comparing progressive muscle–relaxation training to medical management provide persuasive evidence of the efficacy of this approach to stress management.

C. Biofeedback

Initially, biofeedback treatment of IBS attempted to modify colonic motility. Furman (18) used an electronic stethoscope to teach five patients with diarrhea-predominant IBS to alternately increase and decrease bowel sounds. All five patients reported symptom relief as a result of learning to control bowel sounds. However, subsequent investigations (19,20) plus unpublished studies (personal communication) suggested that biofeedback produced relatively weak treatment effects.

Bueno-Miranda et al. (21) used a balloon probe to provide visual feedback on rectal contractions and reported that 14 of 21 IBS patients could learn to reduce contractile activity. However, a follow-up study from the same laboratory (22) showed that a simpler stress-management technique, progressive relaxation training and systematic desensitization training to anxiety-arousing stimuli, produced superior clinical results as compared to pressure biofeedback. On the basis of these studies, biofeedback intended to directly modify colonic motility is no longer recommended for the treatment of IBS and the technique is rarely used.

III. CONSTIPATION DUE TO PELVIC-FLOOR DYSSYNERGIA

A. Description

During defecation, two muscles that are ordinarily tonically contracted, the striated puborectalis and external anal sphincter, must be relaxed to allow the rectum to funnel into the anal canal so that formed stool can pass. Preston and

Lennard-Jones (23) discovered that, in some patients with chronic constipation, during attempts to defecate the puborectalis and external anal sphincter show a paradoxical contraction that obstructs defecation. They called this condition "anismus" (analogous to "vaginismus") but a more appropriate name is pelvic-floor dyssynergia (24). Pelvic-floor dyssynergia is associated with symptoms of straining and feelings of incomplete evacuation. The prevalence of pelvic-floor dyssynergia is unknown. However, published studies (25,26) suggest that pelvic-floor dyssynergia may contribute to complaints of constipation in approximately 50% of chronically constipated patients. In a sample of 74 patients with functional constipation, 74% showed evidence of pelvic-floor dyssynergia (27). In a sample of 18 child patients suffering from constipation and soiling, 78% closed the anal canal during straining by contracting the anal sphincter (28). The symptoms of straining and difficult defecation associated with pelvic-floor dyssynergia are frequently found in patients with anxiety (29) and other types of psychological distress (30).

B. Biofeedback

Clinical investigators were quick to recognize that pelvic-floor dyssynergia, characterized by inappropriate contraction of striated muscles, is the kind of dysfunction for which biofeedback has been very effective. Although additional studies are needed to fully establish the efficacy and the specificity of biofeedback for pelvic-floor dyssynergia, the results of initial studies, summarized below, have been very positive.

The first controlled study was reported by Wald et al. (25), who studied 50 encopretic children. Half of the children with dyssynergia and half of those with normal pelvic-floor responses to straining were randomly assigned to received biofeedback training: the remaining subjects received daily doses of mineral oil. During biofeedback training, which employed a three-balloon rectal tube, patients were instructed to relax and to decrease the pressure in the external-anal-sphincter balloon while straining to defecate. Children with sphincter dyssynergia quickly learned to relax the pelvic-floor muscles during straining. Although the two interventions produced similar outcomes at the end of treatment, at follow-up 6 and 12 months after treatment patients who had exhibited pelvic-floor dyssynergia prior to training tended to benefit more from biofeedback than from mineral oil therapy. Children with other causes of encopresis benefited more from mineral oil than from biofeedback. Because of the small sample size, the differences between groups did not attain statistical significance; nonetheless, these data suggest that biofeedback was an effective treatment for encopresis in children with dyssynergia.

A second controlled study, also with encopretic children, obtained more definitive results. Loening-Baucke (31) randomly assigned encopretic children 5 to 16 years of age—all with pelvic-floor dyssynergia—to one of two treatment groups: conventional laxative treatment (milk of magnesia) or biofeedback combined with laxative therapy. Biofeedback consisted of showing children a polygraph tracing of both anal-canal pressures recorded with a balloon and integrated EMG activity from skin-surface electrodes placed over the external anal sphincter. Eighty-six percent of the children receiving an average of 3.2 biofeedback training sessions learned to relax the external anal sphincter during attempts to defecate. The proportion of children judged to be recovered was significantly greater for the biofeedback group than for the laxative-only group at 7 months follow-up and again at 12 months follow-up. These results suggest that the majority of children with pelvic-floor dyssynergia can learn to produce normal sphincter responses and that such learning is associated with clinical outcomes that are superior to those with laxatives alone.

Loening-Baucke and her associates (32) also evaluated anorectal and psychological factors associated with treatment failure. Of the 38 encopretic children undergoing six biofeedback training sessions, 10 had failed to learn to relax the pelvic floor during straining by a 7-month follow-up, and none of the 10 recovered clinically from constipation. Of 29 children who did learn to relax the pelvic floor during straining, 14 recovered and 15 did not. Nonrecovered patients who learned to relax during straining showed significantly decreased sensitivity to rectal distension compared to the recovered patients during the initial and follow-up anorectal manometric study. At follow-up, the balloon volumes for urge to defecate, rectosphincteric reflex, constant relaxation, and rectal contractions were significantly greater in unrecovered, as compared to recovered, patients. No significant differences were found in age, gender, or frequency of GI and urinary symptoms in successfully biofeedback-treated patients compared to those who did not recover. The Child Behavior Checklist, which contains scales for social competence, behavioral problems, internalizing–externalizing, and other psychological variables, also failed to distinguish children who recovered from those who did not. The authors concluded that correcting abnormal contractions of the pelvic floor by biofeedback treatment cures patients with either normal or mildly impaired rectal and anal sensitivity but not those with severely impaired sensitivity.

Keren et al. (28) reported success in all of 12 constipated and encopretic children treated with biofeedback, but their study included no control group. At the beginning of each session, the children strained to expel a catheter while visual feedback of pressure in the anal canal guided them to relax the anus. After the children learned to relax the anus, the rectal balloon was distended to a perceptible volume, and subjects were instructed to defecate the balloon. Successively, the rectal balloon was distended by gradually decreasing volumes to obtain a defecation response to progressively smaller rectal distensions. The visual feedback was later withdrawn. Therapeutic sessions lasted 45 minutes and were performed once every 2 weeks until defecation was satisfactory. Enemas were tapered off and stopped altogether as defecation improved. The number of sessions required to achieve relaxation of the anal canal on straining, corroborated by manometry, averaged 4.1 sessions. Thereafter patients were followed once every 3–6 months for 7 to 22 months, with an interview and biofeedback session to evaluate the anal response to straining and to reinforce the relaxation response. By the end of the study, all constipated children were considered by their parents to have recovered and no relapses were encountered during follow-up.

Lestar et al. (33) described an uncontrolled study in 16 constipated adults (mean age: 42.5 + 3.5 years). The patients were asked to defecate a simulated stool consisting of a rectal balloon filled with 50 ml of warmed water while they sat on a commode chair. The patient's pressure recordings were displayed on a computer screen, and the physiology of normal defecation and then patient's personal pathology were explained. The balloon was then reinserted and filled with warm water at a rate of 60 ml/min up to a volume that caused a constant desire for defecation. Next, patients were instructed to bear down several times on the bolus without excessive effort while either not increasing anal pressure unduly or decreasing it. Real-time visualization of anal and rectal pressures constituted visual reinforcement; verbal reinforcement helped patients understand pathophysiology and paradoxical striated sphincter contraction. The patients were left alone and instructed to evacuate the balloon. They were given at least two chances. If evacuation was effective, the procedure was repeated, except that the balloon was filled with water at a rate of 50 ml/min. Homee therapy consisted of instructing patients to relax the sphincter during expulsion and to avoid straining. Laxatives, enemas, and digitation to initiate defecation were discouraged. The investigators reported that the treatment was effective in improving function in 11 of 16 of the patients; the gains were maintained at 12-month follow-up in nine of 11 patients, and seven reported easier defecation than before training. Later, 29 new patients were trained using the one-session biofeedback approach. Normalization of defecation occurred in 11 cases, and significant improvement occurred in 16 others; only two patients could not be trained. In the majority of cases, benefits were preserved 6 weeks after treatment.

These observations and others (for example, see Refs. 34–37) suggest that biofeedback is often effective for treating pelvic-floor dyssynergia, especially in children. Clinical observations indicate that adults with constipation related to pelvic-floor dyssynergia respond less consistently to biofeedback treatment than children do. Therefore, additional studies are needed to demonstrate the efficacy and cost-effectiveness of biofeedback for treating constipation related to pelvic-floor dyssynergia in adults.

IV. PROCTALGIA: LEVATOR ANI SYNDROME AND PROCTALGIA FUGAX

A. Description

Levator Ani Syndrome

The levator ani syndrome (also called pyriformis syndrome or diaphragma pelvis spastica) refers to a vague, dull ache or sensation of pressure localized high in the rectum. Associated symptoms include difficult defecation (38), straining, and feelings of incomplete defecation (39). The prevalence of levator ani syndrome in the general population is 6.6% (40). Symptoms are disproportionately common in women (41) and in people between the ages of 40 and 60 (42).

Diagnosis depends primarily on clinical history. Patients report chronic or recurrent anorectal pain or aching for at least 3 months (40). Confidence in the diagnosis increases if posterior traction on the puborectalis reveals tight levator ani muscles and tenderness or pain.

The cause of the syndrome is not known, but accumulating evidence suggests that chronic or recurrent rectal pain, in the absence of any recognized disease process or of symptoms suggestive of IBS, may be due to pelvic-floor muscles that are overly contracted (40). Psychological tension, stress, and anxiety are reported anecdotally to be associated with the syndrome (43), but neither psychiatric evaluations nor systematic investigations have been reported.

Solitary Rectal Ulcer

Solitary rectal ulcer refers to the occurrence of one or more lesions in the rectum near its junction with the anal canal. Symptoms include severe pain and passage of blood and mucus. Little is known about the prevalence of this disorder, but it is believed to be rare. No information is available on associated psychological symptoms or on the role of stress.

The physiological mechanisms responsible for the development of solitary rectal ulcers are incompletely understood. Rectal prolapse or internal intussuception is reported to be present in more than 80% of patients with solitary rectal ulcer (43a,b), suggesting that rectal prolapse contributes to its etiology. High anal-canal pressures and/or pelvic-floor dyssenergia are also reported in a high proportion of patients with this disorder, and one study (43b) suggests that, for those patients who exhibit pelvic-floor dyssynergia, biofeedback may be beneficial.

Proctalgia Fugax

Proctalgia fugax is an idiopathic disorder characterized by recurring attacks of fleeting, intense anorectal pain. These attacks occur at irregular intervals—typically less than six times per year—and last several seconds to 20 minutes before ending (44). Some authors consider the disorder a variant of levator ani syndrome (45). Common precipitators are flatus or defecation for roughly a third of patients and sexual intercourse for 6% (45). Prevalence rates of 13.6% (2) to 18.4% (46) have been reported in healthy adults. The condition is approximately twice as common in females as in males, according to one survey (2) and is rarely reported before puberty (45). Among 148 clinic patients presenting with GI complaints, a 33% prevalence was found, with women outnumbering men by more than three times (51% to 12%) (47).

Diagnostic criteria for proctalgia fugax are as follows (40): recurrent episodes, lasting from seconds to minutes, of midline pain localized to the lower rectum for at least 3 months; no anorectal pain between episodes; and no evidence of another anorectal disease. Generally, the pain is reported as being intense—often sharp or stabbing—and nonradiating, although it may be merely uncomfortable.

The identification of physiological mechanisms has been complicated by the short duration and sporadic, infrequent nature of the disorder. Case reports (primarily from physician self-examinations) have implicated varied possible mechanisms, including a lax anal sphincter, a band of tense tender muscle above the anal shelf attributed to spasms of the levator ani or pubococcygeus muscles, and contractile activity in the sigmoid colon (48–50). Stress, anxiety, and neurotic characteristics were implicated as precipitating attacks in early reports (51–53). Pilling et al. (53), for example, found patients to exhibit neurotic characteristics in an MMPI study: 63% perfectionistic, 73% anxious, 40% hypochondriacal; 52% reported other functional GI disorders whereas 48% reported other functional pain syndromes. These associated symptoms could represent consequence, cause, or unrelated correlate of chronic illness.

B. Relaxation Training, Biofeedback, and Cognitive Behavior-Modification Treatment Approaches

The high percentage of proctalgia patients with functional GI disorders and chronic pain suggests that psychological interventions might be effective treatment strategies. Relaxation training and cognitive behavior modification would be expected to reduce the number and/or intensity of pain episodes in patients who report that stress precipitates or exacerbates the condition. Biofeedback training aimed at teaching patients to reduce anal-canal pressure through pelvic-floor-muscle relaxation should also be an efficacious treatment strategy.

Previously, we emphasized the role of pelvic-floor dyssynergia in constipation and incontinence. Indirect evidence summarized by Whitehead et al. (24) suggests that excessive tension in the pelvic-floor muscles may also be responsible for the functional rectal pain reported in levator ani syndrome and proctalgia fugax. If future research confirms that excessive tension in the pelvic-floor muscles is also responsible for functional rectal pain in levator ani syndrome and proctalgia fugax, biofeedback training to relax the pelvic floor may prove to be beneficial in the relief of proctalgia.

To date, no controlled studies of the efficacy of relaxation training, biofeedback, or cognitive behavior modification for levator ani syndrome or proctalgia fugax have been reported in the literature. Uncontrolled studies and case reports are promising, however. Grimaud and colleagues (54) used visual biofeedback, displaying anal-canal pressures, in 12 consecutive patients with levator ani syndrome. Patients learned to reduce the anal-canal pressures by alternately squeezing and then relaxing the external anal sphincters, capitalizing on the fact that strong contractions tend to be followed by brief periods of relaxation. After an average of 8 weeks of treatment, pain relief was achieved in all 12 patients through relaxation of the pelvic-floor muscles, and it was sustained for 16 months in 11 of the 12 patients. Pain relief was accompanied by reductions in resting pressure in the anal canal. These findings were supported by unpublished data collected by West and her colleagues (personal communication). These investigators used EMG biofeedback recorded from an anal plug to teach 15 patients with levator ani syndrome to relax the pelvic-floor muscles. Pain was eliminated in 70% of patients.

V. INFLAMMATORY BOWEL DISORDER

A. Description

Ulcerative colitis and Crohn's disease are often considered together as inflammatory bowel diseases (IBDs) because they both involve inflammation and ulceration of the bowel and they result in similar symptoms: severe pain and discharge of blood and mucus (55). Family studies show that the two conditions often occur in the same family. However, ulcerative colitis and Crohn's disease differ in histology and in the region of the bowel that is typically affected. Roughly 1.2% of the population will develop ulcerative colitis at some point in their lives; 0.34% of the population will develop Crohn's disease (56,57).

The etiology of the two conditions is unknown. While psychological symptoms and stress have been hypothesized to play a role in the onset and exacerbation of both, the research data are conflicting. Some investigators find little, if any, psychopathology in patients with IBD, and only a few studies suggest that stress is associated with symptom levels (58,59). Ulcerative colitis and Crohn's disease patients consistently exhibit less psychological distress and show less evidence of anxiety and neurosis than do IBS patients (60–63), although their symptoms are more debilitating and can be life-threatening; this argues against a psychosomatic etiology for IBD.

B. Relaxation Training, Biofeedback, and Cognitive Behavior Modification

Mixed findings have emerged from studies of stress management and relaxation training in IBD patients. In an early uncontrolled study, for example, Joachim (64) found that 14 outpatients with IBD experienced greater feelings of control over pain and improved ability to calm themselves after four sessions of deep abdominal breathing exercises and a 45-minute massage. Likewise, when 80 IBD patients were randomly assigned to either treatment (stress management) or control (65), the stress-management group experienced greater improvement in both psychological and physical symptoms as compared to a waiting-list control group. Interpretation of the findings is complicated by the fact that the two groups differed in pretreatment severity of physical symptoms and yet showed similar symptom ratings at the end of treatment, suggesting that the greater treatment gains in the treated subjects may have represented the effects of regression to the mean.

In a second controlled study, Shaw and Ehrlich (66) observed that patients with ulcerative colitis who received relaxation training reported greater reductions in pain than did patients on a waiting list. On the other hand, in a third controlled study, Schwarz and Blanchard (58) found that stress-management training was associated with poorer outcomes than simply remaining on a waiting list. At present, then, the data on relaxation training and IBD are hard to interpret; it is not clear whether relaxation training improves symptomatology in IBD, although patients' subjective sense of well-being appears to improve with treatment.

Autogenic training, a relaxation strategy developed by Schultz (67), was derived from self-hypnosis. Patients assume a passive attitude and repeat phrases that direct their attention to bodily processes associated with relaxation, e.g., "My abdomen is warm." Physiological measurements indicate that the routine repetition of such phrases enables patients to alter blood flow and other functions (68). Several uncontrolled studies suggest that patients with ulcerative colitis can benefit from autogenic training. For example, in one study of 32 patients treated for 1 to 12 years with autogenic training, 29 patients reported either significant improvement or cure (70).

No controlled studies of biofeedback and cognitive behavior-modification treatments of IBD are known to us.

VI. AEROPHAGIA

A. Description

It is estimated that 50–70% of the gas in the GI tract comes from swallowed air (71). Each swallow draws 3–5 ml of air into the stomach (72). The swallowing of excessive amounts of air, or aerophagia, results in symptoms of belching, flatulence, bloating, and abdominal pain. In some cases, excessive swallowing is unconscious;

in other cases, it involves conscious, abnormal swallows in which the head is extended to open the upper-esophageal sphincter and the rib cage is expanded to suck large quantities of air into the esophagus, after which the patient swallows to carry the air into the stomach by peristalsis. The conscious type of aerophagia appears to be confined primarily to institutionalized, retarded individuals, who may engage in it because it produces pleasurable stimulation or attention from caregivers.

Aerophagia may be a relatively common cause of GI symptoms. Approximately 21% of 363 consecutive patients referred to a digestive disease clinic with unexplained upper-GI symptoms swallowed excessively (73). Calloway et al. (74) reported that excessive swallowing was associated with hiatal hernia and peptic ulcer disease. The mechanism for this association is not known, but the authors speculated that distension of the stomach by air may stimulate gastric acid secretion and may promote the ballooning of the stomach through the diaphragm to cause hiatal hernia. Some observers believe that stress and anxiety play roles in precipitating aerophagia (75,76).

B. Relaxation Training, Biofeedback, and Cognitive Behavior Modification

Only one study on the behavioral treatment of aerophagia in individuals with normal intelligence is known to us. The investigators (77) randomly assigned 12 patients with hiatal hernia, who had previously been shown to swallow excessively, to one of two behavioral treatment regimes. Half the patients were taught general relaxation skills using galvanic skin response (GSR) biofeedback; the remaining half were trained to decrease swallowing frequency using auditory biofeedback (a microphone applied to the neck transduced auditory signals). Patients in both groups were instructed to practice twice daily at home following three training sessions. Patients in the auditory biofeedback group were significantly more successful than those in the GSR biofeedback group at reducing their swallowing rate; likewise, a significantly higher proportion of the auditory biofeedback treatment group reported improvement of their GI symptoms as compared to the others. Although the sample size in this study was too small to adequately assess the clinical value of the technique, the results suggest that simple, noninvasive biofeedback techniques may be useful in the management of aerophagia in individuals with normal intelligence. Case reports on behavior-modification treatments of aerophagia in retarded individuals have shown inconsistent results (78–80).

VII. PEPTIC ULCER DISEASE

A. Description

Peptic ulcer disease (PUD) is a disorder characterized by ulcerating lesions in the stomach or duodenum that are thought to be caused by exposure to acid and pepsin (the digestive enzyme that breaks down protein). Infection of the stomach lining by *Helicobacter pylori* is common in the population and is known to predispose people to the development of PUD. PUD is associated with epigastric pain, which is experienced as gnawing hunger. Typically, PUD occurs several hours after eating and is relieved by eating or taking antacids. It is important to note that actual ulcers may be asymptomatic and that pains of the kind described may occur in the absence of ulcers (described in Section VIII below). Approximately 10% of the population can be expected to develop PUD during their lifetime (81,82). While gastric and duodenal ulcers appear to be different in terms of risks, age of onset, genetic predisposition, pathophysiology, and psychological profile, the same treatments have been offered for the two entities; hence, PUD is considered a unitary condition for the purposes of this review.

Numerous investigations have shown associations between psychosocial stress and the development of PUD. Patients with both gastric and duodenal ulcers show elevations in significant life changes preceding symptom flares (83,84); duodenal ulcer patients also report significant life changes preceding disease onset (84–86). Furthermore, medical clinic patients with PUD have been characterized as anxious, depressed, and low in dominance (55). Although psychological factors are associated with the development of PUD, psychological interventions have not proved to be cost-effective alternatives to pharmacological management. Nonetheless, the procedures are of interest for theoretical reasons.

B. Relaxation Training and Cognitive Behavior Modification

The earliest controlled study using a psychological approach to treating PUD was conducted in the middle 1930s and would be considered a type of cognitive behavior modification today (87,88). Through a newspaper article, 52 patients with objectively documented gastric or duodenal ulcer were recruited along with 20 controls. All received frequent feedings on a bland diet, and gastric mucin was administered as an acid neutralizing agent. In addition, the experimental subjects received daily didactic training in small groups 7 days per week for 6 weeks. The controls received no placebo treatment. The experimental treatment included five components:

Education—patients were taught that emotional responses caused peripheral physiological changes. Worrying, especially, was said to be linked to excess acid secretions and to excess motility in the stomach.

Distraction—patients were asked to call to mind a period of life that had been free of stress and to think about this time period when they found themselves worrying.

Extinction of social reinforcement—patients were encouraged to have their families refrain from discussing their illness, a strategy that was also aimed at reducing worrying by the patient.

Positive self-statements—Patients were taught to tell themselves aloud that they were recovering in order to counteract self-perception of sickness and helplessness.

Positive expectation—therapists assured patients daily that they would recover.

At the end of 6 weeks of treatment, 30 of 32 experimental patients were asymptomatic and eating a normal diet whereas only two of 20 controls were doing so. At a follow-up averaging 3 years later, 26 of 28 patients considered themselves healthy, including nine with frequent mild symptoms and five with infrequent mild symptoms. Ten experienced no symptoms during the 3-year period. The controls were monitored for 8 months; at that time the two patients who were improved at the end of the "training" phase had experienced severe recurrences. Although flawed by today's standards of clinical investigation (e.g., no placebo treatment for controls, no endoscopic or radiologic confirmation of ulcer healing), the study does provide evidence of the efficacy of cognitive behavior modification.

Brooks and Richardson (89) reported additional support for the efficacy of behavioral approaches to PUD. They examined the effects of anxiety-management training and assertiveness training on the outcomes of patients with radiologically confirmed duodenal ulcers. The assertiveness training was supposed to remediate inabilities to express anger or aggression that might be contributing to dependency and conformity. During a 2-week period, 11 experimental subjects were seen eight times and compared to 11 controls given three sessions of supportive discussion (a weak placebo). Four sessions of anxiety-management training consisted of 1) identifying irrational anxiety-producing beliefs and worried negative self-verbalizations in connection with stressful daily situations, 2) substitution of positive self-statements for the "irrational" ones, 3) progressive muscle-relaxation training, and 4) practice in coping with stress. Four sessions of assertiveness training were targeted at 1) correcting irrational beliefs about the negative consequences of assertiveness and 2) teaching assertive behavior in frequently encountered situations, using modeling and behavior rehearsal. The data suggested that the experimental intervention was effective and that its benefits lasted over a 42-month follow-up.

C. Biofeedback

During the 1970s, a number of investigators turned to biofeedback to develop treatment strategies for peptic ulcers. Although practical treatment applications did not result, the studies shed light on the regulation of the stomach by the central nervous system. Studies of biofeedback training for decreasing gastric acid secretion by Whitehead et al. (see Ref. 90) and others (91–93) suggested that patients required numerous hours of individualized training (in our experience, roughly 10 to 14 hours) to obtain reliable control over gastric acid secretion; further, the training procedures were technically complex, making gastric acid secretion biofeedback both difficult to implement and costly.

Investigations of biofeedback training to establish control over gastric motility are of potential relevance in PUD treatment because some observers believe that ulcer pain is mediated by abnormal gastric motility (94,95). Research in our laboratory (96) has shown that normal subjects can learn, with relatively little training (4 hours), to increase motility when given feedback in the form of monetary incentives. Our studies do not indicate, however, that this training transfers to no-feedback conditions, and no clinical utility for such training has been demonstrated.

Stress-management training relying on biofeedback has shown promise for relieving symptoms in ulcer patients in uncontrolled studies (97,98). Beaty (98) taught three patients with frequent ulcer pain to relax using forehead EMG biofeedback twice a week and daily relaxation exercises at home. Once they were proficient at relaxing, patients learned to use relaxation to cope with daily stressors. At the end of treatment and at a 6-month follow-up, all three patients reported no pain and no medication use. Aleo and Nicassio (97) provided four patients with radiologically confirmed duodenal ulcers 5 weeks of biweekly EMG biofeedback training accompanied by daily practice of progressive muscle-relaxation exercise. In 7 weeks of biweekly sessions, the patients also imagined themselves using relaxation to cope with stressful situations. Three patients achieved pain elimination and ulcer healing, confirmed radiologically, and the fourth patient attained decreased pain and reduced ulcer size. Since hypnotically induced relaxation has been shown to reliably reduce both basal and betazole-stimulated rates of gastric acid secretion in peptic ulcer patients and controls (99), it appears that relaxation training might contribute to ulcer healing via reduction in gastric acid secretion.

This brief summary suggests that biofeedback, relaxation training, and cognitive behavioral treatment interventions are potentially effective strategies for treating PUD. However, pharmacological management is more cost-effective and has become the treatment of choice for PUD (55).

VIII. FUNCTIONAL DYSPEPSIA

A. Description

Although resembling PUD, functional dyspepsia is considered a distinct clinical syndrome that resembles IBS and is separate from peptic ulcer disease. It is characterized by "chronic or recurrent upper abdominal pain for at least 3 months, or discomfort without x-ray or endoscopic evidence of other disease (e.g., acid-peptic or neoplastic disease of stomach or esophagus, pancreas, or hepatobiliary system) to explain the symptoms" (1, p 164). Sensations of bloating and fullness, belching, boborygmi, nausea, and heartburn are other symptoms often associated with functional dyspepsia (100,48). Somewhere between 50 and 90% of the patients who consult physicians for symptoms suggestive of peptic ulcer disease have no ulcers (101,102); moreover, a prospective study suggests that only 3% of such patients will develop an ulcer within 6 year of initial assessment (103). Dyspepsia accounts for approximately 5% of consultations to internal medical practitioners (104). Prevalence of functional dyspepsia in the community is estimated at 30 to 38% (101,104), but only a minority of those with symptoms, estimated at 28% on the basis of one study (104), consult physicians.

Research linking functional dyspepsia with psychological phenomena is mixed. Dyspepsia sufferers who consult physicians (87%) are more likely to fulfill criteria for a psychiatric disorder (primarily, anxiety disorder) than are controls with an organic basis for their dyspepsia (25%) (105). No relationship has been found, however, between functional dyspepsia and the number of stressful life events recalled for the previous 6 months (106,107).

B. Relaxation Training, Biofeedback, and Cognitive Behavior Modification

To date, no studies have been published evaluating the benefits of relaxation–based therapy, cognitive behavior modification, or biofeedback for functional dyspepsia. Given the size of the population that experiences these problems and the finding that a substantial subsample of them are psychologically distressed and possibly dysfunctional, such research is amply justified.

IX. ESOPHAGEAL MOTILITY DISORDERS AND NONCARDIAC CHEST PAIN

A. Description

Functional disorders of the esophagus are defined as a variable combination of chronic, or recurrent, symptoms attributed to the esophagus that are not readily explained by structural or biochemical abnormalities (108). Usual complaints include heartburn, regurgitation, dysphagia, chest pain, globus sensation, or a combination of these. Heartburn and chest pain are among the most frequent GI symptoms seen by internists (55). Women predominate in the clinic population; and the age range extends from childhood into old age (108). We will be focusing on noncardiac chest pain, for which there is a small body of relevant treatment literature to review.

Noncardiac chest pain is characterized by episodes of midline, angina-like chest pain attributed to the esophagus in the absence of structural abnormalities (108). The prevalence of the condition is unclear. Up to 20 to 30% of coronary angiograms performed due to suspicion of ischemic heart disease are found to be within normal limits (109), and coronary artery spasm is only rarely found to explain the symptoms; prevalence of esophagus-related chest pain is estimated as 20 to 60% of these cases (110). The prevalence in women is only slightly higher than that in men in this group; age of onset ranges between 40 and 60 years (107). Diagnostic criteria include the appropriate symptoms in the absence of cardiac disease (including microvascular angina) and pathological gastroesophageal reflux abnormalities. Subsequent testing is usually directed toward identifying the functional cause of the chest pain, which is likely to be attributable to acid reflux disease, esophageal motility disorders, or lowered visceral pain threshold. Controlled studies suggest that the prevalence of psychosocial factors may be higher in the patient with functional chest pain than in pathology-based esophageal disorders such as achalasia and scleroderma (111,112). Moreover, stressful events have been shown to amplify contraction-wave amplitudes in asymptomatic and symptomatic subjects but not to alter peristalsis (113).

B. Relaxation Training, Biofeedback, and Cognitive Behavior Modification

Uncontrolled case reports (114,115) suggest that behavioral therapy may be helpful for patients with functional chest pain of esophageal origin. In the only controlled study on these conditions published to date, Klimes and colleagues (116) compared a cognitive behavioral treatment group to a waiting-list control group. Thirty-one patients participated, of whom 57% suffered from panic attacks. The treatment focused on modifying poor coping skills and perceived lack of control over unpleasant physical symptoms. Relative to subjects on a treatment waiting list, the treated patients reported significantly greater reductions in chest pain, depressive episodes, symptom severity, and disruption of daily activities. Number of days free of chest pain increased significantly. All changes were maintained at a 6-month follow-up.

Uncontrolled case studies on other esophageal syndromes suggest that relaxation training strategies may be useful in cases in which stress or anxiety is a major component of the disorder (114,115,117). Biofeedback appears to be useful in cases in which voluntary control of specific physiological mechanisms is beneficial. For example, Shay et al. (118) taught a 31-year-old man with a 19-year history of rumination and frequent episodes of heartburn associated with acid gastroesophageal reflux occurring predominantly during the day to relax his abdominal muscles in order to abort or lessen abdominal-muscle contractions associated with the reflux episodes. The treatment resulted in decreased reflux and marked symptomatic improvement. These case studies suggest that behavioral approaches can have beneficial effects on individuals with functional esophageal motility disorders. However, such procedures need to be evaluated in more rigorous studies.

X. CONCLUSION

This review of the research literature on the utility of biofeedback, relaxation training, and cognitive behavior modification for functional GI conditions suggests a number of conclusions. At present, biofeedback is the treatment of choice for the most common types of fecal incontinence, and preliminary studies suggest that biofeedback may become the preferred method for treating patients with constipation attributable to an inability to relax the striated pelvic-floor muscles during attempts to defecate. Whether biofeedback will prove to be generally useful in treating constipation related to dyssynergia or whether its utility will be limited to those with normal or mildly impaired rectal or anal sensitivity remains to be demonstrated. Preliminary data also suggest that biofeedback is a promising treatment for both levator ani syndrome and aerophagia. On the other hand, biofeedback does not appear to be useful for treating IBS, and treatment results have been inconsistent in patients with IBD.

Relaxation training is often combined with nonspecific biofeedback and cognitive behavior modification in treating functional GI disorders. Such multifaceted programs have shown promise in preliminary studies for treating PUD and functional chest pain of esophageal origin.

ACKNOWLEDGMENTS

Preparation of this chapter was supported by grants X05 MH00133 and P-32-AG00120 (Research Training in Gerontology and Geriatrics).

REFERENCES

1. Drossman DA, Thompson WG, Talley NJ, Funch-Jensen P, Janssens J, Whitehead WE. Identification of sub-groups of functional gastrointestinal disorders. Gastroenterol Int 1990; 3:159–172.
2. Thompson WG, Heaton KW. Functional bowel disorders in apparently healthy people. Gastroenterology 1980; 79:283–288.
3. Drossman DA, Sandler RS, McKee DC, Lovitz AJ. Bowel patterns among subjects not seeking health care. Gastroenterology 1982; 83:529–534.
4. Whitehead WE, Winget C, Fedoravicious AS, Wooley S, Blackwell B. Learned illness behavior in patients with irritable bowel syndrome and peptic ulcer. Digest Dis Sci 1982; 27:202–208.

5. Harvey RF, Salih SY, Read AE. Organic and functional disorders in 2,000 gastroenterology outpatients. Lancet 1983; i:632–634.
6. Mitchell CM, Drossman DA. Survey of the AGA membership relating to patients with functional gastrointestinal disorders. Gastroenterology 1987; 92:1228–1245.
7. Whitehead WE, Enck P, Anthony JC, Schuster MM. Psychopathology in patients with irritable bowel syndrome. In: Singer MV, Goebell H, eds. Nerves and the Gastrointestinal Tract. Falk Symposium 50. Lancastar, 1988:465–476.
8. Klein KB. Controlled treatment trials in the inflammatory bowel syndrome: A critique. Gastroenterology 1988; 95:232–241.
9. Bennett P, Wilkinson S. A comparison of psychological and medical treatment of the irritable bowel syndrome. Br J Clin Psychol 1985; 24:215–216.
10. Voirol MW, Hipolito J. Relaxation antroponanalytique dans les syndromes de l'intestin irritable: Resultats à 40 mois. [Anthropoanalytical relaxation in irritable bowel syndrome: Results 40 months later.] Schweizerische Medizinische Wochenschrift 1987; 117:1117–1119.
11. Rumsey N. Group stress management programmes v pharmacological treatment in the treatment of the irritable bowel syndrome. In: Heaton KW, Creed F, Goeting NLM, eds. Current Approaches Towards Confident Management of Irritable Bowel Syndrome. Lyme Regis, England: Lyme Regis Printing, 1991:33–39.
12. Guthrie E, Creed F, Dawson D, Tomenson B. A controlled trial of psychological treatment for the irritable bowel syndrome. Gastroenterology 1991; 100:450–457.
13. Neff DF, Blanchard EB. A multicomponent treatment for irritable bowel syndrome. Behav Ther 1987; 18:70–83.
14. Blanchard EB, Schwarz SP. Adaptation of a multicomponent treatment program for irritable bowel syndrome to a small group format. Biofeedback Self-Reg 1987; 12:63–69.
15. Blanchard EB, Schwarz SP, Suls JM, Gerardi MA, Scharff L, Greene B, Taylor AE, Berreman C, Malamood HS. Two controlled evaluations of a multicomponent psychological treatment of irritable bowel syndrome. Behav Res Ther 1992; 2:175–189.
16. Scwarz SP, Blanchard EB, Neff DF. Behavioral treatment of irritable bowel syndrome: A 1-year follow-up study. Biofeedback Self-Reg 1986; 11:189–198.
17. Lynch PM, Zamble E. A controlled behavioral treatment study of irritable bowel syndrome. Behav Ther 1989; 20:509–523.
18. Furman S. Intestinal biofeedback in functional diarrhea: A preliminary report. J Behav Ther Exper Psychiatry 1973; 4:317–321.
19. Radnitz CL, Blanchard EB. Bowel sound biofeedback as a treatment for irritable bowel syndrome. Biofeedback Self-Reg 1988; 13:169–179.
20. Radnitz CL, Blanchard EB. A 1- and 2-year follow-up study of bowel sound biofeedback as a treatment for irritable bowel syndrome. Biofeedback Self-Reg 1989; 14:333–338.
21. Bueno-Miranda F, Cerulli M, Schuster MM. Operant conditioning of colonic motility in irritable bowel syndrome (IBS) (abstr). Gastroenterology 1976; 70:A867.
22. Whitehead WE. Psychotherapy and biofeedback in the treatment of irritable bowel syndrome. In: Read NE, ed. Irritable Bowel Syndrome. London: Grune & Stratton, 1985:245–266.

23. Preston DM, Lennard-Jones JE. Anismus in chronic constipation. Dig Dis Sci 1985; 34:1168–1172.
24. Whitehead WE, Crowell MD, Schuster MM. Functional disorders of the anus and rectum. Sem Gastrointest Dis 1990; 1:74–84.
25. Wald A, Chandra R, Gabel S, Chiponis D. Evaluation of biofeedback in childhood encopresis. J Pediatr Gastroenterol Nutr 1987; 6:554–558.
26. Loening-Baucke V. Factors determining outcome in children with chronic constipation and faecal soiling. Gut 1989; 30:999–1006.
27. Kuijpers HC. Application of the colorectal laboratory in diagnosis and treatment of functional constipation. Dis Colon Rectum 1990; 33:35–39.
28. Keren S, Wagner Y, Heldenberg D, Golan M. Studies of manometric abnormalities of the rectoanal region during defecation in constipated and soiling children: Modification through biofeedback therapy. Am J Gastroenterol 1988; 83:827–831.
29. Whitehead WE. Illness behavior: Psychological factors in constipation. In: Kamm MA, Lennard-Jones JE, eds. Constipation and Related Disorders. Stroud, England: Wrightson Biomedical Publishing, 1993. In press.
30. Emery Y, Descos L, Meunier P, Louis D, Valancogne G, Weil G. Constipation terminale par asynchronisme abdomino-pelvien: Analyse des données étiologiques, cliniques, manometriques, et des resultats therapeutiques après reeducation par biofeedback. Gastroenterol Clin Biol 1988; 12:6–11.
31. Loening-Baucke V. Modulation of abnormal defecation dynamics by biofeedback treatment in chronically constipated children with encopresis. J Pediatr 1990; 116:214–222.
32. Loening-Baucke V. Persistence of chronic constipation in children after biofeedback treatment. Dig Dis Sci 1991; 36:153–160.
33. Lestar B, Penninckx FM, Kerremans RP. Biofeedback defecation training for anismus. Int J Colorectal Dis 1991; 6:202–207.
34. Wesner SD, Cheape JD, Jorge JMN, Heymen S, Jagelman DG. Prospective assessment of biofeedback for the treatment of paradoxical puborectalis contraction. Dis Colon Rectum 1991; 35:145–150.
35. Dahl J, Lindquist BL, Tysk C, Leissner P, Philipson L, Jarnerot G. Behavioral medicine treatment in chronic constipation with paradoxical anal sphincter contraction. Dis Colon Rectum 1991; 34:769–776.
36. Fleshman JW, Dreznik Z, Meyer K, Fry RD, Carney R, Kodner IJ. Outpatient protocol for biofeedback therapy of pelvic floor outlet obstruction. Dis Colon Rectum 1992; 35:1–7.
37. Kawimbe BM, Papachrysostomou M, Binnie R, Clare N, Smith AN. Outlet obstruction constipation (anismus) managed by biofeedback. Gut 1991; 32:1175–1179.
38. West L, Abell TL, Cutts T. Anorectal manometry and EMG in the diagnosis of the levator ani syndrome (abstr). Gastroenterology 1990; 98:A401.
39. Nicosia JG, Abcarian H. Levator syndrome: A treatment that works. Dis Colon Rectum 1985; 28:406–408.
40. Whitehead WE, Devroede G, Habib FJ, Meunier P, Wald A. Functional disorders of the anorectum. Gastroenterol Int 1992; 5:92–108.

41. Grant SR, Salvati EP, Rubin RJ. Levator syndrome: An analysis of 316 cases. Dis Colon Rectum 1975; 18:161–163.
42. Sinaki M, Merritt JL, Stillwell GK. Tension myalgia of the pelvic floor. Mayo Clin Proc 1977; 109:1271–1275.
43. Billingham RP, Isler JT, Friend WG, Hostetler J. Treatment of levator syndrome using high-voltage electrogalvanic stimulation. Dis Colon Rectum 1987; 30:584–587.
43a. Binnie NR, Papachrysostomou M, Clare N, Smith AN. Solitary rectal ulcer: The place of biofeedback and surgery in the treatment of the syndrome. World J Surg 1992; 16:836–840.
43b. Womack NR, Williams NS, Holmfield JHM, Morrison JFB. Pressure and prolapse: The cause of solitary rectal ulceration. Gut 1987; 28:1228.
44. Thompson WG. Proctalgia fugax. Dig Dis Sci 1981; 26:1121–1124.
45. Thompson WG. Gut Reactions. New York: Plenum, 1989.
46. Panitch NM, Schofferman JA. Proctalgia fugax revisited (abstr). Gastroenterology 1975; 68:1061.
47. Thompson WG. Non-ulcer dyspepsia. Can Med Assoc J 1984; 130:565–569.
48. Douthwaite AH. Proctalgia fugax. Br Med J 1962; 2:164–165.
49. Scott D. Proctalgia fugax. Postgrad Med 1982; 72:44.
50. Harvey RF. Colonic motility in proctalgia fugax. Lancet 1979; ii:713–714.
51. Penny RW. The doctors disease: Proctalgia fugax. Practitioner 1970; 204:843–845.
52. Karras JD, Angelo G. Proctalgia fugax: Clinical observations and a new diagnostic aid. Dis Colon Rectum 1963; 6:130–134.
53. Pilling LF, Swenson WM, Hill JR. The psychologic aspects of proctalgia fugax. Dis Colon Rectum 1972; 8:372–376.
54. Grimaud J-C, Bouvier M, Naudy B, Guien C, Salducci J. Manometric and radiologic investigations and biofeedback treatment of chronic idiopathic anal pain. Dis Colon Rectum 1991; 34:690–695.
55. Whitehead WE, Schuster MM. Gastrointestinal Disorders: Behavioral and Physiological Basis for Treatment. Orlando, FL: Academic Press, 1985.
56. Binder V, Both H, Hansen PK, Hendriksen C, Kreiner S, Torp-Pedersen K. Incidence and prevalence of ulcerative colitis and Crohn's disease in the county of Copenhagen, 1962–1978. Gastroenterology 1982; 83:563–568.
57. Mendeloff AL. The epidemiology of idiopathic inflammatory bowel disease. In: Kirsner JB, Shorter RG, eds. Inflammatory Bowel Disease. Philadelphia: Lea & Febiger, 1975:3–19.
58. Schwarz SP, Blanchard EB. Evaluation of a psychological treatment for inflammatory bowel disease. Behav Res Ther 1991; 29:167–177.
59. Garrett VD, Brantley PJ, Jones GN, McKnight GT. The relation between daily stress and Crohn's Disease. J Behav Med 1991; 14:87–96.
60. Walker EA, Roy-Byrne PP, Katon WJ, Li L, Amos D, Jiranek G. Psychiatric illness and irritable bowel syndrome: A comparison with inflammatory bowel disease. Am J Psychiatr 1990; 147:1656–1661.
61. Fava GA, Pavan L. Large bowel disorders. I. Illness configuration and life events. Psychother Psychosom 1976/1977; 27:93–99.

62. Fava GA, Pavan L. Large bowel disorders. II. Psychopathology and alexithymia. Psychother Psychosom 1976/1977; 27:100–105.
63. Esler MD, Goulston KJ. Levels of anxiety in colonic disorders. N Engl J Med 1973; 288:16–20.
64. Joachim G. The effects of two stress management techniques on feelings of well-being in patients with inflammatory bowel disease. Nursing Papers 1983; 15:5–18.
65. Milne B, Joachim G, Niedhardt J. A stress management programme for inflammatory bowel disease patients. J Adv Nursing 1986; 11:561–567.
66. Shaw L. Ehrlich A. Relaxation training as a treatment for chronic pain caused by ulcerative colitis. Pain 1987; 29:287–293.
67. Schultz JH. Autogenes training. Medizinishe Welt 1929; 47.
68. Luthe W. Atuogenic therapy. Vol IV. Research and theory. New York: Grune & Stratton, 1970.
69. Luthe W, Schultz JH. Autogenic Therapy. Vol ii. Medical Applications. New York: Grune & Stratton, 1969.
70. Schaeffer G. Ergebnisse des autogenen Trainings bei der Colitis ulcerosa. In: Lopez Ibor JJ, ed. IV World Congress of Psychiatry, Madrid, Nov 5–11, 1966. International Congress Series no. 117.48. Amsterdam: Excerpta Medical Foundation.
71. Roth JLA. Aerophagia. In: Linder AE, ed. Emotional Factors in Gastointestinal Illness. Amsterdam: Excerpta Medica, 1973:16–36.
72. Maddock WG, Bell JL, Tremaine MJ. Gastro-intestinal gas. Ann Surg 1949; 130:512–537.
73. Whitehead WE, Chami TN, Crowell MD, Schuster MM. Aerophagia: Association with gastrointestinal and psychological symptoms. Gastroenterology 1991; 100:A508.
74. Calloway SP, Fonagy P, Pounder RE. Frequency of swallowing in duodenal ulceration and hiatus hernia. Br Med J 1982; 285:23–24.
75. Cuevas JL, Cook EW, Richter JE, McCutcheon M, Taub E. Emotional distress, relaxation, and air swallowing rate: A possible etiological mechanism in some gastrointestinal disorders (abstr). Gastroenterology 1993; 104(supp!):A1035.
76. Fonagy P, Calloway SP. The effect of emotional arousal on spontaneous swallowing rate. J Psychosomat Res 1986; 30:183–188.
77. Calloway SP, Fonagy P, Pounder RE, Morgan MD. Behavioural techniques in the management of aerophagia in patients with hiatus hernia. J Psychosom Res 1983; 27:499–502.
78. Barrett RP, McGonigle JJ, Ackles PK, Burkhart JE. Behavioral treatment of chronic aerophagia. Am J Mental Defic 1987; 91:620–625.
79. Holburn CS, Dougher MJ. Effects of response satiation procedures in the treatment of aerophagia. Am J Mental Defic 1986; 91:72–77.
80. Holburn CS, Dougher MJ. Behavioral attempts to eliminate air-swallowing in two profoundly mentally retarded clients. Am J Mental Defic 1985; 89:524–536.
81. Bonnevie O. The incidence of gastric ulcer in Copenhagen County. Scand J Gastroenterol 1975; 10:231–239.
82. Bonnevie O. The incidence of duodenal ulcer in Copenhagen County. Scand J Gastroenterol 1975; 10:385–393.

83. Alp MH, Court JH, Grant AK. Personality pattern and emotional stress in the genesis of gastric ulcer. Gut 1970; 11:773–777.
84. Sapira JD, Cross MR. Pre-hospitalization life change in gastric ulcer (GU) versus duodenal ulcer (DU) (abstr). Psychosom Med 1982; 44:121.
85. Piper DW, Greig M, Shinners J, Thomas J, Crawford J. Chronic gastric ulcer and stress. Digestion 1978; 18:303–309.
86. Thomas J, Greig M, Piper DW. Chronic gastric ulcer and life events. Gastroenterology 1980; 78:905–911.
87. Chappell MN, Stefano JJ, Rogerson JS, Pike FH. The value of group psychological procedures in the treatment of peptic ulcer. Am J Dig Dis Nutr 1936; 3:813–817.
88. Chappell MN, Stevenson TI. Group psychological training in some organic conditions. Ment Hygiene 1936; 20:588–597.
89. Brooks GR, Richardson FC. Emotional skills training: A treatment program for duodenal ulcer. Behav Ther 1980; 11:198–207.
90. Whitehead WE, Renault PF, Goldiamond I. Modification of human gastric acid secretion with operant-conditioning procedures. J Appl Behav Anal 1975; 8:147–156.
91. Welgan PR. Learned control of gastric acid secretions in peptic ulcer patients. Psychosom Med 1974; 36:411–419.
92. Welgan PR. Biofeedback control of stomach acid secretions and gastrointestinal reactions. In: Beatty J, Legewie H, eds. Biofeedback and Behavior. New York: Plenum: 1977; 385–393.
93. Gorman PJ. Cephalic Influences on Human Gastric Acid Secretion and Their Voluntary Control Through Feedback Training. Dissertation, Abstracts International 1976; 36:6413-B. (University Microfilms No. 76-6661.)
94. Ruffin JM, Baylin GJ, Legerton CW, Texter EC Jr. Mechanism of pain in peptic ulcer. Gastroenterology 1953; 23:252–264.
95. Smith HW, Texter EC Jr, Stickley JH, Barborka CJ. Intraluminal pressures from the upper gastrointestinal tract. II. Correlations with gastroduodenal motor activity in normal subjects and patients with ulcer distress. Gastroenterology 1957; 32:1025–1047.
96. Whitehead WE, Drescher VM. Perception of gastric contractions and self-control of gastric motility. Psychophysiology 1980; 17:552–558.
97. Aleo S, Nicassio P. Auto-regulation of duodenal ulcer disease: A preliminary report of four cases. Proceedings of the Biofeedback Society of America (Ninth Annual Meeting). Denver, CO: Biofeedback Society of America, 1978:278–281.
98. Beaty ET. Feedback assisted relaxation training as a treatment for peptic ulcers (abstr). Biofeedback Self-Reg 1976; 1:323–324.
99. Stacher G, Cerner P, Naske R, Schuster P, Bauerr P, Starker H, Schulze D. Effect of hypnotic suggestion of relaxation on basal and Betozole stimulated gastric acid secretion. Gastroenterology 1975; 68:656–661.
100. Talley NJ, Phillips SF. Non-ulcer dyspepsia of unknown cause: Potential causes and pathophysiology. Ann Internal Med 1988; 108:865–879.
101. Krag E. Non-ulcer dyspepsia introduction: Epidemiological data. Scand J Gastroenterol 1982; 17(suppl 79):6–8.
102. Myren J. Review: The natural history of peptic ulcer. Views in the 1980s. Scand J Gastroenterol 1983; 18:993–997.

103. Gregory DW, Davies GT, Evans KT, Rhoade J. Natural history of patients with X-ray negative dyspepsia in general practice. Br Med J 1972; 4:519–520.
104. Jones R, Lydeard B. Prevalence of symptoms of dyspepsia in the community. Br Med J 1989; 298:30–32.
105. Magni G, di Mario F. Bernasconi G, Mastropaolo G. DSM-III diagnoses associated with dyspepsia of unknown causes. Am J Psychiatr 1987; 144:1222–1223.
106. Hui WM, Shiu LP, Lam SK. The perception of life events and daily stress in non-ulcer dyspepsia. Am J Gastroenterol 1991; 86:292–296.
107. Talley NJ, Piper DW. The association between non-ulcer dyspepsia and other gastrointestinal disorders. Scand J Gastroenterol 1985; 20:896–900.
108. Richter JE, Bald F, Clouse RE, Diamant NE, Janssens J, Staiano A. Functional esophageal disorders. Gastroenterol Int 1992; 5:3–17.
109. Kemp HG, Vokonas PS, Cohn PF, et al. The anginal syndrome associated with normal coronary arteriogram: Report of a six-year experience. Am J Med 1973; 54:735–742.
110. Richter JE, Bradley LA, Castell DO. Esophageal chest pain: Current controversies in pathogenesis, diagnosis and therapy. Ann Intern Med 1989; 110:66–78.
111. Richter JE, Obrecht WF, Bradley LA, Young ID, Anderson KO. Psychological comparison of patients with nutcracker esophagus and irritable bowel syndrome. Dig Dis Sci 1986; 31:131–138.
112. Clouse RE, Lustman PJ. Psychiatric illness and contraction abnormalities of the esophagus. N Engl J Med 1983; 309:1337–1342.
113. Anderson KO, Dalton CB, Bardley LA, Richter JE. Stress induces alteration of esophageal pressures in healthy volunteers and non-cardiac chest pain patients. Dig Dis Sci 1989; 34:83–91.
114. Levenkron JC, Goldstein MG, Adamides O, et al. Chronic chest pain with normal coronary arteries: A behavioral approach to rehabilitation. J Cardiopulm Rehab 1985; 5:475–479.
115. Shabsin HS, Katz PO, Schuster MM. Behavioral treatment in intractible chest pain in a patient with vigorous achalasia. Am J Gastroenterol 1988; 83:970–973.
116. Klimes I, Mayou RA, Pearce MJ, et al. Psychological treatment for atypical non-cardiac chest pain: A controlled observation. Psychol Med 1990; 20:605–611.
117. McDonald-Haile J, Bradley LA, Bailey MA, Schan CA, Richter JE. Relaxation training reduces symptom reports and acid exposure in patients with gastroesophageal reflux disease. Gastroenterology 1994; 107:61–69.
118. Shay SS, Johnson LF, Wong RKH, Curtis DJ, Rosenthal R, Lamott JR, Owensby LC. Rumination, heartburn, and daytime gastroesophageal reflux. J Clin Gastroenterol 1986; 8:115–126.

17

Individual and Group Psychotherapy of Functional GI Disorders

Kevin W. Olden
University of California, San Francisco
and St. Mary's Medical Center
San Francisco, California

Thomas N. Wise
Georgetown University School of Medicine
and Fairfax Hospital
Falls Church, Virginia

Richard L. Goldberg
Georgetown University School of Medicine
Washington, D.C.

I. INTRODUCTION

Humans have always been fascinated by what they eat, what they excrete and the disorders that upset their gastrointestinal (GI) tracts. Ancient Egyptian rulers appointed a "Shepherd of the Anus" to manage GI problems, and the ancient Ebhers Papyrus focused on problems of the GI system (1). Current culture also emphasizes the relationship between emotions and GI disease. Common advertisements link stress with abdominal discomfort and the need for antacids (2). Over a century ago, DaCosta and other clinical observers noted that irritable bowel syndrome (IBS) was often seen in patients with neurasthenic vulnerability, and Osler described the syndrome of alternating constipation and diarrhea as a "secretory neurosis" (3). In the first modern description of irritable bowel, in 1928, Bockus et al. (4) labeled what we now know as IBS "neurogenic mucous colitis" to emphasize its psychological dimensions.

Contemporary gastroenterology has increasingly focused on psychological factors as having a role in the understanding of functional GI syndromes, such as IBS, non-ulcer dyspepsia, and esophageal spasm (5). Recent research has corroborated the links between emotional phenomena, stress, life events, and GI physiology (6). Early childhood trauma such as sexual abuse has been found to be correlated with the seeking of care for IBS. In 1990 Drossman et al. (7) showed that 46% of women presenting for treatment of a functional GI disorder were found to have a history of physical or sexual abuse, in either childhood or adulthood. This prevalence of abuse history was significantly different from that of age-matched controls presenting to the same clinic with organic disorders. This work has been validated by Walker et al. (8) and Felitti (9), among others. Likewise, histories of childhood physical and sexual abuse have been associated with a wide variety of excessive health care utilization (10) and other poor health care outcomes (11). In addition, a history of sexual and/or physical abuse can generate psychiatric disorders associated with GI symptoms, e.g., eating disorders (12). Childhood physical and sexual abuse has also been associated with impaired sexual functioning, often accompanied by chronic pelvic pain and dissociation (13). Finally, there is a significantly greater prevalence of psychiatric disorders, particularly depression (14), anxiety disorders (14), and personality disorders (15), among patients who have suffered abuse.

Functional GI disorders are extremely common. Over 50% of the gastroenterologist's clinical activities are devoted to complaints that are primarily functional (16). Many patients with functional GI disorders never seek medical consultation for their complaints—even though 85% of patients who seek help obtain relief, through standard medical management of their diets and perhaps antispasmodic therapy (17). However, approximately 15% of GI patients will be relatively refractory to medical treatment, and many of them will become high utilizers of health care (10). For these individuals, psychotherapy as an adjunct to standard medical treatment may well prove both useful and cost-effective. Prior to commencing adjunctive psychotherapy, the therapist must have a clear concept of functional GI disorders from multiple perspectives.

II. MULTIPLE PERSPECTIVES

It is important to distinguish whether a GI problem is a direct reaction to physiological dysfunction that could cause reactive dysphoria or a somatic idiom of distress called *somatization* (18). In either situation, the psychiatrist must understand that multiple perspectives are necessary in managing these patients. These perspectives have been outlined by Drs. Paul McHugh and Philip Slavney in two books that discuss the differences between the approaches (19,20).

A. The Disease Approach

The *disease approach* is based on a medical model in which syndromic categorization, defined by signs and symptoms, identifies a discrete category and then searches for a pathophysiological causal factor. Syndromes are developed via the five phases of diagnostic validity and careful clinical descriptions utilizing demographic and clinical factors and laboratory studies, to distinguish them from other established disorders. Long-term follow-up studies can help to ascertain the natural history of the disorder, as well as the response to various treatments. Family studies that look at both genetic and environmental causes are also important (21).

The disease approach can help explain, for example, chest pain resulting from abnormalities in esophageal motility. The astute clinician considering a history of chest pain in combination with symptoms of difficulty in swallowing solids, heartburn, or regurgitation will recognize that these symptoms are commonly found in individuals who have esophageal motility disorders. Esophageal motility studies may then be performed to document patterns of dysmotility associated with stress (22). For example, an elevated prevalence of anxiety disorders, depression, and other psychiatric disorders has been found among individuals with esophageal motility disorders (23). Similarly, recent studies by Leroi and colleagues (24) have shown that the anorectal motility disorder anismus is closely associated with a history of physical and sexual abuse. Leroi has proposed linking an anorectal motility study to psychosocial history-taking to detect the underlying social pathology that led to physical/sexual abuse and its psychopathological sequelae. Likewise, studies have shown that anxious individuals may in fact exacerbate their GI symptoms by swallowing more air (25). This is called *aerophagy*, and it can be etiological to upper-GI functional complaints (26). Psychosocial and medical history-taking and evaluation clearly can play complementary roles.

Chronic abdominal pain, one of the more refractory functional GI disorders, has a strong correlation with severe psychosocial dysfunction. A thorough history of the onset and course of abdominal pain must be obtained. Drossman (27) reviewed his experience with patients with chronic abdominal pain and found them particularly resistant to psychiatric referral. Patients with abdominal pain may also tend to be more refractory to psychotherapeutic intervention (28a,b). Likewise, Walker et al. (14) showed that patients with chronic pelvic pain of functional etiology were much more likely to have psychiatric disorders, as compared to patients with chronic pelvic pain of organic etiology. Walker also documented a significant history of physical and sexual abuse in his patient group. The approach to treating these patients must be governed by patience, prudence, and extraordinary sensitivity to the psychosocial aspects of their complaints (29). Focusing on a purely biomedical model has been shown to be less than ideal in working with these patients (30).

B. Life-History Methodology

Another perspective, the *life-history methodology* (31), treats the individual as a unique subject—in contrast to the disease approach, which views the individual as a biological organism. Via empathic listening, the physician gains an understanding of the patient's reactions to his or her current predicament in the context of the patient's developmental vicissitudes and life history (32). Examples of such connections can be found in Drossman's study (7), which found that 46% of the patients with a functional diagnosis in a GI clinic had been physically or sexually abused, and that patients with functional bowel disorders had a greater prevalence of physical abuse than those with clearly organic disorders. The ability to form an empathic bond with the patient in a nonthreatening manner creates an environment in which the patient can divulge information that may never have been previously revealed. Indeed, in Drossman's study, only 17% of the patients who had been physically or sexually abused had ever reported such abuse to their physicians. It is therefore essential for the physician to carefully inquire about early life events and understand their relationship to present issues. The ability to make meaningful connections between a patient's life history and current feeling states and behaviors can help determine if psychotherapeutic intervention is indicated. Family history is equally important. For example, a patient with a strong family history of colon carcinoma may repeatedly seek medical care for minor lower-GI complaints, whereas a patient with a strong family history of coronary artery disease may misinterpret heartburn as the onset of a myocardial infarction.

C. The Dimensional Approach

The third perspective is the *dimensional approach*. Traits and characteristics exist along a dimensional continuum: An individual is more or less prone to anxiety and worry, or more or less outgoing, energetic, and high-spirited. For the purposes of this approach, personality is best understood in terms of trait-dimensional description (33). The five-factor model of personality offers a clinically valid, heuristically useful approach to measuring an individual's enduring patterns and elucidates the correlation between the stress-provoking mechanism and the patient's typical response pattern (34). The five factors are:

Neuroticism—a tendency to worry, feel self-conscious and vulnerable, and be susceptible to affects of anxiety, depression, and hostility

Extroversion—a tendency to be high-spirited, fun-loving, passionate, and talkative
Openness to experience—the tendency toward a creative, original, and curious cognitive and personal style
Agreeableness—the tendency to be lenient, good-natured, trusting, and generous
Conscientiousness—tending to be hard-working, organized, goal-directed, and ambitious

The clinician should be especially attuned to the dimensions of neuroticism, extroversion, and openness to experience. Neuroticism as a general tendency toward emotional distress and instability has been elucidated by both the five-factor model of personality and Eysenck's approach to such trait taxonomy (35). Neurotic patients also tend to focus on somatic complaints. Openness to experience is an important construct that can determine whether a patient with functional bowel complaints is capable of making cognitive readjustments about the etiology of the disorder. Personality traits can be determined by administering a brief form of the five-factor inventory and discussing the results with the patient. Miller (36) has recently described utilization of this inventory in clinical work.

In addition to the five factors, there is another personality trait, *alexithymia*, that clinicians should be alert to. The term was first used by Sifneos in 1972 (37). Drawing from Greek, Sifneos defined this characteristic of somatic patients as being "without words for mood" (37). Lesser et al. (38) described this trait as an "emotional illiteracy." Patients with alexithymia have great difficulty expressing emotional distress. They tend to generate physical complaints as the equivalent of their emotional distress. These patients tend not to be psychologically minded, and to be rigid and have difficulty dealing with abstract terms. They often have "operational thinking," which means they think in very concrete terms and are comfortable with tangible aspects of their well-being but are not in touch with the emotional dimensions to their overall wellness or illness. Patients with alexithymia and somatization tend to be of lower socioeconomic status. Patients with functional GI complaints as well as other somatization phenomena are often found to have this trait (39–41), characterized by a tendency to express emotional distress through somatic complaints (42). Alexithymia can be a primary personality characteristic or a secondary phenomenon in mood disorders. Insight-oriented psychotherapy with alexithymic patients is difficult because they have difficulty expressing feelings, preferring to focus on somatic issues instead. Behavioral approaches such as behavioral analysis via diaries and relaxation techniques are useful in highly alexithymic individuals (44).

D. Motivated Behaviors

The final perspective is that of *motivated behaviors*, activities directed toward a specific bodily event such as consumption of alcohol or other addictive substances, gluttony, or orgastic release in sexual acting out (19). For example, it is essential to rule out substance abuse and eating disorders in patients with abdominal pain. Patients often present with physical symptoms that mask underlying, completely hidden behavioral disorders. Examples are patients who present with bleeding from Mallory-Weiss tears secondary to bulimic purging and patients who suffer rebound constipation from laxative abuse. Likewise, patients presenting with pancreatitis or hepatitis of unclear etiology may be in significant denial of covert alcohol dependence. Clinicians must be especially vigilant for the presence of substance abuse and eating disorders because they are often denied on initial history.

E. Summary

The utility of these perspectives in managing the patient with functional GI disease is illustrated by understanding the discrete psychiatric disorders commonly found in association with functional bowel disorders, as well as the personality traits that can make such patients resistant to treatment. Patients with functional GI disorders often have comorbid affective or anxiety disorders, including panic disorder (45), which must be identified and treated. In one study, Lydiard and colleagues (46) showed a high prevalence of panic disorder, obsessive-compulsive disorder, depressive disorders, and somatization in patients with functional GI disorders. In a study of a group of patients with functional bowel disease, Ford and colleagues (6) discovered that only anxiety-provoking life events produced increased GI symptomatology. "Anxiety-provoking" is a relative term: One individual may be calm in the face of certain events while another may react to similar events with anxiety or depression and subsequently become somatically preoccupied with functional irritable bowel symptomatology. Drossman (47) has reported that many patients with symptoms of IBS never seek medical care and simply tolerate their bowel habits, whereas others, feeling a greater sense of vulnerability, attribute their symptoms to illness and seek medical care.

It is clear that patients who seek medical care for their functional GI complaints are different from symptomatic patients who choose not to seek health care. In one study, Whitehead (48) compared a population of churchgoers to patients presenting to a GI clinic in a university setting. All patients were screened for lactose malabsorption. This was done because the symptoms of lactose malabsorption, i.e., diarrhea, bloating, abdominal pain, and discomfort, are similar to symptoms of a functional GI disorder. Patients were also screened psychologically, using the SCL-90 to measure psychological distress. Whitehead showed that patients with IBS who sought care were much more likely to have elevated scores on the SCL-90 than were controls or patients with lactose malabsorption. Thus, a GI patient with high trait neuroticism may begin to ruminate about life changes, and may not only develop a functional GI disorder but also display significantly different health-care-seeking behavior. The interaction among these perspectives leads to a final common pathway: the clinical presentation of the patient's symptoms and complaints. It is the task of the psychiatrist to consider all four perspectives and utilize each appropriately.

III. EVALUATION OF THE PATIENT

Michael Balint (49) suggests that the most important "drug" in medical care is the doctor himself. Patients often come to a doctor with preconceived ideas about the nature and cause of their discomfort even though no illness has been formally diagnosed. At this point, abnormal illness beliefs may be not only evident but actually formed. By carefully drawing out patients' belief systems and any misinformation, fears, and ideas about the nature of their complaints, the physician can help structure patients' understanding of their disorder. Initially, the clinician should focus on the patient's somatic understanding of their disorder. Initially, the clinician should focus on the patient's somatic complaints: when they occur, where, and how often. The doctor should obtain data on self-remedies employed to alleviate discomfort—as mentioned, patients generally have ideas about the nature of their difficulties and try self-help remedies prior to seeing the doctor. The physician can attempt to determine a patient's illness beliefs by using the dimensions formulated by Pilowsky (50). These include a sense of whether the patient generally feels his or her illnesses are serious and has a hypochondriacal style or whether the patient believes psychological or somatic factors are primary causes. Is there a tendency to deny emotional and family difficulties? Are there affective disturbances, due primarily to depression or anxiety? Is the patient particularly irritable or angry? Finally, does the patient appear alexithymic or inhibited in affect?

The physician's intuitions, however, are not enough. A careful mental-status examination must be performed to rule out formal psychiatric disorders. Psychiatric or psychological consultation may be helpful. Patients with non-ulcer dyspepsia whose presentation includes chest pain and heartburn have been shown to have an increased incidence of anxiety disorders and depression (51). Magni and coworkers (52) studied 30 patients with a diagnosis of functional dyspepsia. They found that 86.7% of their patients with dyspepsia of unknown cause presented with an Axis I diagnosis, with generalized anxiety disorder being the most common. Anxiety disorders in general were more common. IBS sufferers have been shown to have an increased prevalence of generalized anxiety disorder and depression, and panic disorder has been known to present with symptoms similar to those of irritable bowel (28,53,54). Creed and Whorwell (55) have demonstrated that patients with functional bowel disease often have symptoms in other organ systems and frequently have somatization disorder. Any psychiatric disorder discovered through the mental-status exam must be treated with appropriate methods.

Because GI complaints can be temporally related to intake of certain types of food, a careful history of dietary provokers of symptoms should be elicited. Within this history, it is important to understand the nature of family food preferences as well as the individual's. Developmental data such as the patient's childhood experiences with various foods—what he liked, what he was forced to eat, and what he did not have to eat—are important in understanding his life history. Many GI patients believe that food allergies cause their indigestion, nausea, or flatulence. They may also attribute their discomfort to "malabsorption" or "enzyme deficiencies" (56). Lactose intolerance, which can cause a variety of GI symptoms, can be easily diagnosed utilizing the lactose hydrogen breath test (57). Consumption of dietetic foods and fruit that contain sorbitol may induce osmotic diarrhea, which can simulate functional GI symptoms. Fatty foods, chocolate, and peppermint can decrease lower-esophageal sphincter pressure and foster gastroesophageal reflux. Interestingly, however, of patients who believe they have food allergies, in only a minority do objective data confirm a sensitivity to the putative dietary agent. Investigators have found that many patients with food allergies do not have definable sensitivity reactions (47). False disease convictions can lead patients to seek alternative treatments rather than focus on the issues of abnormal illness belief. Following a detailed self-report history of the somatic complaint and an investigation of the biopsychosocial issues, the clinician must coordinate his or her care with that of other physicians involved with the care of the patient by obtaining their views of the problem.

The next phase in assessment is behavioral analysis via record-keeping by the patient (44). It is helpful to have patients clearly document the symptoms that cause the most distress. The time and place, as well as the duration and intensity of the discomfort, can provide helpful clues. Any events or social situations that provoke the patient's symptoms should be noted. The behavioral analysis should include diet and all medications taken. Patients often do not associate consumption of so-called therapeutic foods with symptoms such as bloating or gas, and an ongoing match of dietary intake and consequent symptoms can identify such culprits. Dietary fiber, for example, is widely advertised as being healthy, but excessive use can make diarrhea-predominant IBS patients much worse. Careful documentation of symptoms and the context in which they occur may provide better understanding of the symptoms themselves.

IV. EVIDENCE FOR THE EFFECTIVENESS OF PSYCHOTHERAPEUTIC TREATMENT

A considerable body of data collected from various studies indicates that psychotherapy directed toward relieving functional GI symptoms by helping the patient face underlying psychological disturbances can be quite effective. Much of this research has been performed on patients with IBS. Early studies on these disorders offered scant information on patient selection and did not use standardized outcome measures. However, this research has become more sophisticated and includes randomizing patients to treatment and control groups and utilizing standardized outcome measures evaluated by blind raters.

In an early study, Schonecke and Schuffel (45) compared the effects of three 20-minute interviews that focused on life problems versus a tranquilizer for the treatment of IBS. Both were equally effective in treating the symptoms of abdominal distress. The authors of the study surmised that the pharmacological management of patients involved considerable interaction between the patient and physician, and that perhaps this doctor–patient relationship shared by both treatment modalities accounted for positive symptom change. However, in another study that looked more specifically at hypnotherapy for the treatment of functional GI disorders, Whorwell et al. (52a) allowed time for an untrained psychotherapist to work with IBS patients in psychotherapy. In this study, there was no apparent benefit from intervention by an untrained psychotherapist, but improvement occurred when treatment was performed by a skilled hypnotherapist. Comparison of the results of psychotherapeutic intervention in this study with those of other studies suggests that psychotherapy's impact on functional GI complaints relies more on the skills of an experienced psychotherapist performing the psychotherapeutic task than on the nonspecific supportive aspects of a good doctor–patient relationship.

Hislop (52b) studied the effects of psychotherapy directed toward exploring the connection between life stresses and GI symptoms on patients with GI complaints secondary to IBS. This study found that psychotherapy had a positive effect on GI symptoms, particularly in patients who were able to express their feelings in an open fashion. Unfortunately, this study did not utilize a control group and reported outcome data in a nonstandardized manner.

In a later study, Svedlund (51) recruited 101 IBS patients from a medical clinic and randomly assigned them to either standard medical treatment alone or standard medical treatment combined with individual psychotherapy. Psychotherapy consisted of 10 1-hour sessions directed toward identifying stress responses and their relationship to bowel symptoms. Patients were also taught coping strategies. Ratings of GI symptomatology as well as coping skills were performed by the patients and independent evaluators before randomization, after 3 months, and after 1 year. The group of patients receiving psychotherapy demonstrated greater improvement in abdominal pain and bowel symptoms at 3 months, and an even greater improvement after 1 year. Self-confidence and coping skills improved significantly in the patients receiving the combined treatment. Confounding variables such as life events and drinking habits did not contribute to the different outcomes of the groups. Patients who appeared to have a periodic versus constant course of IBS seemed best suited to change with psychotherapy.

Research by Guthrie et al. (28b) further supports the effectiveness of psychotherapy in the treatment of IBS. These investigators recruited 102 of 115 eligible patients with IBS from a medical clinic and assigned them randomly to either a group that received only standard medical treatment for IBS or a group that received psychotherapy combined with relaxation therapy and standard medical treatment. Only patients who had not improved after 6 months of standard medical treatment were selected for this study. Assessments of GI symptoms, depression, and anxiety were performed at baseline, after 3 months, and after 1 year. Physician evaluators were blinded to which group the patients were enrolled in. Psychotherapy consisted of an initial interview and six weekly follow-up visits. Many individuals in the control group that received standard medical treatment were offered psychotherapeutic treatment after the first 3 months of follow-up. At 3 months, the treatment group showed significantly greater improvement in several GI symptoms, such as diarrhea and abdominal pain. Anxiety and depression scores also improved. Constipation changed little for patients in both groups. Patients with overt psychiatric symptoms and intermittent IBS symptoms were greatly helped; patients with constant pain benefited the least. This study demonstrated that psychotherapy was effective in improving both bowel symptomatology and emotional well-being in two-thirds of IBS patients who did not respond to standard treatment alone.

In a second study, Guthrie and colleagues (28a) studied 102 patients with refractory IBS who were randomized to a course of short-term dynamic psychotherapy in addition to conventional medical therapy versus a control group of medical therapy plus "supportive listening." The supportive listening group consisted of a physician meeting with patients and letting them expound on their life circumstances but offering no formal psychiatric intervention. Patients were recruited consecutively, and only those with a history of unresponsiveness to medical treatment were included. Patients with psychiatric illness were not excluded. The only psychiatric exclusion criterion was active suicidal ideation. Patients in both groups were subjected to independent physical and psychological assessments, which were carried out both at the entry into the study and at the end of the 12-week trial period. Fifty-three patients were allocated to the treatment group and 49 patients to the control. The form of psychotherapy employed by Guthrie and colleagues was the "conversational model," as described by Hobson (58). The treatment group received an initial intake psychotherapeutic session of 3–4 hours followed by six psychotherapy sessions of 45 minutes each over 12 weeks. At the end of the 12–week trial in women, psychotherapy was found to be superior than supportive listening, in terms of both physical and emotional symptoms. This trend was similar for men, but it was not statistically significant compared to the results in the non-treatment group. Dropping out of psychotherapy at 1 year was associated with a return of symptoms and increase in functional bowel complaints. It was important to note that Guthrie's patients were not seeking psychotherapy; i.e., they had not considered this as a therapeutic option. Their major characteristic was chronic abdominal complaints that were refractory to traditional medical treatment.

Greene and Blanchard (59) treated 20 IBS patients with individual and cognitive therapy consisting of 10 sessions over 8 weeks versus eight weeks of brief visits to monitor GI symptoms. Ratings of GI symptomatology in the treatment group before and after treatment were significantly different, demonstrating improvement directly related to the cognitive therapy. Eighty percent of the cognitive therapy group showed significant clinical improvement in GI symptoms whereas only 10% of the control group reported any improvement. Greene and Blanchard proposed that cognitive therapy is particularly efficacious for functional GI complaints because of its "ability to decrease negative automatic thoughts" as well as stimulation of more positive thinking. It is significant to note, however, that the patients in this study were actively seeking psychotherapy; the fact that they were already motivated for psychotherapeutic intervention may have introduced bias.

Blanchard and coworkers (60) have also studied the use of relaxation training in IBS. They studied 16 patients who were randomized either to an 8-week course of progressive muscle relaxation (PMR) or to a group that received no treatment but was monitored monthly to track GI symptoms as reported by patient diaries. Treatment patients who completed the study experienced a significant decrease in abdominal pain, constipation, flatulence, belching, and nausea, as compared to the controls. The prevalence of diarrhea did not decrease, however. Blanchard and others concluded that relaxation training alone could be a useful treatment for IBS, particularly for abdominal pain and possibly constipation.

Effective psychotherapy for functional GI disorders need not be on an individual basis. Wise et al. (53) studied 20 IBS patients who underwent six weekly sessions of group psychotherapy that incorporated behavioral and didactic techniques. Psychometric follow-up revealed a significant reduction in dysphoric emotions despite the persistence of somatic complaints. This study demonstrates that group treatment delivered in a time-limited approach may provide symptomatic relief to IBS patients. In another study, Harvey et al. (54), utilized group hypnotherapy techniques and compared their effectiveness with that of individual hypnotic techniques in the treatment of IBS patients. The results indicated that a group approach was equally effective in reducing functional GI symptoms.

These findings are not surprising. Other investigators have shown the effectiveness of psychotherapy in dealing with somatizing patients. Smith and coworkers (61) followed 56 patients with somatization disorder and demonstrated that psychiatric consultation, including psychotherapeutic intervention, could result in a 32.9% reduction in the annual cost of medical care for these patients. Wilhelmsen et al., studying patients with peptic ulcer, (62) also showed that short-term cognitive psycotherapy delivered in 10 sessions over 4 months, in combination with standard medical treatment, did not produce any change in ulcer relapse rate but did produce significant reductions in symptoms of abdominal pain and discomfort in the therapy group, compared to controls. Also, neuroticism, as measured by the Eysenck Personality Questionnaire, and anxiety, as measured by the Spielberger Trait Anxiety Scale, was also significantly improved in the therapy group over controls. It is clear that psychotherapeutic intervention plays an important role in the treatment of somatizing patients, and certainly in patients with significant functional GI complaints. This has been reviewed eloquently by Kelner (63). It is not clear which patients are the best candidates nor which modalities are most efficacious. Further research is needed to address these questions.

V. INGREDIENTS OF SUCCESSFUL PSYCHOTHERAPY FOR FUNCTIONAL GI DISORDERS

For psychotherapy to be truly useful in the treatment of patients with functional GI disorders, it should be cost-effective. Likewise, it is important that patients be carefully selected. It should certainly be offered to those who have failed to respond to standard medical treatment. Patients who present with intermittent abdominal pain seem to have better response than do patients with constant pain, although in most studies abdominal pain seems to be less responsive in general to psychotherapeutic intervention and has been associated with poor outcome (28,55). Psychiatric symptoms that are present at treatment onset are not predictive of outcome (28,54,56,57).

Once patients are selected for psychotherapy, their primary-care physician should refer them to a therapist who is available to see the patient promptly, to counteract any resistance that might emerge in response to such a referral (28). The psychotherapist should instruct the patient about the process. The primary aims of psychotherapy for functional GI patients are enhancement of quality of life and functional improvement in activities of daily living. Both physician and patient need to understand that these can be achieved even if some level of GI symptomatology persists.

In psychotherapy, symptom relief is achieved by helping the patient face underlying psychological conflicts and emotional disturbances. GI patients should also be actively educated about their bowel problems. Attempts should be made to link their difficulties in coping with stress with the physiological vulnerability of their GI tract. Patients need to be informed at treatment onset about boundary issues related to time, money, and role differentiation between the psychotherapist and the primary-care physician. Another important goal for the psychotherapist working with such patients is, by decreasing abnormal illness behavior, to reduce the risk of exposure to unnecessary and potentially harmful medical or surgical interventions (47).

The psychotherapist must develop a strong working alliance with these patients. Although the goal of psychotherapeutic treatment should be to link psychological phenomena with GI symptoms, it is important, at least initially, for patients to have an opportunity to talk to an empathic therapist about their somatic complaints. To help engage these patients in an active alliance, the therapist might ask them to keep diaries that chronicle the changing frequency and severity of such symptoms as abdominal pain and bowel habits. A symptom diary can also be an important tool for thc psychotherapist in keeping track of treatment progress.

Successful case management for the patient with a functional GI disorder will include a combination of techniques. For example, a psychotherapist will employ both cognitive and didactic strategies to help patients learn new coping skills (48). Combining homework assignments of relaxation therapy with the psychodynamic interventions seems particularly useful (60,43). The psychotherapist may also want to refer GI patients to self-help groups as an adjunct to individual psychotherapy. These self-help groups, similar to professionally led groups, educate patients about their disorders and help them recognize that their symptoms are not unique or esoteric. The group cohesion created by successful self-help and professionally led groups allows patients to overcome their sense of isolation as they struggle to come to terms with their disorders. Data are emerging that this "combined-treatment" approach, using psychodynamic and cognitive-based approaches in conjunction with relaxation training and patient education, can be particularly helpful (64).

Patients with functional GI disorders frequently present with a history of prior psychiatric illness. As mentioned above, some of these patients will reveal history of early sexual trauma (4). When a history of prior psychiatric illness is present, psychotherapy must address those issues, and, when indicated, a medical psychotherapist should not hesitate to combine psychopharmacological and psychotherapeutic interventions.

The studies cited above indicate that psychotherapy can be an effective intervention with GI patients, including those with long-standing functional disorders. Indeed, the literature supporting psychotherapeutic intervention in functional GI disorders is more definitive than the literature supporting purely medical intervention. A psychotherapist who is interested in exploring the connections between psychological and somatic GI complaints will find work with these patients both rewarding and productive, as well as gratifying. Moreover, methodological approaches to studying the impact of psychotherapy on functional GI patients have improved greatly, creating a fertile environment for future research on the usefulness of psychotherapeutic modalities in psychosomatic gastroenterology.

REFERENCES

1. Ghalioungui P. Magic and Medical Science in Ancient Egypt. London: Hodder and Stoughton, 1961.
2. Clouse RE. Anxiety and gastrointestinal illness. Psychiatric Clin North Am 1988; 11:399–417.
3. DaCosta J. Mucous enteritis. Medicine and Medical Science 1871; 83:321–335.
4. Bockus HL, Bauk J, Wilkinson SA. Neurogenic mucous colitis. Am J Med Sci 1928; 176:813–829.
5. Folks DG, Kinney FC. The role of psychological factors in gastrointestinal conditions: a review pertinent to DSM-IV. Psychosomatics 1992; 33:257–270.
6. Ford JM, McMiller P, Eastwood P, et al. Life events, psychiatric illness and the irritable bowel syndrome. Gut 1987; 28:160–165.
7. Drossman DA, Leserman J, Nachman G, et al. Sexual and physical abuse in women with functional or organic gastrointestinal disorders. Ann Intern Med 1990; 113:828–833.
8. Walker EA, Katon WJ, Roy-Byrne PP, et al. Histories of sexual victimization in patients with irritable bowel syndrome or inflammatory bowel disease. Am J Psychiatry 1993; 150:1502–1506.
9. Felitti V. Long-term medical consequences of incest, rape and molestation. South Med J 1991; 84:328–331.
10. Arnold R, Rogers D, Cook D. Medical problems of adults who were sexually abused in childhood. Br Med J 1990; 300:705–708.
11. Schofferman J, Anderson D, Hines R, et al. Childhood psychological trauma correlates with unsuccessful lumbar spine surgery. Spine 1992; 17:S138–S144.
12. Fallon BA, Sadik C, Saoud JB, et al. Childhood abuse, family environment, and outcome in bulimia nervosa. J Clin Psychiatry 1994; 55:424–428.
13. Walker EA, Katon WJ, Neraas K, et al. Dissociation in women with chronic pelvic pain. Am J Psychiatry 1992; 149:534–537.
14. Walker EA, Roy-Byrng PP, Katon WJ. irritable bowel syndrome and psychiatric illness. Am J Psychiatry 1990; 147:565–572.
15. Herman JL, Perry J, Van der Kolk B. Childhood trauma in borderline personality disorder. Am J Psychiatry 1989; 146:490–495.
16. Camilleri M, Prather CM. The irritable bowel syndrome: mechanisms and a practical approach to management. Ann Intern Med 1992; 116:1001–1008.
17. Harvey RF, Mauad EC, Brown Am. Prognosis in the irritable bowel syndrome: a 5-year prospective study. Lancet 1987; 963–965.
18. Lipowski ZJ. Somatization, a borderline between medicine and psychiatry. Can Med Assoc J 1986; 135:609–614.
19. McHugh PR, Slavney PR. The Perspectives in Psychiatry. Baltimore: Johns Hopkins University Press, 1986.
20. Slavney PR, McHugh PR. Psychiatric Polarities. Baltimore: Johns Hopkins University Press, 1987.
21. Robins E, Guze SB. Establishment of diagnostic validity in psychiatric illness. Am J Psychiatry 1984; 126:107–111.
22. Camilleri M, Neri M. Motility disorders and stress. Dig Dis Sci 1989; .:1777–1786.

23. Clouse RE, Costman PJ. Psychiatric illness and contraction abnormalities of the esophagus. N Engl J Med 1982; 309:1337–1342.
24. Leroi AM, Berkelmans I, Denis P, et al. Anismus as a marker of sexual abuse: consequences of abuse on anorectal motility. Dig Dis Sci 1995; 40:1411–1416.
25. Fonagy P, Calloway SP. The effect of emotional arousal on spontaneous swallowing rates. J Psychosom Res 1986; 30:183–188.
26. Talley NJ, Phillips SF. Non-ulcer dyspepsia: potential causes and pathophysiology. Ann Intern Med 1988; 108:865–879.
27. Drossman DA. Patients with psychogenic abdominal pain. Am J Psychiatry 1982; 139:1549–1557.
28a. Guthrie E., Creed FH, Dawson D. A controlled trial of psychological treatment for the irritable bowel syndrome. Gastroenterology 1991; 100:450–457.
28b. Guthrie E, Creed FH, Dawson D, et al. A randomised controlled trial of psychotherapy in patients with refractory irritable bowel syndrome. Br J Psychiatry 1993; 163:315–321.
29. Drossman DA, Talley NJ, Leserman J, et al. Sexual and physical abuse and gastrointestinal illness: review and recommendations. Ann Intern Med 1995. 123:782–794.
30. Klein K. Controlled treatment trials in the irritable bowel syndrome: a critique. Gastroenterology 1988; 95:232–241.
31. Slavney PR, McHugh PR. Life stories and meaningful connections: reflections on a clinical method in psychiatry and medicine. Perspectives Biol Med 1984; 27:279–288.
32. Jaspers K. General Psychopathology. Chicago: University of Chicago Press, 1972:301–363.
33. Slavney PR. Perspectives in Hysteria. Baltimore: Johns Hopkins University Press, 1990.
34. McCrae RR, Costa PT. Personality in Adulthood. New York: Golford, 1990.
35. Eysenck HJ, Eysenck SB. Personality Structure and Measurement. San Diego: Knapp, 1969.
36. Miller TR. Personality: a clinician's experience. J Personality Assess 1991; 57:415–433.
37. Sifneos PE. Short Term Psychotherapy and Emotional Crises. Cambridge, MA: Harvard University Press, 1972.
38. Lesser IM, Ford CV, Friedman C. Alexithymia in the somaticizing patient. Gen Hosp Psychiatry 1979; 1:256–261.
39. Taylor GJ. Alexithymia: concept measurement and implications for treatment. Am J Psychiatry 1984; 141:725–732.
40. Taylor GJ, Bagby RM, Ryan DD, Parker JDA. Validation of the alexithymia construct, a measurement based approach. Can J Psychiatry 1990; 35:290–297.
41. Lesser IM, Lesser BZ. Alexithymia: examining the development of a psychological concept. Am J Psychiatry 1983; 140:305–308.
42. Fava GA, Paran L. Large bowel disorders. II: Psychopathology and alexithymia. Psych Ther Psychosom 1976; 27:100–105.
43. Wise TN, Mann LS, Mitchell JD, Ryvniak M. Secondary alexithymia: an empirical validation. Comprehen Psychiatry 1990; 311–316.
44. Kanfer FH, Saslow G. Behavioral analysis. Arch Gen Psych 1965; 12:529–538.

45. Schonecke OW, Schuffel W. Evaluation of combined pharmacological and psychotherapeutic treatment in patients with functional abdominal disorders. Psychother Psychosom 1975; 26:86–92.
46. Lydiard RB, Greenwald S, Weissman MM, et al. Panic disorder and gastrointestinal symptoms: findings from the NIMH Epidemiologic Catchment Area project. Am J Psychiatry 1994; 151:64–70.
47. Drossman DA. Illness behavior in the irritable bowel syndrome. Gastroenterol Int 1991; 4:77–81.
48. Whitehead WE. Behavioral medicine approaches to gastrointestinal disorders. J Consult Clin Pyschol 1992; 4:605–612.
49. Balint M. The doctor, his patient and the illness. Lancet 1955; 683–688.
50. Pilowsky I, Spence N, Cobb J. The Illness Behavior Questionnaire as an aid in clinical assessment. Gen Hosp Psychiatry 1984; 6:123–130.
51. Svedlund J. Psychotherapy in irritable bowel syndrome: a controlled outcome study. Acta Psychiatr Scand 1983; 67:1–86.
52. Magni G, DiMario F, Bernasconi G, et al. DSM-III diagnoses associated with dyspepsia of unknown cause. Am J Psychiatry 1987; 144:1222–1223.
52a. Whorwell PJ, Prior A, Fafagher EBI. Controlled trial of hypnotherapy in the treatment of severe refractory irritable bowel syndrome. Lancet 1984; ii:1232–1234.
52b. Hislop IG. Effect of very brief psychotherapy on the irritable bowel syndrome. Med J Aust 1980; 2:620–623.
53. Wise TN, Cooper JN, Ahmed S. The efficacy of group therapy for patients with irritable bowel syndrome. Psychosomatics 1982; 23:465–469.
54. Harvey RF, Gunary RM, Hinton RA, et al. Individual and group hypnotherapy in treatment of refractory irritable bowel syndrome. Lancet 1989; 424–425.
55. Creed F, Whorwell PJ. Hypnotherapy in the irritable bowel syndrome. Lancet 1984; ii:1232–1234.
56. Whorwell PJ. Hypnotherapy in the irritable bowel syndrome. Stress Med 1987; 3:5–7.
57. Lancaster-Smith MJ, Prout BJ, Pinto T, et al. Influence of drug treatment on the irritable bowel syndrome and its interaction with psychoneurotic morbidity. Acta Psychiatr Scand 1982; 66:33–41.
58. Hobson RF. Forms of Feeling. London: Tavistock, 1985.
59. Greene B, Blanchard EB. Cognitive therapy for irritable bowel syndrome. J Consult Clin Psychol 1994; 62:576–582.
60. Blanchard EB, Greene B, Scharff L, et al. Relaxation training as a treatment for irritable bowel syndrome. Biofeed Self-Reg 1993; 18:125–132.
61. Smith GR, Rost K, Kashner TM. A trial of the effect of a standardized psychiatric consultation on health outcomes and costs in somatizing patients. Arch Gen Psychiatry 1995; 52:238–243.
62. Wilhelmsen I, Tangen Haug T, Ursin H, et al. Effect of short-term cognitive psychotherapy on recurrence of duodenal ulcer: a prospective randomized trial. Psychosom Med 1994; 56:440–448.
63. Kellner R. Diagnosis and treatment sof hypochondriacal syndromes. Psychosomatics 1992; 33:278–289.
64. Toner BB. Cognitive-behavioral treatment of functional somatic syndromes: integrating gender issues. Cog Behav Pract 1994; 1:157–178.

Appendix: Patient Support Organizations

The following patient support and advocacy organizations for patients with functional bowel and motility disorders have been set up and are run by lay people. These organizations can be a valuable source of information and assistance for both physicians and patients. In addition to providing newsletters and other patient education materials these groups serve as a point of contact for information and education and as advocates at the national level for those suffering from functional GI disorders.

International Foundation for Bowel Dysfunction (IFBD)
P.O. Box 17864
Milwaukee, WI 53217

Intestinal Disease Foundation, Inc. (IDF)
1323 Forbes Ave., Suite 200
Pittsburgh, PA 15219

American Society of Adults with Pseudo-Obstruction, Inc. (ASAP)
19 Carroll Road
Woburn, MA 01801

American Pseudo-Obstruction and Hirschsprung's Society, Inc. (APHS)
P.O. Box 772
Medford, MA 02155

Index

About the Editor

Kevin W. Olden is Assistant Clinical Professor of Medicine and Psychiatry at the University of California, San Francisco, and Director of the Gastroenterology Training Program at St. Mary's Medical Center, San Francisco, California. He is also Coordinator of the Functional GI Clinic of the University of California, San Francisco. The author or coauthor of numerous professional publications, Dr. Olden serves as a reviewer for several medical journals, including *Gastroenterology* and the *Journal of the American Medical Association.* He is a Fellow of the Academy of Psychosomatic Medicine, the American College of Physicians, and the American College of Gastroenterology. He is also a member of the American Gastroenterological Association and the American Psychiatric Association, among others. He received the A.B. degree (1971) in sociology from New York University, New York, New York, and the M.D. degree (1976) from State University of New York Downstate Medical Center, Brooklyn, New York.